D1784698

Fundamentals of Musculoskeletal Pain

Mission Statement of IASP Press®

IASP brings together scientists, clinicians, health care providers, and policy makers to stimulate and support the study of pain and to translate that knowledge into improved pain relief worldwide. IASP Press publishes timely, high-quality, and reasonably priced books relating to pain research and treatment.

Fundamentals of Musculoskeletal Pain

Editors

Thomas Graven-Nielsen, Dr Med Sci, PhD
Department of Health Sciences and Technology, Center for Sensory-Motor Interaction, Aalborg University, Aalborg, Denmark

Lars Arendt-Nielsen, Dr Med Sci, PhD
Department of Health Sciences and Technology, Center for Sensory-Motor Interaction, Aalborg University, Aalborg, Denmark

Siegfried Mense, Dr Med
Institute of Anatomy and Cell Biology, University of Heidelberg, Heidelberg, Germany

IASP PRESS® • SEATTLE

Library of Congress Cataloging-in-Publication Data

Fundamentals of musculoskeletal pain / editors, Thomas Graven-Nielsen, Lars Arendt-Nielsen, Siegfried Mense.
     p. ; cm.
  Includes bibliographical references.
  Summary: "Basic scientists and clinicians explain the fundamentals of musculoskeletal pain and describe current research that can benefit clinical strategies. Part I reviews the peripheral and central mechanisms of muscle pain. Part II describes key factors in pain sensitivity, including sex-related and genetic factors. Part III describes the effects of muscle pain on motor function."--Provided by publisher.
  ISBN 978-0-931092-72-5 (hardcover : alk. paper)
 1. Myalgia. I. Graven-Nielsen, Thomas, 1970- II. Arendt-Nielsen, Lars, 1958- III. Mense, Siegfried. IV. International Association for the Study of Pain.
  [DNLM: 1. Musculoskeletal Diseases--physiopathology. 2. Pain--physiopathology. WE 140 F981 2008]
  RC935.M77.F86 2008
  616.7'42--dc22

                        2008014881

Published by:

IASP Press
International Association for the Study of Pain
111 Queen Anne Ave N, Suite 501
Seattle, WA 98109-4955, USA
Fax: 206-283-9403
www.iasp-pain.org

Printed in the United States of America

Contents

Part III Effects of Muscle Pain on Motor Function

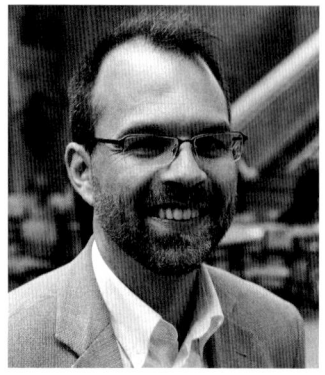

Thomas Graven-Nielsen, Dr Med Sci, PhD, is Professor in Pain Neuroscience at the Center for Sensory-Motor Interaction, Department of Health Science and Technology, and Head of the International Doctoral Program in Biomedical Science and Engineering, Aalborg University, Denmark. His research interests focus on mechanisms of muscle pain, referred pain, deep-tissue hyperalgesia, and interactions between muscle pain, fatigue, and motor control. Dr. Graven-Nielsen has published more than 150 papers and reviews (including over 110 peer-reviewed papers) on new electrophysiological methods and basic muscle pain physiology. He has a background of extensive national and international collaborations on muscle pain research. He reviews papers on a regular basis for highly ranked journals.

Lars Arendt-Nielsen, Dr Med Sci, PhD, is Professor at the Center for Sensory-Motor Interaction, Department of Health Science and Technology, Aalborg University, Denmark. He is founder and head of the Pain Research Unit at Aalborg University and has worked extensively in the area of human experimental and clinical pain research, with a focus on induction and assessment of pain from skin, muscles, and viscera. He has published more than 500 peer-reviewed papers in the field and serves on the IASP Council (2005–2010). He serves on the editorial board for *Pain, European Journal of Pain, The Journal of Pain,* and *Experimental Brain Research.*

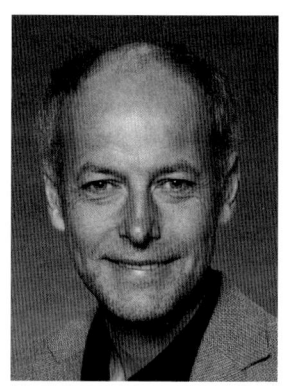

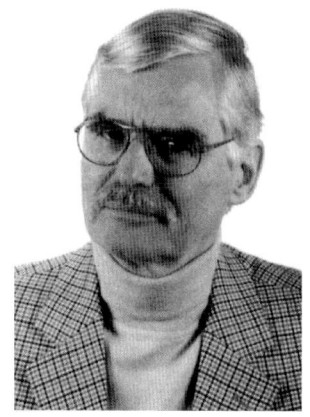

Siegfried Mense, Dr Med Habil, is Professor at the Department of Anatomy and Cell Biology, University of Heidelberg, Heidelberg, Germany. He is professionally educated as physician, physiologist, and anatomist. His research interests lie within the neuroanatomy and neurophysiology of muscle pain. Dr. Mense has published more than 180 scientific articles, including book contributions, and is the author of two books and editor of two books. He is a member of the editorial boards for *Journal of Musculoskeletal Pain* and *European Journal of Pain.* He has served as council member of the German Chapter of IASP (1981–1996) and as chair of the German Pain Foundation (since 1994).

Contributing Authors

Randi Abrahamsen, DDS *Department of Clinical Oral Physiology, School of Dentistry, University of Aarhus, Aarhus, Denmark*

Giannapia Affaitati, MD *Pathophysiology of Pain Laboratory, Ce.S.I, "G. D'Annunzio" Foundation, Department of Medicine and Science of Aging, "G. D'Annunzio" University of Chieti, Italy*

Per Alstergren, DDS, PhD *Department of Clinical Oral Physiology, Institute of Odontology, Karolinska Institute, Huddinge, Sweden*

Lars Arendt-Nielsen, Dr Med Sci, PhD *Department of Health Sciences and Technology, Center for Sensory-Motor Interaction, Aalborg University, Aalborg, Denmark*

Henning Bliddal, DMSc *The Parker Institute, Frederiksberg Hospital, Frederiksberg, Denmark*

Laurence A. Bradley, PhD *Division of Clinical Immunology and Rheumatology, University of Alabama at Birmingham, Birmingham, Alabama, USA*

Brian E. Cairns, PhD, ACPR, RPh *Faculty of Pharmaceutical Sciences, The University of British Columbia, Vancouver, British Columbia, Canada*

Norman F. Capra, PhD *Department of Biomedical Sciences and Program in Neuroscience, University of Maryland Baltimore School of Dentistry, Baltimore, Maryland, USA*

Raffaele Costantini, MD, PhD *Department of General Surgery, "G. D'Annunzio" University of Chieti, Italy*

Michele Curatolo, MD, PhD *Department of Anesthesiology, University of Bern, and Department of Anesthesiology, Division of Pain Therapy, Inselspital, Bern, Switzerland*

Erin A. Dannecker, PhD, ATC *University of Missouri-Columbia, Department of Physical Therapy, Columbia, Missouri, USA*

Anthony H. Dickenson, PhD *Department of Pharmacology, University College London, London, United Kingdom*

Mats Djupsjöbacka, PhD *Center for Musculoskeletal Research, University of Gävle, Umeå, Sweden*

Xudong Dong, BDS, MSc, PhD *Faculty of Pharmaceutical Sciences, The University of British Columbia, Vancouver, British Columbia, Canada*

Malin Ernberg, DDS, PhD *Department of Clinical Oral Physiology, Institute of Odontology, Karolinska Institute, Huddinge, Sweden*

Deborah Falla, PhD *Center for Sensory-Motor Interaction, Department of Health Science and Technology, Aalborg University, Aalborg, Denmark*

Dario Farina, PhD *Center for Sensory-Motor Interaction, Department of Health Science and Technology, Aalborg University, Aalborg, Denmark*

Maria Adele Giamberardino, MD *Pathophysiology of Pain Laboratory, Ce.S.I, "G. D'Annunzio" Foundation, Department of Medicine and Science of Aging, "G. D'Annunzio" University of Chieti, Italy*

Richard H. Gracely, PhD *Departments of Medicine-Rheumatology and Neurology, University of Michigan Health System, Ann Arbor, Michigan, USA*

Thomas Graven-Nielsen, Dr Med Sci, PhD *Department of Health Sciences and Technology, Center for Sensory-Motor Interaction, Aalborg University, Aalborg, Denmark*

Paul W. Hodges, MedDr, PhD, BPhty(Hons) *NHMRC Centre of Clinical Research Excellence in Spinal Pain, Injury and Health, School of Health and Rehabilitation Sciences, The University of Queensland, Brisbane, Queensland, Australia*

Ulrich Hoheisel, Dr Rer Nat, *Institute of Pharmacology and Toxicology, Charité, Humboldt University, Berlin, Germany*

Sigvard Kopp, DDS, PhD *Department of Clinical Oral Physiology, Institute of Odontology, Karolinska Institute, Huddinge, Sweden*

Stefan Lautenbacher, PhD *Department of Physiological Psychology, University of Bamberg, Bamberg, Germany*

Pascal Madeleine, PhD *Laboratory for Work-Related Pain and Biomechanics, Center for Sensory-Motor Interaction, Department of Health Science and Technology, Aalborg University, Aalborg, Denmark*

William Maixner, DDS, PhD *Center for Neurosensory Disorders, School of Dentistry, University of North Carolina, Chapel Hill, North Carolina, USA*

Radi Masri, BDS, PhD *Department of Endodontics, Prosthodontics and Operative Dentistry, and Program in Neuroscience, University of Maryland Baltimore School of Dentistry, Baltimore, Maryland, USA*

Siegfried Mense, Dr Med *Institute of Anatomy and Cell Biology, University of Heidelberg, Heidelberg, Germany*

Kazue Mizumura, MD, PhD *Department of Neuroscience II, Research Institute of Environmental Medicine, Nagoya University, Nagoya, Japan*

Wahida Rahman, PhD *Department of Pharmacology, University College London, London, United Kingdom*

Jin Y. Ro, PhD *Department of Biomedical Sciences and Program in Neuroscience, University of Maryland Baltimore School of Dentistry, Baltimore, Maryland, USA*

Barry J. Sessle, MDS, PhD, DSc(hc), FRSC *Faculty of Dentistry and Centre for the Study of Pain, Toronto, Ontario, Canada*

Kathleen A. Sluka, PT, PhD *Physical Therapy and Rehabilitation Science Graduate Program, Pain Research Program, University of Iowa, Iowa City, Iowa, USA*

Peter Svensson, DDS, PhD, Dr Odont *Department of Clinical Oral Physiology, School of Dentistry, University of Aarhus, Aarhus, Denmark; Department of Oral and Maxillofacial Surgery, Aarhus University Hospital, Aarhus, Denmark; Orofacial Pain Laboratory, Center for Sensory-Motor Interaction, Aalborg University, Aalborg, Denmark*

Toru Taguchi, PhD *Department of Neuroscience II, Research Institute of Environmental Medicine, Nagoya University, Nagoya, Japan*

Irmgard Tegeder, Dr Med *Pharmazentrum Frankfurt, Institute of Clinical Pharmacology/ZAFES, Clinic of the Johann Wolfgang Goethe University, Frankfurt am Main, Germany*

Roxanne Y. Walder, PhD *Physical Therapy and Rehabilitation Science Graduate Program, Pain Research Program, University of Iowa, Iowa City, Iowa, USA*

Preface

The clinical importance of pain from musculoskeletal structures is obvious. Musculoskeletal pain is a diagnostic and therapeutic problem, and further insights into the peripheral and central neurobiological mechanisms are needed to improve diagnosis, therapy, and the implementation of mechanism-based treatment regimes. It has become increasingly evident that muscle hyperalgesia, referred pain, referred hyperalgesia, and widespread hyperalgesia play an important role in chronic musculoskeletal pain. Besides the sensory consequences of musculoskeletal pain, the motor control systems are also affected, changing the drive to the muscles and the related biomechanics.

This book integrates the research findings within the field of musculoskeletal pain into a comprehensive publication that will update the reader on novel mechanisms involved in the sensory and motor characteristics of such pain. The authors attempt to translate findings from basic animal studies, and from human experimental pain studies, into potential clinical mechanisms.

The historical perspective of muscle pain investigations is extensive. Articular and muscular forms of rheumatism had been differentiated by the 18th century. Muscular rheumatism was defined as pain and stiffness in muscle and soft tissue. Other authors note the use of alternative terms: Muskelschwiele (muscle callus; defined in 1843), "muscular rheumatism" (1900), fibrositis (1915), Myogelose (muscle gelling; 1919), Muskelhärten (muscle hardenings; 1925), myalgia (1942), myogelosis (1942), nonarticular rheumatism (1951), and myofascial pain (1952) (Reynolds MD. The development of the concept of fibrositis. J Hist Med Allied Sci 1983;38:5–35; Simons DG. Muscular pain syndromes. In: Fricton JR, Awad E, editors. Myofascial pain and fibromyalgia. New York: Raven Press; 1990, pp 1–41). In the 1930s, Lewis and Kellgren pioneered the experimental approach to the study of muscle hyperalgesia and referred pain in humans and introduced the concept of experimentally induced muscle pain. Some of the first systematic recordings from thin-caliber muscle afferent fibers in animals were made in the early 1960s by Paintal (J Physiol 1960;152:250–270) and Iggo (J Physiol 1961;155:52–53), who reported responsiveness to noxious and innocuous stimuli. The next major breakthrough in muscle pain physiology was in the mid-1970s, when Mense, Kniffki, and Schmidt thoroughly characterized a subgroup of thin-afferent nerve fibers as muscle nociceptors. This work was later followed by numerous animal investigations addressing the central consequences of peripheral muscle nociception. For over a decade there has been extensive work on translating the basic animal findings to clinical manifestations, especially in experimental muscle pain studies in humans. Over the last 10 years the relative publication rate per year within the field of musculoskeletal pain has been higher than for pain in general. This trend reflects the need to develop new pharmacological targets for chronic musculoskeletal pain (including fibromyalgia), which is now a major focus of many pharmaceutical companies.

This volume includes contributions mainly based on presentations from the 7th IASP Research Symposium, "Fundamentals of Musculoskeletal Pain," which took place in May 2007 at Aalborg University's Center for Sensory-Motor Interaction and was organized by Profs. Thomas Graven-Nielsen and Lars Arendt-Nielsen. More than 180 clinicians and basic scientists participated in the 3-day symposium. The symposium attracted participants from Europe and from 18 countries outside Europe, including Australia, Brazil, Canada, Egypt, Israel, Japan, New Zealand, Russia, and Switzerland. Twenty-seven plenary lectures were given by invited international speakers, and there were also poster presentations and oral presentations based on peer-reviewed accepted abstracts.

The present book is organized in three main sections: (I) Basic Mechanisms of Muscle Pain, (II) Key Factors Determining Muscle Pain Sensitivity, and (III) Effects of Muscle Pain on Motor Function. The first section focuses on morphology and functional types of peripheral muscle nociceptors; on central neurophysiological mechanisms involved in nociception, such as central sensitization and descending modulation of spinal mechanisms; and on cortical representation of muscle nociception. The potential human correlates are outlined. The next section presents factors that can influence muscle nociceptive mechanisms, including genetics, gender, chronic pain, analgesics, and pain from other tissues. Part III outlines the effects of musculoskeletal pain on muscle function in contributions covering lower back, neck, and jaw muscle systems together with advanced neurophysiological assessments of muscle function, from proprioceptive afferents to motor units. Each section emphasizes the translational aspects and includes contributions from animal studies, human experimental studies, and clinical findings. All authors are sincerely acknowledged for meeting our publication deadlines with their enthusiastic contributions of high-quality manuscripts and for their help with peer reviews.

PROF. THOMAS GRAVEN-NIELSEN, DR MED SCI, PHD
AALBORG UNIVERSITY, DENMARK

PROF. LARS ARENDT-NIELSEN, DR MED SCI, PHD
AALBORG UNIVERSITY, DENMARK

PROF. SIEGFRIED MENSE, DR MED
UNIVERSITY OF HEIDELBERG, GERMANY

Acknowledgments

The organizers of the Fundamentals of Musculoskeletal Pain symposium would like to acknowledge IASP (which provided a Research Symposium Grant), Mundipharma, Norpharma, and the International Doctoral School in Biomedical Science and Engineering, Aalborg University, Denmark, for supporting the symposium on which this volume is based. Furthermore, the professional organizing assistance from the Center for Sensory-Motor Interaction (SMI), Aalborg University, and especially all the work by Ms. Susanne Nielsen, Head of Section, is greatly appreciated. We sincerely thank her for the work she did in organizing the practical aspects related to the symposium and this book. The highly professional people at IASP Press are acknowledged for their capable work in preparing the book for publication. In particular we thank Associate Editor Elizabeth Endres, IASP Press, who did comprehensive and valuable edits of the original manuscripts to make them easily readable for a wide audience.

PROF. THOMAS GRAVEN-NIELSEN, DR MED SCI, PHD
AALBORG UNIVERSITY, DENMARK

PROF. LARS ARENDT-NIELSEN, DR MED SCI, PHD
AALBORG UNIVERSITY, DENMARK

Part I

Basic Mechanisms of Muscle Pain

Morphology and Functional Types of Muscle Nociceptors

Siegfried Mense[a] and Ulrich Hoheisel[b]

[a]Institute of Anatomy and Cell Biology, University of Heidelberg, Heidelberg, Germany;
[b]Institute of Pharmacology and Toxicology, Charité, Humboldt University, Berlin, Germany

The term "nociceptor" (from the Latin word "noxius" for damaging or harmful) denotes a sensory ending that detects actual or potential tissue damage. The stimulation threshold of nociceptors is just below tissue-damaging intensity, because their main function is not to signal existing tissue damage, but to alert the central nervous system of possible danger.

It has long been known that small-diameter afferent fibers must be activated in order to elicit muscle pain. These fibers conduct at a velocity of below 30 m/s in the cat. Histologically, they comprise thin myelinated (group III) and unmyelinated (group IV) fibers, according to the roman numeral nomenclature suggested by Lloyd (1943) for muscle afferent fibers. The conduction velocity of group IV fibers is 0.5–2.5 m/s.

Studies in cats and rats have detected unmyelinated afferent units that have receptive fields in two different tissues. Some units had one receptive field in deep somatic tissues (muscle, joint, or periosteum) and another in the skin distal to the deep receptive field (Mense et al., 1981). The anatomical basis of this feature probably involves branching of the afferent fiber close to its termination.

Fundamentals of Musculoskeletal Pain
edited by Thomas Graven-Nielsen, Lars Arendt-Nielsen, and Siegfried Mense
IASP Press, Seattle, © 2008

3

Nociceptive afferent fibers are equipped with tetrodotoxin-resistant (TTX-r) sodium channels. The neurotoxin TTX blocks conduction in nerve fibers that possess TTX-sensitive sodium channels (mostly large-diameter fibers), but it does not affect nociceptive fibers. Two TTX-r Na$^+$ channels that are important for nociception are the voltage-gated sodium channels (Na$_V$) 1.9 and 1.8. Na$_V$1.9 has been found exclusively on nociceptive primary afferent neurons, whereas Na$_V$1.8 occurs in both nociceptive and non-nociceptive neurons (see Djouhri and Lawson, 2004, for review). Afferent fibers from high-threshold mechanosensitive (HTM, presumably nociceptive) muscle receptors are not blocked by TTX, which indicates that they have TTX-r sodium channels (Steffens et al., 2003).

Morphological Features of Nociceptive Afferent Units from Muscle

In comparison to cutaneous pain, which is more localized, muscle pain is more diffuse. At the level of the peripheral nociceptive neuron, possible reasons for this difference are the larger receptive fields of single nociceptive fibers and the lower innervation density of muscle tissue. The receptive fields of cutaneous polymodal nociceptors are less than 2 mm^2 in cats (Bessou and Perl, 1969) and 6–32 mm^2 in rabbits (Kenins, 1988). For muscle nociceptors the size of the receptive field is difficult to determine. The reported size of superficially located receptive fields or the projections of deep fields on the muscle surface range from spotlike to more than 1 cm^2 in the gastrocnemius-soleus (GS) muscle of the cat and dog (Kumazawa and Mizumura, 1977; Mense and Meyer, 1985).

Morphologically, nociceptors are free nerve endings. This term indicates that when seen under a light microscope, the nerve ending lacks a visible (corpuscular) receptive structure (Stacey, 1969). Free nerve endings are not free in the strict sense, because most of them are ensheathed by Schwann cells. Under a light microscope, the nerve ending looks like a string of beads of relatively wide diameter (known as "varicosities") connected by very thin stretches of axon. The diameter of a branch of a free nerve ending is 0.5–1.0 μm (Fig. 1A,B).

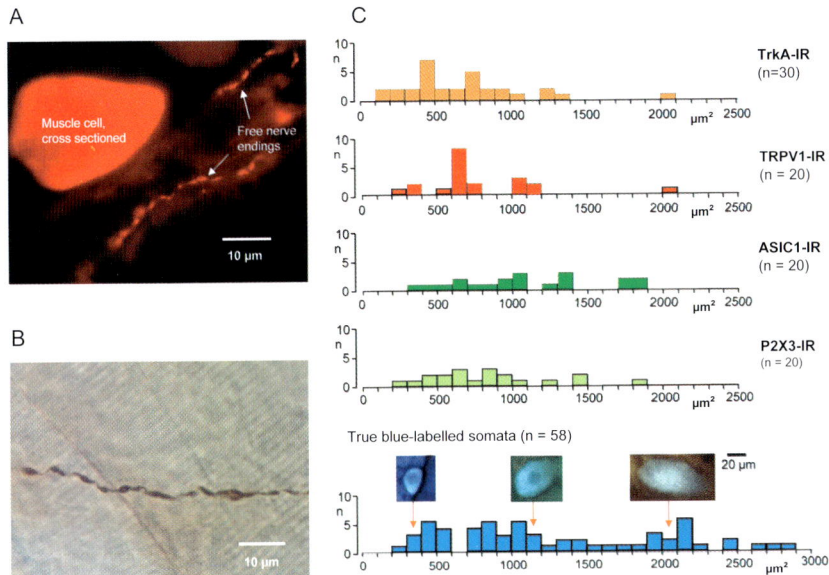

Fig. 1. (A) Two free nerve endings in the rat gastrocnemius-soleus (GS) muscle visualized with fluorescent antibodies to substance P (SP). (B) A preterminal axon in the rat multifidus muscle stained with antibodies to calcitonin gene-related peptide (CGRP). Panels A and B show the varicosities connected by very thin stretches of axon. (C) Size distribution of rat dorsal root ganglion (DRG) cells exhibiting immunoreactivity to various receptor molecules. Only cells are shown that projected to the GS muscle. For comparison, the lowermost panel shows the size distribution of all DRG cells retrogradely marked by injections of true blue into the GS muscle. Most of the cells with immunoreactivity to receptor molecules were small. Data for TrkA are from Hoheisel and Mense (unpublished data); TRPV1, ASIC1, P2X3: modified from Hoheisel et al. (2004).

In addition to nociceptors, thermoreceptors and some low-threshold mechanoreceptors are also free nerve endings, and so far no features are known by which these functionally different endings can be distinguished by light or electron microscopy. The same applies to the various functional types of nociceptor (e.g., mechano- or polymodal nociceptors), which cannot be recognized by their microscopic appearance.

The first comprehensive report on the morphology of free nerve endings in skeletal muscle was published by Stacey (1969). He used the silver impregnation technique in sympathectomized cats and focused on endings supplied by group III and IV fibers. Most of the latter had a diameter of 0.35 µm, the unmyelinated afferents outnumbering the myelinated ones by a factor of 2. The predominant location of free nerve endings supplied by group IV fibers was the adventitia of arterioles and venules. Group III afferents generated not only free nerve endings but also paciniform corpuscles, whereas group IV fibers terminated exclusively in free nerve endings (see also Barker, 1967). Thus, the number of free nerve endings is much higher than that of muscle spindles and pacinian corpuscles together.

The electron microscope shows that free nerve endings have a rather complete sheath of Schwann cells, with only small patches of the axonal membrane uncovered. These exposed areas are separated from the interstitial fluid by the basal lamina (Andres et al., 1985; Heppelmann and al., 1990a,b; Messlinger, 1997). The varicosities contain mitochondria and vesicles and show other structural specializations characteristic of receptive structures. The exposed membrane areas are assumed to be the sites where external stimuli act (Fig. 2). Electron microscopic features that are considered characteristic for nociceptive free nerve endings are an axoplasmic reticulum (probably derived from the smooth endoplasmic reticulum), vesicle aggregates embedded in a granular axonal matrix, and exposed membrane areas (Andres and v. Düring, 1973; Kruger et al., 2003a,b). Often, nociceptive endings exhibit dense core vesicles that contain neuropeptides. The function of the round clear vesicles in the peripheral ending is still obscure, but they may contain the same transmitters as the central synaptic terminal (e.g., glutamate).

In skeletal muscle of sympathectomized cats, the terminals of group III fibers were found to be generally larger than those of group IV fibers, and they contained more mitochondria (Düring and Andres, 1990). The authors suggested that those terminals that had a close spatial relation to mast cells were nociceptors.

Neuropeptide Content of Muscle Nociceptors

No neuropeptide or combination of peptides has been found that can be considered specific for afferent fibers from muscle. Dorsal root ganglion (DRG) cells projecting in a muscle nerve contain substance P (SP),

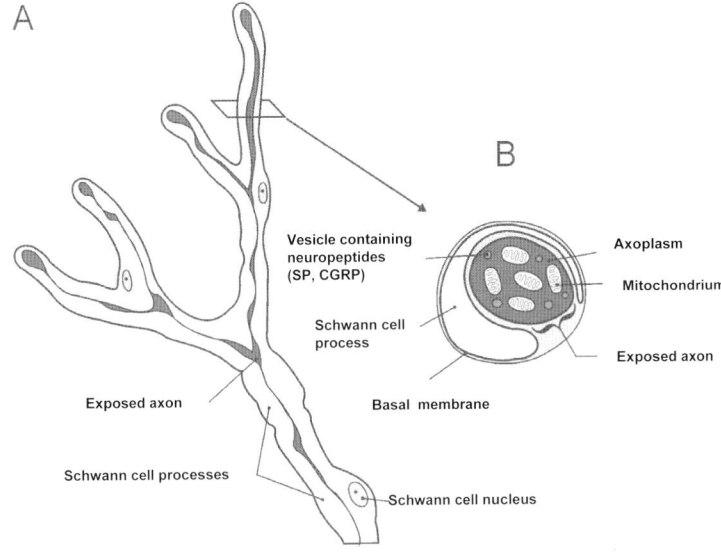

Fig. 2. (A) Scheme of a free nerve ending reconstructed from electron microscopic sections. The ending is almost completely ensheathed by Schwann cell processes, with only small patches of axon uncovered (exposed axon areas). (B) Cross-section through a branch of the ending.

calcitonin gene-related peptide (CGRP), and somatostatin and thus present a peptide pattern similar to that of cutaneous nerves (Molander et al., 1987; O'Brien et al., 1989). Muscle nerves contain less SP than skin nerves. A possible teleological reason for this difference is that the edema caused by the release of SP from muscle afferents would lead to very high pressure in muscles that are surrounded by a tight fascia. The high pressure may damage muscle cells.

In DRG cells, SP-like immunoreactivity (SP-LI)—and to a lesser extent, CGRP-LI—occurs predominantly in nociceptive units (Lawson et al., 1997; Djouhri and Lawson, 2004). However, there is also evidence against a relationship between nociceptive function and the presence of SP. For instance, Leah et al. (1985) found that 10 out of 12 individually identified nociceptive DRG cells did not exhibit SP-LI. The presence of CGRP does not distinguish between high- and low-threshold mechanosensitive receptors with group IV afferent fibers, because the neuropeptide was found in both types of receptor (Hoheisel et al., 1994).

One hypothesis states that there are two immunohistochemically distinct types of nociceptors: peptidergic and lectin-positive. Lectin-positive endings, which are largely peptide free, bind the plant isolectin B4 (IB4). Many IB4-positive endings express the purinergic P2X3 receptor. In contrast, peptidergic endings are equipped with the vanilloid receptor TRPV1 (Snider and McMahon, 1998; Stucky and Lewin, 1999). The peptidergic endings express trkA receptors, are dependent on nerve growth factor (NGF) in their development, and express predominantly TTX-sensitive Na^+ channels, whereas the nonpeptidergic, IB4-positive endings depend on glial-cell-derived neurotrophic factor (GDNF) in their development and express more TTX-resistant Na^+ channels than do IB4-negative fibers (Wu and Pan, 2004). So far, this hypothesis has not been tested in muscle nociceptors.

The marked sensitivity of free nerve endings to chemical stimuli, particularly to those released during ischemia and inflammation, may be related to their location in or close to the wall of blood vessels. A quantitative evaluation of neuropeptide-immunoreactive (-ir) free nerve endings in the rat GS muscle found that most endings were near small blood vessels (arterioles or venules) (Reinert et al., 1998). CGRP-ir endings were most numerous, followed by endings with immunoreactivity for SP, vasoactive intestinal polypeptide (VIP), nerve growth factor (NGF), and growth-associated protein (GAP) 43. Many endings exhibited immunoreactivity for more than one peptide, e.g., for SP and CGRP or for SP and VIP.

After 12 days of experimental myositis, the innervation density of the muscle with neuropeptide-ir free nerve endings increased significantly. The effect was particularly marked for endings with SP immunoreactivity (Reinert et al., 1998). The density of NGF-ir and GAP-43-ir fibers was likewise higher in inflamed muscle, which may indicate that sprouting had occurred, because NGF and GAP-43 are strongly expressed in growth cones.

Experiments in which single DRG cells with receptive endings in muscle were first functionally identified and then injected with a dye have shown CGRP-LI in at least some cell bodies whose peripheral axons terminated in HTM (presumably nociceptive) receptors (Hoheisel et al., 1994). However, immunoreactivity to SP, CGRP, and other neuropeptides occurred not only in nociceptive units but also in other types of muscle receptors, including muscle spindles and other low-threshold mechano-sensitive (LTM) units.

Functional Properties of Muscle Nociceptors

In mammalian skin, the following types of nociceptor are generally distinguished (data from monkeys, after Djouhri and Lawson, 2004):

- Type I A mechano-heat (AMH) receptors. They are supplied by myelinated A fibers, either thick (Aβ) or thin myelinated (Aδ) fibers.
- Type II A mechano-heat (AMH) nociceptors. These receptors have thin myelinated (Aδ) afferent fibers.
- C-fiber mechano-heat (CMH) nociceptors, which are supplied by unmyelinated C fibers.
- Cold nociceptors, which are excited by very low temperatures.
- Polymodal nociceptors, which respond to all types of noxious stimuli—mechanical as well as chemical and thermal.

For muscle nociceptors, no generally accepted classification is available. Most studies have used graded mechanical stimuli and intramuscular injection of algesic substances to roughly characterize the endings. Fig. 3A shows the determination of the mechanical threshold of a single muscle group IV unit using a pneumatic forceps. The forceps delivered pressure stimuli of increasing intensity to the GS muscle (stimulus trace in the lower panel). The first clear excitation occurred at a stimulus intensity of 2 bar (upper panel, intensity given on the ordinate axis). In behavioral tests, this intensity was the pressure pain threshold of nonanesthetized rats. When a hand-held forceps was used for classification (Fig 3B), two groups were distinguished—LTM units that responded to innocuous deformation of the muscle and HTM units that were excited only by noxious squeezing of the muscle. The latter stimulus was perceived as painful when applied to the experimenters' thenar muscle. As can be seen from Fig. 3B, the distribution of the mechanical thresholds of the two groups (determined with the pneumatic forceps) shows two clear peaks that characterize the majority of LTM and HTM units classified by hand.

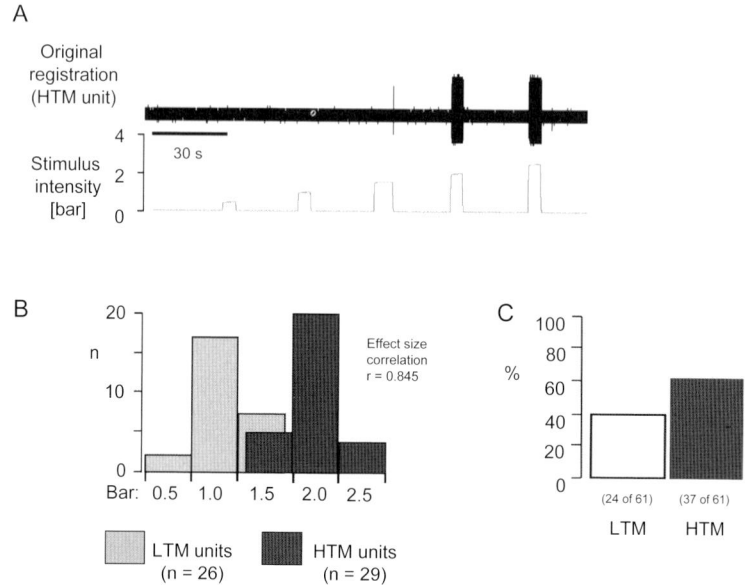

Fig. 3. High-threshold mechanosensitive (HTM, presumably nociceptive) and low-threshold mechanosensitive (LTM, presumably non-nociceptive) group IV afferent units from rat GS muscle. (A) Identification of an HTM receptor with mechanical stimuli delivered by a pneumatic forceps. The ending had a threshold of 2 bar. (B) distribution of the mechanical thresholds of 55 group IV muscle receptors. The classification of the units into LTM and HTM was made with a hand-held forceps, and then the objective thresholds were determined with a pneumatic forceps. The two mechanosensitive populations are clearly separate with a small overlap at a stimulation intensity of 1.5 (bar). The effect size correlation is the measure of the strength of the relationship between two variables. It is indicative of the overlap of two (treatment) groups (0: total overlap; −1 or 1: no overlap). (C) Relative proportions of LTM and HTM units among 61 group IV units of the rat GS muscle. Modified after Hoheisel et al. (2005).

High-threshold mechanosensitive (HTM) receptors. As stated above, HTM receptors have a high stimulation threshold to local pressure stimulation and require tissue-threatening stimuli for excitation. They are supplied by group III or group IV afferent fibers. These nociceptors do not respond to everyday stimuli such as physiological movements or gentle muscle stretching (Mense and Meyer, 1985; Mense, 1997). The proportion of pure mechanonociceptors among group III–IV units is difficult to assess, because if a unit has a high mechanical threshold and does not respond to chemical stimuli, it is possible either that the injected material did not reach the ending or that the receptor does not possess the proper receptor molecules. In a recent study of our group, approximately 60% of all mechanosensitive group IV endings had a high mechanical threshold (Hoheisel et al., 2005; Fig. 3C). Among group III muscle afferent units, the proportion of HTM receptors was smaller.

Chemonociceptors. Often, endings are encountered that respond to algesic agents but not to mechanical stimuli. Examples are receptors that are strongly excited by ischemic contractions but not (or only weakly) by contractions alone (Kaufman et al., 1984). All receptors that showed strong reactions to ischemic contractions had group IV afferent fibers (Mense and Stahnke, 1983). Therefore, the pain of intermittent claudication may be a type of pain that is exclusively due to activity in group IV afferent units. In the cat, the proportion of these units was approximately 10% of the group IV units (Mense and Stahnke, 1983).

Polymodal nociceptors. These units respond to high-intensity pressure stimulation and algesic substances (noxious heat is difficult to test in muscle). When free nerve endings in muscle are tested with a defined set of mechanical and chemical stimuli, they show all possible response combinations (Kniffki et al., 1978). Microneurographic recordings in human muscles have demonstrated receptors that respond to both noxious squeezing and injection of algesic substances (e.g., capsaicin; Marchettini et al., 1996). The chemical sensitivity of group IV endings is often restricted to only some of the algesic agents. For instance, intramuscular injection of an acidic buffer solution (pH 6) excited about 60% of the group IV units tested (Hoheisel et al., 2004). The only chemical stimulus that excited every unit tested was hypertonic saline. Some investigators consider all muscle nociceptors to be polymodal (Kumazawa and Mizumura, 1976; Kumazawa, 1996).

Studies in cats have found nociceptors in the joints that initially did not respond to mechanical stimuli, but became mechanosensitive after induction of an experimental arthritis (Schaible and Schmidt, 1988). Whether such silent or "sleeping" nociceptors are also present in skeletal muscle has yet to be determined.

Not all muscle group IV afferent fibers are nociceptors. In the rat GS muscle, approximately 40% are LTM receptors (Fig. 3C; Mense and

Meyer, 1985; Light and Perl, 2003; Hoheisel et al., 2005). Many of them can be excited by weak innocuous pressure stimuli but not by physiological stretching. These endings probably mediate subjective pressure sensations (Graven-Nielsen et al., 2004). Another non-nociceptive type of group IV afferent unit is the ergoreceptor. Some ergoreceptors are activated by physiological contractions and strong stretching, and others by metabolites; they are assumed to mediate the adjustment of respiration and circulation during physical exercise (McCloskey and Mitchell, 1972; Kalia et al., 1981).

Receptor Molecules in the Membrane of a Nociceptive Ending

No specific data are available on the receptor molecules that are present in the membrane of muscle nociceptors. Judging from the responsiveness of these endings to injections of algesic agents the following receptor molecules are likely to be relevant for muscle pain (Mense and Meyer, 1985; Caterina and Julius, 1999; 2001; McCleskey and Gold, 1999; Mense, 2007).

Receptors for inflammatory substances. Bradykinin, serotonin (5-hydroxytryptamin, 5-HT), and prostaglandin E_2 (PGE_2) have long been known to excite or sensitize muscle nociceptors (Kumazawa and Mizumura, 1977; Mense and Meyer, 1985). Bradykinin is ubiquitously present in the body, because it is released from plasma proteins by the action of the enzyme kallikrein. Receptors for bradykinin are the B_1 and B_2 receptor, for 5-HT the $5-HT_3$ receptor, and for prostaglandin E_2 the prostanoid (EP_2) receptor. In intact tissue, bradykinin influences the ending through the B_2 receptor; when a tissue is inflamed, B_1 receptors are synthesized and mediate the effects of bradykinin (Perkins and Kelley, 1993). This is an example of a neuroplastic change in the nociceptive ending.

Receptors for protons. Besides acid-sensing ion channels (e.g., ASIC1 and 3), the vanilloid receptor (TRPV1; Caterina and Julius, 1999; 2001) has been found in DRG cells that supply receptive endings in skeletal muscle (Fig. 1C; Hoheisel et al., 2004). Capsaicin is the specific ligand of the TRPV1 receptor; it is also sensitive to hydrogen ions and heat. In a recent study, capsaicin activated approximately 54% of muscle group IV units (Hoheisel et al., 2004). Circumstances in which the pH of the tissue is low (exhausting muscle work, ischemia, and inflammation) are likely to activate the proton-sensitive receptors. In a rat study, approximately 60% of group IV muscle receptors were excited by intramuscular injections of a buffer solution at a pH of 6 (Hoheisel et al., 2004). The proton-sensitive nociceptors may be of particular importance for chronic muscle pain conditions. Repeated intramuscular administration of acidic solutions have been reported to induce a long-lasting hyperalgesia (Sluka et al., 2001).

   Purinergic receptors. These receptors bind adenosine triphosphate (ATP) and the products of ATP degradation. P2X3 receptors (Burnstock, 2000; Cook and McCleskey, 2002) are present in cutaneous nociceptors; they have also been found in DRG cells supplying the rat GS muscle (Fig. 1C). ATP is present in all cells of the body and is released when cells or their membranes are damaged. In the rat GS muscle, group IV receptors responded to ATP in concentrations that occur in muscle cells (Reinöhl et al., 2003). When injected into human muscle, ATP causes pain (Mörk et al., 2003).

   Receptors for growth factors. Data from our group (Hoheisel et al., 2005) showed that NGF (the ligand of the TrkA receptor) excites exclusively HTM muscle receptors (presumable nociceptors). NGF is the only substance known so far that has such an exclusive action on nociceptive endings. DRG cells supplying rat GS muscle express TrkA receptors (Fig. 1C).

   Receptors for excitatory amino acids. Evidence from experiments in rats indicates that nociceptors in muscle are equipped with glutamate receptors (Cairns et al., 2002; Lam et al., 2005). Likewise, nociceptors in the deep tissues around the temporomandibular joint are activated by glutamate (Cairns et al., 1998). Since glutamate is the main neurotransmitter of nociceptors at the spinal level, it could also be released from the receptive ending. However, in experimental muscle pain tests, no increased release was found (Ashina et al., 2005).

Among the algesic agents that probably activate muscle nociceptors without binding to specific receptor molecules are hypertonic Na^+ solutions. Large increases in extracellular Na^+ do not occur under physiological (or pathophysiological) conditions but can be induced in clinical studies on muscle pain mechanisms when hypertonic saline is injected or infused intramuscularly (Graven-Nielsen et al., 1997). In these experiments, the high Na^+ concentration—and not the hypertonicity of the solution—appears to be the effective stimulus (Mense, 2007). Theoretically, the receptive ending could shrink in the hypertonic environment, and stretch-sensitive Na^+-channels could open. However, nothing is known about the water permeability of nociceptive endings, and the high mechanical stimulation threshold of muscle nociceptors speaks against this mechanism. Hypertonic saline may also excite muscle nociceptors indirectly by releasing glutamate (Tegeder et al., 2002; Svensson et al., 2003).

One of the characteristic properties of a mechanonociceptor is its high mechanical stimulation threshold. The high mechanical threshold is surprising, considering the fact that a free nerve ending is a delicate structure with a semifluid membrane. One factor that may be responsible for the high mechanical threshold is a special mechanosensitive ion channel, the TRPV4 channel (Liedtke, 2005).

Of the receptor molecules mentioned above, three are probably particularly relevant for clinical cases of muscle pain. One is the P2X3 receptor for ATP. The concentration of ATP is relatively high in muscle, and therefore ATP released from muscle cells is an important factor for all cases that are associated with lesions of muscle cells (e.g., acute trauma or chronic conditions with muscle cell necrosis). The second type of membrane receptor includes those that are sensitive to protons (TRPV1, ASICs). In almost all pathological muscle conditions myositis, tonic contractions, and myofascial trigger points, tissue pH is lowered to an extent that can activate the proton-sensitive channels. The third receptor is TrkA, which binds NGF. NGF appears to be particularly important for chronic muscle pain conditions, because it is a powerful sensitizing agent at both the peripheral and spinal level. It is probably involved in most cases of allodynia and hyperalgesia seen in patients with chronic muscle pain. However, it has to be kept in mind that in clinical pain conditions, many of the pronociceptive substances are released together in various combinations. Therefore, it is difficult to name key substances.

References

Andres KH, Düring MV. Morphology of cutaneous receptors. In: Iggo A, editor. Handbook of sensory physiology, Vol. II, Somatosensory system. Berlin: Springer, 1973. p 3–28.

Andres KH, Düring MV, Schmidt RF. Sensory innervation of the Achilles tendon by group III and IV afferent fibers. Anat Embryol 1985;172:145–156.

Ashina M, Jorgensen M, Stallknecht B, Mork H, Bendtsen L, Pedersen JF, Olesen J, Jensen R. No release of interstitial glutamate in experimental human model of muscle pain. Eur J Pain 2005;9:337–343.

Barker D. The innervation of mammalian skeletal muscle. In: DeReuck AVS, Knight J, editors. CIBA Foundation Symposium on myotatic, kinesthetic and vestibular mechanisms. Boston: Little, Brown, 1967. p. 3–19.

Bessou P, Perl ER. Response of cutaneous sensory units with unmyelinated fibers to noxious stimuli. J Neurophysiol 1969;32:1025–1043.

Burnstock G. P2X receptors in sensory neurones. Br J Anaesth 2000;84:476–488.

Cairns BE, Sessle BJ, Hu JW. Evidence that excitatory amino acid receptors within the temporomandibular joint region are involved in the reflex activation of the jaw muscles. J Neurosci 1998;18:8056–8064.

Cairns BE, Gambarota G, Svensson P, Arendt-Nielsen L, Berde CB. Glutamate-induced sensitization of rat masseter muscle fibers. Neuroscience 2002;109:389–399.

Caterina MJ, Julius D. Sense and specificity: a molecular identity for nociceptors. Curr Opin Neurobiol 1999;9:525–530.

Caterina MJ, Julius D. The vanilloid receptor: a molecular gateway to the pain pathway. Ann Rev Neurosci 2001;24:487–517.

Cook SP, McCleskey EW. Cell damage excites nociceptors through release of cytosolic ATP. Pain 2002;95:41–47.

Djouhri L, Lawson SN. Aβ-fiber nociceptive primary afferent neurons: a review of incidence and properties in relation to other afferent A-fiber neurons in mammals. Brain Res Rev 2004;46:131–145.

Düring MV, Andres KH. Topography and ultrastructure of group III and IV nerve terminals of the cat's gastrocnemius-soleus muscle. In: Zenker W, Neuhuber WL, editors. The primary afferent neuron. New York: Plenum Press, 1990. p. 35–41.

Graven-Nielsen T, Arendt-Nielsen L, Svensson P, Jenssen TS. Experimental muscle pain: a quantitative study of local and referred pain in humans following injection of hypertonic saline. J Musculoskel Pain 1997;5:49–69.

Graven-Nielsen T, Mense S, Arendt-Nielsen L. Painful and non-painful pressure sensations from human skeletal muscle. Exp Brain Res 2004;59:273–283.

Heppelmann B, Messlinger K, Neiss W, Schmidt RF. Ultrastructural three-dimensional reconstruction of group III and group IV sensory nerve endings (free nerve endings) in the knee joint capsule of the rat: evidence for multiple receptive sites. J Comp Neurol 1990a;292:103–116.

Heppelmann B, Messlinger K, Neiss WF, Schmidt RF. The sensory terminal tree of 'free nerve endings' in the articular capsule of the knee. In: Zenker W, Neuhuber WL, editors. The primary afferent neuron. New York: Plenum Press, 1990b. p. 73–85.

Hoheisel U, Mense S, Scherotzke R. Calcitonin gene-related peptide-immunoreactivity in functionally identified primary afferent neurones in the rat. Anat Embryol 1994;189:41–49.

Hoheisel U, Reinöhl J, Unger T, Mense S. Acidic pH and capsaicin activate mechanosensitive group IV muscle receptors in the rat. Pain 2004;110:149–157.

Hoheisel U, Unger T, Mense S. Excitatory and modulatory effects of inflammatory cytokines and neurotrophins on mechanosensitive group IV muscle afferents in the rat. Pain 2005;114:168–176.

Kalia M, Mei SS, Kao FF. Central projections from ergoreceptors (C-fibers) in muscle involved in cardiopulmonary responses to static exercise. Circ Res 1981;48:148–162.

Kaufman MP, Rybicki KJ, Waldrop TG. Effect of ischemia on responses of group III and IV afferents to contraction. J Appl Physiol 1984;57:644–650.

Kenins P. The functional anatomy of the receptive fields of rabbit C polymodal nociceptors. J Neurophysiol 1988;59:1098–1115.

Kniffki K, Mense S, Schmidt RF. Responses of group IV afferent units from skeletal muscle to stretch, contraction and chemical stimulation. Exp Brain Res 1978;31:511–522.

Kruger L, Light AR, Schweizer FE. Axonal terminals of sensory neurons and their morphological diversity. J Neurocytol 2003a;32:205–216.

Kruger L, Kavookjian AM, Kumazawa T, Light AR, Mizumura, K. Nociceptor structural specialization in canine and rodent testicular "free" nerve endings. J Comp Neurol 2003b;463:197–211.

Kumazawa T. The polymodal receptor; bio-warning and defense system. In: Kumazawa T, Kruger L, Mizumura K, editors. Progress in Brain Research, Vol.113. Amsterdam: Elsevier Science, 1996. p. 3–18.

Kumazawa T, Mizumura K. The polymodal C-fiber receptor in the muscle of the dog. Brain Res 1976;101:589–593.

Kumazawa T, Mizumura K. Thin-fibre receptors responding to mechanical, chemical and thermal stimulation in the skeletal muscle of the dog. J Physiol 1977;273:179–194.

Lam DK, Sessle BJ, Cairns BE, Hu JW. Peripheral NMDA receptor modulation of jaw muscle electromyographic activity induced by capsaicin injection into the temporomandibular joint of rats. Brain Res 2005;1046:68–76.

Lawson SN, Crepps BA, Perl ER. Relationship of substance P to afferent characteristics of dorsal root ganglion neurons in guinea-pig. J Physiol 1997;505:177–191.

Leah JD, Cameron AA, Snow PJ. Neuropeptides in physiologically identified mammalian sensory neurones. Neurosci Lett 1985;56:257–263.

Liedtke WB. TRPV4 plays an evolutionary conserved role in the transduction of osmotic and mechanical stimuli in live animals. J Physiol 2005;567:53–58.

Light AR, Perl ER. Unmyelinated afferent fibers are not only for pain anymore. J Comp Neurol 2003;461:137–139.

Lloyd DPC. Neuron patterns controlling transmission of ipsilateral hind limb reflexes in cat. J Neurophysiol 1943;6:293–315.

Marchettini P, Simone DA, Caputi G, Ochoa JL. Pain from excitation of identified muscle nociceptors in humans. Brain Res 1996;40:109–116.

McCleskey EW, Gold MS. Ion channels of nociception. Annu Rev Physiol 1999;61:835–856.

McCloskey DI, Mitchell JH. Reflex cardiovascular and respiratory responses originating in exercising muscle. J Physiol 1972;224:173–186.

Mense S. Pathophysiologic basis of muscle pain syndromes. Phys Med Rehab Clin N Am 1997;8:23–53.

Mense S. Muscle nociceptors and their neurochemistry. In: Schmidt RF, Willis WS. Encyclopedic Reference of Pain. Heidelberg: Springer; 2007. p 1203–1207.

Mense S, Light AR, Perl ER. Spinal terminations of subcutaneous high-threshold mechanoreceptors. In: Brown AG, Réthelyi M, editors. Spinal cord sensation. Edinburgh: Scottish Academic Press; 1981, p. 79–86.

Mense S, Meyer H. Different types of slowly conducting afferent units in cat skeletal muscle and tendon. J Physiol 1985;363:403–417.

Mense S, Stahnke M. Responses in muscle afferent fibres of slow conduction velocity to contractions and ischaemia in the cat. J Physiol 1983;342:383–397.

Mörk H, Ashina M, Bendtsen L, Olesen J, Jensen R. Experimental muscle pain and tenderness following infusion of endogenous substances in humans. Eur J Pain 2003;7:145–153.

Messlinger K. Was ist ein Nozizeptor? Schmerz 1997;5:353–367.

Molander C, Ygge I, Dalsgaard CJ. Substance P-, somatostatin-, and calcitonin gene-related peptide-like immunoreactivity and fluoride resistant acid phosphatase-activity in relation to retrogradely labeled cutaneous, muscular and visceral primary sensory neurons in the rat. Neurosci Lett 1987;74:37–42.

O'Brien C, Woolf CJ, Fitzgerald M, Lindsay RM, Molander C. Differences in the chemical expression of rat primary afferent neurons which innervate skin, muscle or joint. Neuroscience 1989;32:493–502.

Perkins MN, Kelly D. Induction of bradykinin-B1 receptors in vivo in a model of ultraviolet irradiation-induced thermal hyperalgesia in the rat. Br J Pharmacol 1993;110:1441–1444.

Reinert A, Kaske A, Mense S. Inflammation-induced increase in the density of neuropeptide-immunoreactive nerve endings in rat skeletal muscle. Exp Brain Res 1998;121:174–180.

Reinöhl J, Hoheisel U, Unger T, Mense S. Adenosine triphosphate as a stimulant for nociceptive and non-nociceptive muscle group IV receptors in the rat. Neurosci Lett 2003;338:25–28.

Schaible HG, Schmidt RF. Time course of mechanosensitivity changes in articular afferents during a developing experimental arthritis. J Neurophysiol 1988;60:2180–2195.

Sluka KA, Kalra A, Moore SA. Unilateral intramuscular injections of acidic saline produce a bilateral long-lasting hyperalgesia. Muscle Nerve 2001;24:37–46.

Snider WE, McMahon SB. Tackling pain at the source: new ideas about nociceptors. Neuron 1998;20:629–632.

Stacey MJ. Free nerve endings in skeletal muscle of the cat. J Anat 1969;105:231–254.

Steffens H, Eek B, Trudrung P, Mense S. Tetrodotoxin block of A-fibre afferents from skin and muscle: a tool to study pure C-fibre effects in the spinal cord. Pflugers Arch 2003;445:607–613.

Stucky CL, Lewin GR. Isolectin B_4-positive and -negative nociceptors are functionally distinct. J Neurosci 1999;19:6497–6505.

Svensson P, Cairns BE, Wang K, Hu JW, Graven-Nielsen T, Arendt-Nielsen L, Sessle BJ. Glutamate-evoked pain and mechanical allodynia in the human masseter muscle. Pain 2003;101:221–227.

Tegeder L, Zimmermann J, Meller ST, Geisslinger G. Release of algesic substances in human experimental muscle pain. Inflamm Res 2002;51:393–402.

Wu ZZ, Pan HL. Tetrodotoxin-sensitive and –resistant Na^+ channel currents in subsets of small sensory neurons of rats. Brain Res 2004;1029:251–258.

Correspondence to: Prof. Dr. med. S. Mense, Institut für Anatomie und Zellbiologie III, Universität Heidelberg, Im Neuenheimer Feld 307, 69120 Heidelberg, Germany. Tel: 49-6221-544193; fax: 49-6221-546071; email: mense@urz.uni-heidelberg.de.

Physiological Properties of Thin-Fiber Muscle Afferents: Excitation and Modulatory Effects

Brian E. Cairns

Faculty of Pharmaceutical Science, The University of British Columbia, Vancouver, British Columbia, Canada

Skeletal muscle is innervated by large, myelinated fibers as well as thinly myelinated (group III or Aδ fibers) and unmyelinated (group IV or C fibers) afferent fibers that have nonspecialized endings and can respond to noxious mechanical and/or chemical stimuli (Graven-Nielsen and Mense, 2001). Physiologically, group III and group IV fibers are differentiated on the basis of conduction velocity, such that in larger mammals, conduction velocities for group III fibers are 2.5–35 m/s and group IV fibers less than 2.5 m/s (Graven-Nielsen and Mense, 2001; Djouhri and Lawson, 2004). In smaller mammals such as rats and guinea pigs, muscle nerve-evoked compound action potentials suggest that the range of conduction velocities for group III fibers and group IV fibers are about 2–10 m/s and <2 m/s, respectively (Brunetti et al., 2003; Djouhri and Lawson, 2004). This chapter reviews the response characteristics of thinly myelinated and unmyelinated afferent fibers that innervate skeletal muscle and discusses the functional significance of these characteristics with an emphasis on their role as muscle nociceptors.

Fundamentals of Musculoskeletal Pain
edited by Thomas Graven-Nielsen, Lars Arendt-Nielsen, and Siegfried Mense
IASP Press, Seattle, © 2008

Mechanoreceptive Properties

Although important advances have been made in the last 15 years, the exact mechanisms whereby mechanical stimuli are converted into action potentials in mechanoreceptive afferent fibers are not yet fully elucidated. In vitro, it has been shown that mechanical (pressure or distension) or osmotic deformation of the membrane of dorsal root ganglion neurons results in the opening of nonselective cation channels that depolarize the ganglion neuron, leading to the generation of action potentials (Cho et al., 2002; Drew et al., 2002). Some evidence suggests the existence of two or more subtypes of mechanically activated cation channels that respond to lower and higher threshold mechanical stimuli (Cho et al., 2002; Drew et al., 2002). There is also evidence for both rapidly adapting and slowly adapting mechanically activated currents, which parallels the characteristics of mechanically activated afferent discharge in vivo (Drew et al., 2002). Although the exact receptor mediating these currents has not been identified, potential candidate channels include members of the transient receptor potential (TRP) family (Levine and Alessandri-Haber, 2007). It is important to recognize that these findings are based on the response of ganglion neurons in culture, and thus it is uncertain whether these same mechanisms contribute to transduction of mechanical stimuli at the peripheral terminals of afferent fibers that innervate skeletal muscle.

Anatomical and electrophysiological studies in animals suggest that slowly conducting muscle afferent fibers from the leg muscles (e.g., gastrocnemius) project to lamina I and laminae IV/V of the spinal cord (Hoheisel et al., 1989; Panneton et al., 2005), whereas slowly conducting muscle afferent fibers that innervate the masticatory muscles project to the two most caudal subnuclei (interpolaris and caudalis) of the trigeminal sensory nuclear complex (Capra and Wax, 1989; Cairns et al., 2002; Wang et al., 2006). The majority of group III fibers that innervate the gastrocnemius muscle of the cat respond to pressure stimuli with an estimated threshold of 30–200 kPa (Paintal, 1960). In the rat, however, mechanically activated group III afferent fibers are much less commonly encountered than group IV fibers in the gastrocnemius muscle (Diehl et al., 1993). Most pressure-activated gastrocnemius muscle afferent fibers adapt rapidly (within 2 seconds) to mechanical stimuli, with only a few exhibiting slowly adapting discharge (Paintal, 1960). In contrast, in uninjured rat masseter muscle, pressure stimuli activate predominantly group III fibers, although some group IV fibers are also activated (Cairns et al., 2002). About one-third of these pressure-activated masseter muscle afferent fibers that project to the caudal trigeminal sensory nuclear complex have mechanical thresholds that exceed the human pressure pain threshold (200–300 kPa) for the masseter muscle (Fig. 1) (Cairns et al., 2002). Most group III and group IV fiber mechanoreceptors in the masseter muscle exhibit slowly adapting responses to sustained suprathreshold mechanical stimulation and are not activated by jaw opening (Cairns et al., 2002).

Chemoreceptive Properties

Group III and group IV fibers that innervate skeletal muscle can be excited by changes in interstitial osmolarity and pH as well as by increases in the interstitial concentrations of a number of compounds associated

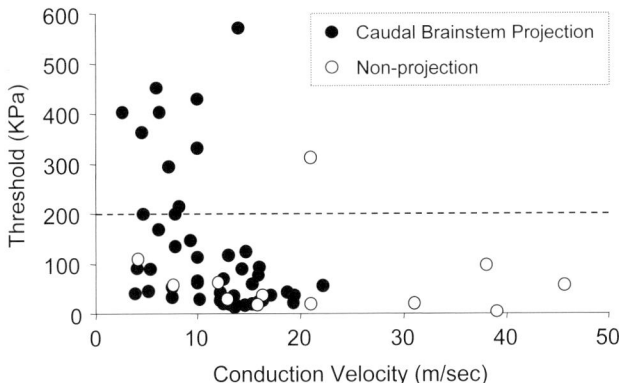

Fig. 1. The relationship between mechanical threshold and conduction velocity of rat masseter muscle afferent fibers. The dotted line indicates an approximate human pressure pain threshold (PPT) for the masseter muscle. Adapted from Cairns et al. (2002), with permission from Elsevier.

with tissue injury, such as potassium chloride (KCl), adenosine triphosphate (ATP), biogenic amine and amino acid neurotransmitters, and inflammatory mediators such as bradykinin and various cytokines. The following sections review the effect of some of the more commonly used algogenic compounds on the excitability of slowly conducting muscle afferent fibers.

Hypertonic Saline

One of the most commonly used chemical stimulants of thin-fiber muscle afferents in experimental research is hypertonic saline (HS), a solution of 4–6% sodium chloride. Injection or infusion of HS into the skeletal muscle evokes nociceptor activity and nocifensive behavior (paw shaking) in acutely anesthetized rats and causes localized muscle pain in human subjects (Svensson et al., 1995; Ro et al., 2003). Hypertonic saline solutions, when injected into the muscle, reliably evoke group III and group IV fiber discharge, and the magnitude of this discharge is inversely related to the conduction velocity of the afferent fiber (Paintal, 1960; Kumazawa and Mizumura, 1977; Mense, 1977; Cairns et al., 2003) (Fig. 2). This relationship suggests that injected HS solutions are reasonably selective in their activation of slowly conducting afferent fibers. It is not yet clear exactly how HS activates nociceptors, although researchers have theorized that the osmotic strength of HS solutions shrinks the terminal endings of sensory fibers; this effect might excite the nociceptors by opening mechanosensitive cation channels or cause the release of other excitants (Hamill and Martinac, 2001).

pH

Lowered muscle pH is also thought to play a role in muscle pain. For example, surgical trauma to the gastrocnemius muscle may cause the pH to fall to around 6.5 (Woo et al., 2004). In humans, injection of pH 5.2 buffer solution intramuscularly results in localized muscle pain (Steen et al., 2001). In rats, injection of a pH 6.0 buffer into the gastrocnemius-soleus muscle excites ~50% of mechanosensitive C fibers (Hoheisel et al., 2004).

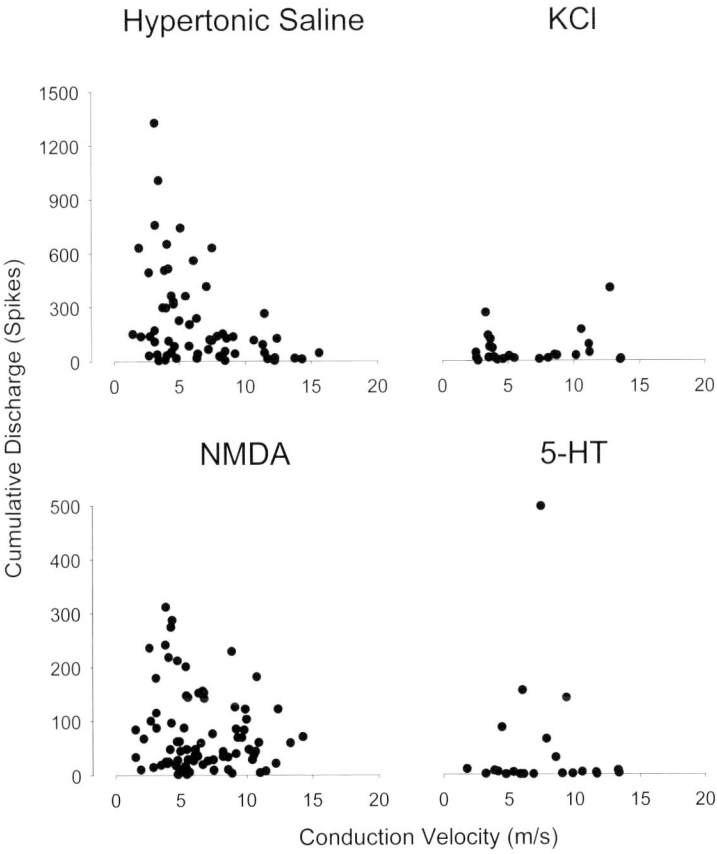

Fig. 2. The relationship between evoked discharge and conduction velocity of afferent fibers after injection of hypertonic saline, KCl, NMDA, or 5-HT into the rat masseter muscle. Note the inverse relationship between conduction velocity and cumulative discharge for hypertonic saline and NMDA, but not for KCl or 5-HT.

These effects of increased tissue proton concentrations are thought to be mediated by a family of nonselective cation channels called acid-sensing ion channels (ASICs), of which ASIC1 and ASIC3 are found in muscle afferent fibers (Sluka et al., 2003; Hoheisel et al., 2004). The ASIC1 subtypes are rapidly desensitizing cation channels that are activated at a pH of less than 6.9, whereas the ASIC3 subtype has a sustained current and is activated around pH 6.0 (Wemmie et al., 2006). In vitro, application of a pH 5–6 buffer solution evokes a large inward current that has both rapidly deactivating and sustained components in subpopulations of both gastrocnemius and masseter muscle ganglion neurons (Sluka et al., 2003; Connor et al., 2005).

Potassium Chloride

Another salt that has been used to excite muscle group III and group IV fibers is KCl. Injection of a high concentration of KCl is thought to depolarize afferent fibers by reversing the K equilibrium potential, which leads to an inward K current (O'Shaughnessy et al., 1993). In humans, injection of KCl into craniofacial muscle has been reported to be as painful as injection of HS (Jensen and Norup, 1992). In animals, close arterial injection of KCl excites both group III and group IV fibers of the gastrocnemius muscle (Fock and Mense, 1976; Kumazawa and Mizumura, 1977; Mense, 1977). However, when used to excite masseter muscle afferent fibers, KCl (2 M) is a much less effective excitant of masticatory muscle afferent fibers than HS (1 M), and it is not particularly selective for slowly conducting afferent fibers (Fig. 2).

Bradykinin

Bradykinin alone is only mildly painful when injected into human skeletal muscles (Jensen et al., 1990; Babenko et al., 1999). It is, however, a potent and selective excitant of both group III and group IV fibers in somatic muscle (Kaufman et al., 1982; Mense and Meyer, 1988). Bradykinin appears to induce small inward or outward currents in some ganglion neurons, but appears to act via the B_2 receptor to enhance the responses of other receptors involved in inflammatory responses, for example the serotonin (5-HT$_3$) receptor (Hu et al., 2005).

Serotonin

Interstitial concentrations of 5-HT may be elevated in women with fibromyalgia, and injection of 5-HT into human muscle results in brief episodes of modest muscle pain (Ernberg et al., 1999). 5-HT excites group

III and C muscle fibers that innervate the gastrocnemius and masseter muscles, but these discharges are usually brief and appear to be a result of the activation of $5HT_3$ receptors (Fock and Mense, 1976; Mense, 1977; Sung et al., 2008). Indeed, 5-HT evokes a brief, rapidly desensitizing inward current in ganglion neurons through activation of $5\text{-}HT_3$ receptors (Hu et al., 2005).

Adenosine Triphosphate

Interstitial concentrations of ATP are elevated after muscle trauma and can activate a family of cation channels expressed by trigeminal and dorsal root ganglia known as P2X receptors, in particular the P2X2 and P2X3 receptors that appear to be expressed peripherally on slowly conducting muscle afferent fibers (Ambalavanar et al., 2005). Infusion of ATP into the trapezius muscle of humans results in reports of taut muscle pain (Mørk et al., 2003). Injection of ATP or its analogues intramuscularly or by close interarterial injection can excite somatic muscle group IV fibers but is not very effective in exciting Aδ fibers (Reinohl et al., 2003; Hanna and Kaufman, 2004). Nevertheless, about two-thirds of masseter muscle ganglion neurons are depolarized by ATP, and inward currents are both rapidly and slowly adapting (Connor et al., 2005).

Glutamate

Some evidence associates certain muscle pain conditions with elevation of interstitial levels of the excitatory amino acid glutamate (Rosendal et al., 2004). In humans, injection of glutamate into skeletal muscles is associated with the development of muscle pain, and in rats, glutamate excites slowly conducting afferent fibers that innervate masticatory muscles (Svensson et al., 2005). These effects of glutamate appear to result from the activation of peripheral *N*-methyl-D-aspartate (NMDA) receptors that are expressed by masseter ganglion neurons (Cairns et al., 2003; Dong et al., 2007). The magnitude of afferent discharge evoked by peripheral NMDA-receptor activation is inversely related to the conduction velocity of the afferent fiber (Fig. 2).

Capsaicin

Injection of capsaicin into human muscle causes intense pain (Graven-Nielsen and Mense, 2001). Capsaicin strongly excites a subpopulation of group III and group IV fibers that innervate the skeletal muscle (Kaufman et al., 1982; Hoheisel et al., 2004), presumably through activation of the transient receptor potential vanilloid 1 (TRPV1) receptor. About 50% of dorsal root ganglion neurons that innervate the gastrocnemius muscle express TRPV1 receptors, and about the same percentage of trigeminal ganglion neurons that innervate the masseter muscle are depolarized by capsaicin (Hoheisel et al., 2004; Connor et al., 2005).

Modulation of Mechanical Response Properties

Injection of certain chemicals can alter the mechanical response properties of group III and C fibers that innervate skeletal muscle. For example, injection of bradykinin into the gastrocnemius muscle increases the response of slowly conducting afferent fibers to graded mechanical stimulation, which is an indication of mechanical sensitization (Mense and Meyer, 1988). Elevation of interstitial glutamate concentration in the masseter muscle also decreases the mechanical threshold of rat masseter muscle afferent fibers through activation of peripheral NMDA receptors (Cairns et al., 2002, 2007). Indeed, a two- to threefold elevation in interstitial glutamate levels in the rat masseter muscle from their usual baseline of ~ 25 µM is sufficient to induce afferent mechanical sensitization (Cairns et al., 2007). However, this mechanical sensitization does not appear to be related to either afferent conduction velocity or mechanical threshold, which suggests that it is not specific for slowly conducting, putative nociceptive afferent fibers. In contrast, injection of other excitants, such as HS and 5-HT, does not significantly alter the mechanical threshold of slowly conducting muscle fibers (Mok et al., 2005; Sung et al., 2008). Moreover, capsaicin has been reported to desensitize slowly-conducting skeletal muscle afferent fibers to mechanical stimulation

(Hoheisel et al., 2004). These findings suggest that chemically induced mechanical sensitization is not merely a result of excitation of fibers by these substances but depends on the recruitment of specific peripheral receptor mechanisms, such as activation of peripheral bradykinin or NMDA receptors.

Various cytokines have also been reported to mechanically sensitize slowly conducting afferent fibers. Close arterial injection of arachidonic acid, the precursor of prostaglandins, into the femoral artery increased the response of slowly conducting fibers to static muscle contractions of the triceps surae (Rotto et al., 1990). Injection of human nerve growth factor into the masseter muscle mechanically sensitized slowly conducting masseter afferent fibers for a period exceeding 3 hours after injection (Mann et al., 2006). On the other hand, tumor necrosis factor alpha (TNF-α) caused a significant, but short-lasting desensitization of slowly conducting afferent fibers after injection into the gastrocnemius muscle (Hoheisel et al., 2005).

Functional Role of Slowly Conducting Afferent Fibers

The findings presented above indicate that many pressure-activated group III and group IV fibers that innervate skeletal muscle have high mechanical thresholds and slowly adapting responses that are consistent with a role for these fibers in mechanical nociception. In addition, almost all of these mechanically (pressure) responsive slowly conducting afferent fibers can also be excited by a variety of chemicals known to produce pain when injected into human skeletal muscle, which suggests that they are also chemonociceptors. Finally, a small subpopulation of slowly conducting muscle afferent fibers also respond to innocuous and noxious thermal stimuli (Kumazawa and Mizumura, 1977; Mense and Meyer, 1988). Taken together, these results suggest that a significant percentage of group III and group IV fibers that innervate skeletal muscle serve as polymodal nociceptors.

A second proposed role for slowly conducting afferent fibers is as metabolic state and vascular tone sensors whose function is to activate cardiovascular reflexes and help regulate motor function under conditions of muscle fatigue. In particular, group III and group IV fibers—which respond to muscle contractions and have low to moderate mechanical thresholds to pressure stimuli—increase their response to contraction after the experimental induction of muscle fatigue, and they are further modulated by ischemia (Haouzi et al., 2004). However, group III fibers that have high mechanical thresholds to pressure stimuli and lack a response to muscle contractions do not appear to be affected by muscle ischemia (Paintal, 1960). Many skeletal muscle group IV fibers and some group III fibers appear to have their afferent endings in close association with blood vessels, and about one-third of mechanically activated group IV fibers respond to changes in vascular tone (Haouzi et al., 2004). This subpopulation of "low-threshold" mechanoreceptive slowly conducting afferent fibers appear, therefore, to monitor vascular tone and/or muscle metabolic state and may play an important role in regulating cardiovascular response to muscle fatigue.

The evidence presented suggests that vascular/metabolic sensors and nociceptors represent two distinct and separate populations of slowly conducting skeletal muscle afferent fibers. While this remains a distinct possibility, it is also conceivable that there is overlap in the performance of these functions, such that the same slowly conducting afferent fibers that sense alterations in vascular tone or metabolic state associated with muscle fatigue and ischemia also act as nociceptors. Exercise-induced muscle fatigue is often associated with low to moderate levels of muscle pain in humans, which may result from the activation of slowly conducting afferent fibers that sense alterations in vascular tone or metabolic state (Adreani and Kaufman, 1998; Haouzi et al., 2004). On the other hand, the activity of many slowly conducting afferent fibers in skeletal muscle with high mechanical thresholds can be modulated by elevated levels of chemicals that are also associated with muscle fatigue, which suggests that some of these fibers may also play a role in sensing muscle metabolic demand (Kumazawa and Mizumura, 1977; Kaufman et al., 1982).

A final point to consider is the relative contribution of group III and group IV fibers to muscle nociception. It is thought that group IV fibers may be more important for skeletal muscle nociceptive input, whereas group III fibers may play a much less important role in this function. In the rat (but not the cat), group IV fibers make up a majority of the mechanical nociceptors in the gastrocnemius muscle of the leg, although in rat masticatory muscles, group III mechanonociceptors appear to be more common (Paintal, 1960; Diehl et al., 1993; Cairns et al., 2002). While this discrepancy most likely reflects significant anatomical and functional differences between these two muscles in rats, it also illustrates an important caveat in the interpretation of scientific literature with regard to muscle nociception; for the most part the leg and masticatory muscles are the only skeletal muscles in which the physiological properties of nociceptors have been extensively investigated. Thus, it is important to broaden research to examine physiological properties of slowly conducting afferent fibers and their role in nociceptive mechanisms in other skeletal muscles, particularly those muscles which are the most common causes of pain in human musculoskeletal pain conditions.

Clinical Relevance

Resolving the peripheral mechanisms that underlie the transmission of muscle pain to the central nervous system may yield direct benefits for patients with muscle pain. Understanding which chemical mediators and receptor mechanisms are important for muscle nociceptor activation and muscle-specific differences in these mechanisms could lead to the development of more specific analgesic agents for the treatment of different types of muscle pain. Indeed, this approach is already being tried, for example in clinical trials to access the efficacy of the $5HT_3$ antagonist granisetron to treat masticatory muscle pain (Christidis et al., 2007). Thus, unraveling nociceptive mechanisms in skeletal muscles is the first step on the path toward improved treatment of muscle pain.

Acknowledgments

The author would like to acknowledge research support provided by a Canadian Pain Society/Astra-Zeneca Research Award, PHS grant DE15420 (NIDCR), and CIHR grant MOP-77538 (IMHA). The author is the recipient of a Canada Research Chair.

References

Adreani CM, Kaufman MP. Effect of arterial occlusion on responses of group III and IV afferents to dynamic exercise. J Appl Physiol 1998;84:1827–1833.

Ambalavanar R, Moritani M, Dessem D. Trigeminal P2X3 receptor expression differs from dorsal root ganglion and is modulated by deep tissue inflammation. Pain 2005;117:280–291.

Babenko V, Graven-Nielsen T, Svensson P, Drewes AM, Jensen TS, Arendt-Nielsen L. Experimental human muscle pain and muscular hyperalgesia induced by combinations of serotonin and bradykinin. Pain 1999;82:1–8.

Brunetti O, Della Torre G, Lucchi ML, Chiocchetti R, Bortolami R, Pettorossi VE. Inhibition of muscle spindle afferent activity during masseter muscle fatigue in the rat. Exp Brain Res 2003;152:251–262.

Cairns BE, Dong XD, Mann MK, Svensson P, Sessle BJ, Arendt-Nielsen L, McErlane KM. Systemic administration of monosodium glutamate elevates intramuscular glutamate levels and sensitizes rat masseter muscle afferent fibers. Pain 2007;132:33–41.

Cairns BE, Gambarota G, Svensson P, Arendt-Nielsen L, Berde CB. Glutamate-induced sensitization of rat masseter muscle fibers. Neuroscience 2002;109:389–399.

Cairns BE, Svensson P, Wang K, Hupfeld S, Graven-Nielsen T, Sessle BJ, Berde CB, Arendt-Nielsen L. Activation of peripheral NMDA receptors contributes to human pain and rat afferent discharges evoked by injection of glutamate into the masseter muscle. J Neurophysiol 2003;90:2098–2105.

Capra NF, Wax TD. Distribution and central projections of primary afferent neurons that innervated the masseter muscle and mandibular periodontium: a double-label study. J Comp Neurol 1989;279:341–352.

Cho H, Shin J, Shin CY, Lee SY, Oh U. Mechanosensitive ion channels in cultured sensory neurons of neonatal rats. J Neurosci 2002;22:1238-1247.

Christidis N, Nilsson A, Kopp S, Ernberg M. Intramuscular injection of granisetron into the masseter muscle increases the pressure pain threshold in healthy participants and patients with localized myalgia. Clin J Pain 2007;23:467–72.

Connor M, Naves LA, McCleskey EW. Contrasting phenotypes of putative proprioceptive and nociceptive trigeminal neurons innervating jaw muscle in rat. Mol Pain 2005;1:31–41.

Diehl B, Hoheisel U, Mense S. The influence of mechanical stimuli and of acetylsalicylic acid on the discharges of slowly conducting afferent units from normal and inflamed muscle in the rat. Exp Brain Res 1993;92:431–140.

Djouhri L, Lawson SN. Aβ-fiber nociceptive primary afferent neurons: a review of incidence and properties in relation to other afferent A-fiber neurons in mammals. Brain Res Rev 2004;46:131– 145.

Dong XD, Mann MK, Kumar U, Svensson P, Arendt-Nielsen L, Hu JW, Sessle BJ, Cairns BE. Sex-related differences in glutamate evoked rat muscle nociceptor discharge result from estrogen-mediated modulation of peripheral NMDA receptors. Neuroscience 2007;146:822–832.

Drew LJ, Wood JN, Cesare P. Distinct mechanosensitive properties of capsaicin-sensitive and -insensitive sensory neurons. J Neurosci 2002;22:1–5.

Ernberg M, Hedenberg-Magnusson B, Alstergren P, Kopp S. The level of serotonin in the superficial masseter muscle in relation to local pain and allodynia. Life Sci 1999;65:313–325.

Ernberg M, Hedenberg-Magnusson B, Kurita H, Kopp S. Effects of local serotonin administration on pain and microcirculation in the human masseter muscle. J Orofac Pain 2006;20:241–248.

Fock S, Mense S. Excitatory effects of 5-hydroxytryptamine, histamine and potassium ions on muscular group IV afferent units: A comparison with bradykinin. Brain Res 1976;105:459–469.

Graven-Nielsen T, Mense S. The peripheral apparatus of muscle pain: evidence from animal and human studies. Clin J Pain 2001;17:2–10.

Hamill OP, Martinac B. Molecular basis of mechanotransduction in living cells. Physiol Rev 2001;81:685–740.

Hanna RL, Kaufman MP. Activation of thin-fiber muscle afferents by a P2X agonist in cats. J Appl Physiol 2004;96:1166–1169.

Haouzi P, Chenuel B, Huszczuk A. Sensing vascular distension in skeletal muscle by slow conducting afferent fibers: neurophysiological basis and implication for respiratory control. J Appl Physiol 2004;96:407–418.

Hoheisel U, Lehmann-Willenbrock E, Mense S. Termination patterns of identified group II and III afferent fibres from deep tissues in the spinal cord of the cat. Neuroscience 1989;28:495–507.

Hoheisel U, Reinohl J, Unger T, Mense S. Acidic pH and capsaicin activate mechanosensitive group IV muscle receptors in the rat. Pain 2004;110:149–157.

Hoheisel U, Unger T, Mense S. Excitatory and modulatory effects of inflammatory cytokines and neurotrophins on mechanosensitive group IV muscle afferents in the rat. Pain 2005;114:168–176.

Hu WP, Li XM, Wu JL, Zheng M, Li ZW. Bradykinin potentiates 5-HT3 receptor-mediated current in rat trigeminal ganglion neurons. Acta Pharmacol Sin 2005;26:428–434.

Jensen K, Norup M. Experimental pain in human temporal muscle induced by hypertonic saline, potassium and acidity. Cephalalgia 1992;12:101–106.

Jensen K, Tuxen C, Pedersen-Bjergaard U, Jansen I, Edvinsson L, Olesen J. Pain and tenderness in human temporal muscle induced by bradykinin and 5-hydroxytryptamine. Peptides 1990;11:1127–1132.

Kaufman MP, Iwamoto GA, Longhurst JC, Mitchell JH. Effects of capsaicin and bradykinin on afferent fibers with ending in skeletal muscle. Circ Res 1982;50:133–139.

Kumazawa T, Mizumura K. Thin-fibre receptors responding to mechanical, chemical, and thermal stimulation in the skeletal muscle of the dog. J Physiol (Lond) 1977;273:179–194.

Levine JD, Alessandri-Haber N. TRP channels: Targets for the relief of pain. Biochim Biophys Acta 2007;1772:989–1003.

Mann MK, Dong XD, Svensson P, Cairns BE. Influence of intramuscular nerve growth factor injection on the response properties of rat masseter muscle afferent fibers. J Orofacial Pain 2006;20:325–336.

Mense S. Nervous outflow from skeletal muscle following chemical noxious stimulation. J Physiol (Lond) 1977;267:75–88.

Mense S, Meyer H. Bradykinin-induced modulation of the response behaviour of different types of feline group III and IV muscle receptors. J Physiol (Lond) 1988;398:49–63.

Mok E, Mann MK, Dong XD, Cairns BE. Local anaesthetic-like effects of diclofenac on muscle nociceptors. Pain Res Manage 2005;10:95.

Mørk H, Ashina M, Bendtsen L, Olesen J, Jensen R. Experimental muscle pain and tenderness following infusion of endogenous substances in humans. Eur J Pain 2003;7:145–153.

O'Shaughnessy CT, Connor HE, Feniuk W. Extracellular recordings of membrane potential from guinea-pig isolated trigeminal ganglion: lack of effect of sumatriptan. Cephalalgia 1993;13:175–179.

Paintal JS. Functional analysis of group III afferent fibres of mammalian muscles. J Physiol (Lond) 1960;152:250–270.

Panneton WM, Gan Q, Juric R. The central termination of sensory fibers from nerves to the gastrocnemius muscle of the rat. Neuroscience 2005;134:175–87.

Reinohl J, Hoheisel U, Unger T, Mense S. Adenosine triphosphate as a stimulant for nociceptive and non-nociceptive muscle group IV receptors in the rat. Neurosci Lett 2003;338:25–28.

Ro JY, Capra N, Masri R. Development of a behavioral assessment of craniofacial muscle pain in lightly anesthetized rats. Pain 2003;104:179–185.

Rosendal L, Larsson B, Kristiansen J, Peolsson M, Søgaard K, Kjær M, Sørensen J, Gerdle B. Increase in muscle nociceptive substances and anaerobic metabolism in patients with trapezius myalgia: microdialysis in rest and during exercise. Pain 2004;112:324–334.

Rotto DM, Hill JM, Schultz HD, Kaufman MP. Cyclooxygenase blockade attenuates responses of group IV muscle afferents to static contraction. Am J Physiol 1990;259:H745–750.

Sluka KA, Price MP, Breese NM, Stucky CL, Wemmie JA, Welsh MJ. Chronic hyperalgesia induced by repeated acid injections in muscle is abolished by the loss of ASIC3, but not ASIC1. Pain 2003;106:229–239.

Steen KH, Wegner H, Meller ST. Analgesic profile of peroral and topical ketoprofen upon low pH-induced muscle pain. Pain 2001;93:23–33.

Sung D, Dong X, Ernberg M, Kumar U, Cairns BE. Serotonin (5-HT) excites rat masticatory muscle afferent fibers through activation of peripheral 5-HT3 receptors. Pain 2008;134:41–50.

Svensson P, Arendt-Nielsen L, Nielsen H, Larsen JK. Effect of chronic and experimental jaw muscle pain on pain-pressure thresholds and stimulus-response curves. J Orofac Pain 1995; 9:347–356.

Svensson P, Wang K, Arendt-Nielsen L, Cairns BE, Sessle BJ. Pain effects of glutamate injections into human jaw or neck muscles. J Orofac Pain 2005; 19:109–118.

Wang H, Wei F, Dubner R, Ren K. Selective distribution and function of primary afferent nociceptive inputs from deep muscle tissue to the brainstem trigeminal transition zone. J Comp Neurol 2006; 498:390–402.

Wemmie JA, Price MP, Welsh MJ. Acid-sensing ion channels: advances, questions and therapeutic opportunities. Trends Neurosci 2006; 29:578–586.

Woo YC, Park SS, Subieta AR, Brennan TJ. Changes in tissue pH and temperature after incision indicate acidosis may contribute to postoperative pain. Anesthesiology 2004; 101:468–475.

Correspondence to: Brian E. Cairns, PhD, ACPR, RPh, Faculty of Pharmaceutical Sciences, The University of British Columbia, 2146 East Mall, Vancouver, BC, Canada, V6T 1Z3. Tel: 1-604-822-7715; fax: 1-604-822-3535; email: brcairns@ interchange.ubc.ca.

Functional Role of Peripheral Glutamate Receptors in Craniofacial Muscle Pain and Hyperalgesia

Jin Y. Ro

Department of Biomedical Sciences, Program in Neuroscience, University of Maryland Baltimore School of Dentistry, Baltimore, Maryland, USA

A large body of evidence attests to the role of peripheral excitatory amino acid (EAA) receptors in nociception and inflammation. Immunohistochemical studies show that all glutamate receptor types are localized on cutaneous unmyelinated axons (Carlton et al., 1995; Coggeshall and Carlton, 1998; Bhave et al., 2001). Activation of any of the glutamate receptor subtypes induces nociceptive behaviors that are attenuated by peripheral injection of appropriate receptor antagonists (Jackson et al., 1995; Zhou et al., 1996; Davidson et al., 1997; Bhave et al., 2001; Walker et al., 2001). Glutamate injection into the rat glabrous skin induces excitation and sensitization of nociceptors (Du et al., 2001, 2003). EAA concentrations in the rat skin or knee joint increase significantly after experimentally induced inflammation (Omote et al., 1998; Lawand et al., 2000), suggesting that endogenous release of glutamate in peripheral tissue following tissue injury or inflammation can exacerbate the inflammatory condition and modulate functional properties of primary afferent neurons. This chapter summarizes recent findings on the role of peripheral EAA receptors in muscular pain and hyperalgesia, from data obtained primarily in the trigeminal system.

Glutamate-Induced Activation
of Muscle Nociceptors

A small volume of glutamate (0.5 M), which produces pain in human subjects, activates a group of primary afferent neurons in the trigeminal ganglia (TG) when administered directly in the masseter muscle (Cairns et al., 2001). These neurons were determined to be masseteric nociceptive afferents because they could be activated by noxious mechanical and electrical stimulations of the muscle receptive field. The nociceptive function of these glutamate-sensitive muscle afferents is also indirectly supported by their projection to the subnucleus caudalis (Vc), an area known to receive small-diameter afferent input from the masseter (Shigenaga et al., 1988). A higher concentration of glutamate (1.0 M) injected into the masseter not only activates TG muscle afferents but also produces sensitization to mechanical stimulation (Cairns et al., 2002). Cairns et al. proposed that the glutamate effect is mediated by EAA receptors in the masseter muscle because a broad-spectrum EAA receptor antagonist, kynurenate, coadministered in the masseter, effectively prevented the glutamate-induced activation and sensitization of TG muscle afferents. Subsequent electrophysiological studies further demonstrated that peripherally located N-methyl-D-aspartate (NMDA) receptors are involved in activating and sensitizing masseter nociceptive afferents (Cairns et al., 2003). Interestingly, the NMDA-mediated effects could not be clearly demonstrated in TG afferents that innervate temporalis muscle (Dong et al., 2006), suggesting tissue-specific EAA receptor contributions, even among muscles with similar or synergistic function.

These studies provide evidence that peripheral NMDA receptors might be associated with muscle nociception and muscle hypersensitivity. However, studies demonstrating modulatory effects of endogenously released glutamate on muscle nociceptors will further strengthen the functional role of peripheral NMDA receptors in muscle pain and hyperalgesia. Contributions from other EAA receptors such as α-amino-3-hydroxy-5-methyl-4-isoxazole propionate (AMPA), kainate, and metabotropic glutamate receptors (mGluR) in activation and sensitization of muscle nociceptors have yet to be elucidated.

Role of Peripheral Excitatory Amino Acid Receptors in Muscle Pain and Hyperalgesia

Human Studies

Intramuscular injections of glutamate into human masseter, splenius, and trapezius muscles produce intense pain that lasts 5–10 minutes (Ge et al., 2005; Svensson et al., 2005). The duration of perceived pain in human subjects appears to correlate well with the masseter afferent activity following glutamate injection in rats (Cairns et al., 2001). Repeated injections of glutamate significantly decreased the pressure pain threshold (PPT) of injected muscles in the studies mentioned above. Glutamate injected into the splenius muscle, but not the masseter muscle, produces referral of muscle pain (Svensson et al., 2005), again suggesting potential tissue-related differences in peripheral glutamate effect on nociceptive processing. However, it is also possible that this difference depends on central mechanisms related to the two muscles. Glutamate-evoked muscle pain and mechanical sensitization are significantly attenuated when local NMDA receptors are blocked with ketamine (Cairns et al., 2003, 2006). Thus, in consistency with electrophysiological data, human experimental studies suggest that peripheral NMDA receptors are involved in localized muscle pain, mechanical allodynia, and referred pain.

Animal Studies

One of the limiting factors in studying pathophysiological mechanisms of orofacial muscle pain has been the lack of reliable animal models. Hence, animal behavioral models that were recently developed for assessing temporomandibular joint (TMJ) and masseter pain provide important tools for evaluating mechanistic hypotheses of orofacial deep tissue pain and hyperalgesia (Ren, 1999; Harper et al., 2000; Ro et al., 2003; Ro, 2005; Ro and Capra, 2006; Thut et al., 2007). In our model using lightly anesthetized rats, we have shown that algesic chemical injection into the masseter muscle evokes vigorous shaking of the hindpaw that diminishes over several minutes (Ro et al., 2003). The shaking behavior is directed to the injected site as an attempt to rub or scratch the affected region, which is a stereotypical nocifensive behavior in intact animals. The same stimulus in awake rats produces prolonged and intense bouts of scratching over the injected muscle with a duration consistent with the hindpaw shaking in lightly anesthetized animals. We performed a series of experiments to quantify and validate the behavior as an appropriate index of craniofacial muscle nociception (Ro et al., 2003).

First we investigated the functional role of NMDA receptors in masseter muscle pain in animals. Intramuscular injection of the inflammatory irritant mustard oil, produces an immediate and intense ipsilateral paw-shaking behavior that lasts for several minutes, with the peak number of shakes occurring within the first minute. MK-801 (0.3 mg/kg), which blocks NMDA-receptor noncompetitively, injected locally into the masseter muscle significantly attenuated the peak and overall magnitude of the nocifensive responses, while a vehicle control did not. This effect is not due to widespread systemic effects of MK-801 since the same dose of MK-801 injected into the biceps muscle prior to mustard oil injection did not have a significant effect on the magnitude or duration of the paw-shaking behavior. Similarly, pretreating the masseter muscle with MK-801 dose-dependently attenuated nocifensive responses induced by prolonged infusion of 5% hypertonic saline (HS) into the masseter muscle (Ro et al., 2007). These data provide evidence that endogenously released glutamate following algesic stimulation of muscle tissue evokes acute nociception by activating NMDA receptors localized on muscle afferents. However, in a previous rat study, masseter afferent activity induced by a bolus injection of HS was not blocked by NMDA-receptor antagonists (Cairns et al., 2003). This discrepancy could be due to the difference in HS injection protocols (single injection versus continuous infusion).

We developed another animal behavioral model to assess inflammation-induced changes in craniofacial muscle tissue sensitivity on a more long-term basis (e.g., over several days). This model utilizes bite-force measurement from rats trained under an operant behavioral paradigm, which involves more than simple reflex responses to noxious stimulation of the muscle. The inflammation-induced reduction of bite force is used as an index of muscle hyperalgesia. The methodology of this model has been described elsewhere (Nies and Ro, 2004; Ro, 2005). Bilateral intramuscular injections of complete Freund's adjuvant (CFA) significantly reduced bite performance (measured as success rate) and mean bite force at days 1, 2, and 3; these parameters gradually returned to baseline within 14 days after CFA treatment (Ro, 2005). Intramuscular administration of AP5, a competitive NMDA-receptor antagonist that does not readily cross the blood-brain barrier (Wong et al., 1991), dose-dependently attenuated CFA-induced muscular hyperalgesia. Pretreatment with AP5 reversed the overall magnitude of reduction in mean bite force and success rate in CFA-inflamed rats, and it significantly facilitated the recovery of these measures to preinjection levels. However, AP5 treatment 1 day after the CFA injection had little effect on CFA-mediated changes in bite force measurements. These data suggest that peripheral NMDA receptors may play a critical role in the development, but not in the maintenance, of persistent muscle hyperalgesia (Ro et al., 2005).

Despite the accumulating evidence on the role of peripherally located type I mGluRs in mediating pain and hyperalgesia under a variety of painful conditions (Dogrul et al., 2000; Bhave et al., 2001; Walker et al., 2001; Zhu et al., 2005), the potential contribution from these G-protein-coupled EAA receptors in muscle pain has not been extensively studied. Typically, activation of type I mGluRs (mGluR 1 and 5) increases neuronal excitability via post-translational modulation of various ion channels and receptors, which may underlie hypersensitivity in the peripheral nociceptive system (Bhave and Gereau, 2004).

The role of mGluRs in the development of activity-dependent changes in mechanical sensitivity of the masseter muscle was investigated with the lightly anesthetized hindpaw model. Masseter injections with widely used algogenic agents, such as capsaicin, bradykinin, or glutamate, transiently (but reliably) evoke the nocifensive hindpaw responses and time-dependently increase the sensitivity of muscle tissue to mechanical stimulation (Ro and Capra, 2006). This behavioral model offers a simple, convenient, and reliable means of measuring muscle tissue sensitivity in lightly anesthetized rats that can be utilized to investigate underlying mechanisms of experimental and clinical conditions in which muscular hyperalgesia or allodynia develop.

To determine whether the activation of peripheral mGluRs modulates sensitivity of muscle tissue, we compared the mechanical thresholds that evoked the nocifensive hindpaw responses before and after intramuscular injections with the mGluR agonist DHPG (Lee and Ro, 2007). DHPG induces mechanical hypersensitivity in the injected muscle in a time- and dose-dependent manner (Fig. 1A,B). This effect is specific to DHPG-injected muscle; neither the vehicle injection nor DHPG injected in the muscle contralateral to the mechanical sensitivity testing produced hypersensitivity. Pretreatment with MPEP, an mGluR5 antagonist,

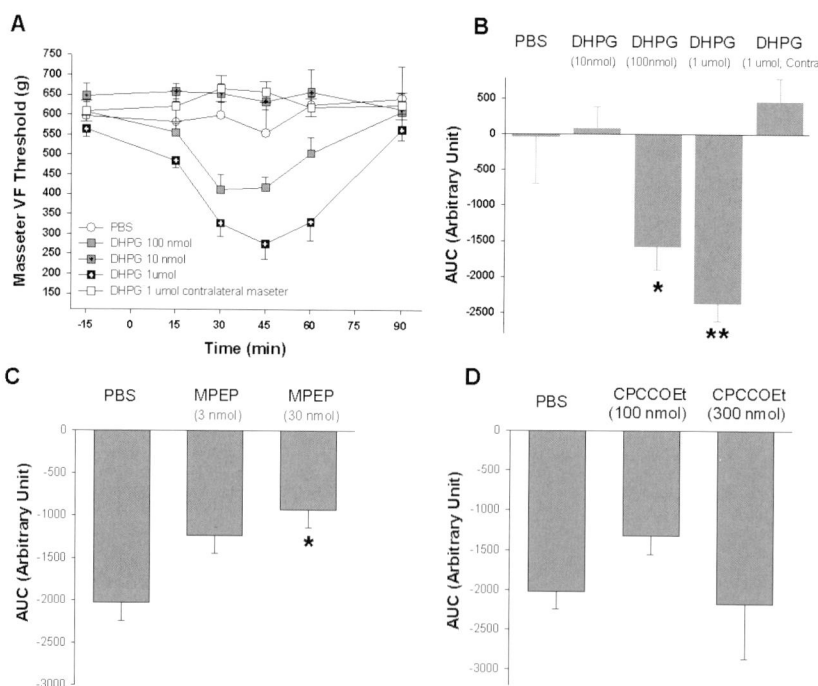

Fig. 1. (A) Line graphs show time-dependent changes in noxious mechanical thresholds following treatment with the mGluR agonist DHPG. (B) Dose-dependent effect of DHPG on the overall magnitude of mechanical sensitivity change was assessed by calculating area-under-the-curve (AUC) values of the rats treated with different doses of DHPG. DHPG injected into the contralateral masseter muscle failed to produce mechanical hypersensitivity, ruling out the possibility of widespread systemic effects of DHPG. (C,D) Pretreatment with MPEP, a selective mGluR5 antagonist, prevented DHPG-induced mechanical hypersensitivity, whereas pretreatment with a selective mGluR1 antagonist, CPCCOEt, did not. $^{*} P < 0.05$; $^{**} P < 0.01$.

significantly blocked DHPG-induced mechanical hypersensitivity (Fig. 1C). In contrast, DHPG-induced mechanical sensitivity changes were not effectively blocked by the mGluR1-specific antagonist CPCCOEt (Fig. 1D), suggesting that peripheral mGluR5, but not mGluR1, mediates the development of mechanical hypersensitivity in the masseter muscle. A recent study, independently conducted in another laboratory, also demonstrated the contribution of peripheral mGluR5, but not mGluR1, in masseter nociception and inflammation (Lee et al., 2006). The predominance of a specific subtype of mGluRs in nociceptor sensitization is not unique to muscle tissue or to trigeminal afferents. Data on modulation of cutaneous thermal sensitivity by peripheral mGluRs also show predominance of either mGluR1 or 5 (Dogrul et al., 2000; Bhave et al., 2001; Zhou et al., 2001), suggesting that the relative contribution of mGluR subtypes in nociceptive processing may depend on pharmacological agents, target tissues, species, and types of sensory testing.

Type I mGluRs primarily act on the phospholipase C-coupled second-messenger pathway, resulting in activation of protein kinase C (PKC) and other kinases (Conn and Pin, 1997; De Blasi et al., 2001). Whereas second-messenger pathways involving PKC activation have been widely shown to produce nociceptor sensitization (Gold and Flake, 2005), peripheral mGluR-mediated PKC activation in the development of muscle tissue hypersensitivity has not been demonstrated. It has recently been demonstrated that both PKC-α and PKC-ε inhibitors (GF109203X and εV1-2 [EAVSLKPT], respectively) significantly and dose-dependently reverse DHPG-induced masseter hypersensitivity when injected directly injected into the masseter muscle prior to DHPG administration in the same muscle (Lee and Ro, 2007). The role of PKC-ε in chronic hyperalgesia has been amply demonstrated (Aley et al., 2000, 2001). Bradykinin-induced sensitization to heat stimuli is principally mediated by PKC-ε, but not by other PKC isoforms, in cultured DRG neurons (Cesare et al., 1999). In contrast, a recent study demonstrated a predominant activation of PKC-α, a conventional PKC isoform, over PKC-ε following phorbol ester stimulation in the mouse paw (Ferreira et al., 2005). The data from the trigeminal system suggest that activation of peripheral mGluRs in craniofacial muscle tissue activates both PKC-α and PKC-ε

and thus contributes to the induction of nociceptor sensitization and muscle hypersensitivity.

Taken together, these animal studies provide strong evidence for the functional role of peripheral glutamate in acute muscle nociception as well as in muscle hyperalgesia. They clearly point to the involvement of both ionotropic and metabotropic glutamate receptors in muscle pain processing in the trigeminal system.

Activation of Peripheral NMDA Receptors and Central Neurons

Activation of nociceptors induces an activity-dependent neuronal plasticity that modifies the excitability of central neurons by exaggerating or prolonging their responses to subsequent stimuli (Ji and Woolf, 2001). It is possible that activation of muscle nociceptors under inflammatory conditions could trigger the release of glutamate from primary afferent endings via the axon reflex (Rees et al., 1994; Lawand et al., 2000). The result would be prolonged autogenic activation of glutamate receptors, which would then contribute to the initiation and maintenance of sensitization in central trigeminal neurons. Such prolonged nociceptive input may facilitate activation of transcription factors that contribute to long-lasting changes in the function of central neurons that underlie the persistent hyperalgesia found in chronic pain conditions (Dubner and Ruda, 1992; Woolf and Salter, 2000). Consistent with this hypothesis, blockade of peripheral NMDA receptors in the masseter significantly reduced the total number of mustard oil- and HS-induced neuronal activations,

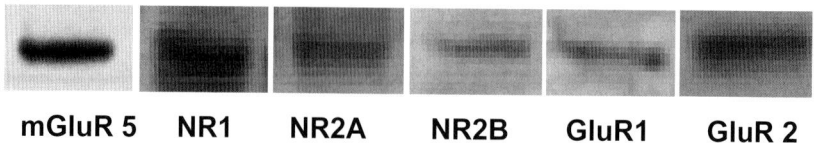

mGluR 5   NR1   NR2A   NR2B   GluR1   GluR 2

Fig. 2. Western blot analyses show protein expression of mGluR5 and ionotropic EAA receptor subunits from trigeminal ganglia (TG) in naive rats. mGluR1 protein was not reliably detected from TG. Blots shown in this figure are assembled from separate experiments run for each protein.

assessed by Fos protein immunoreactivity, in the trigeminal sensory nuclear complex (Ro et al., 2004, 2007).

Peripheral blockade of NMDA receptors prevents sensitization of the spinal cord dorsal horn neurons induced by subcutaneous injection of bee venom (Chen et al., 1999; You et al., 2002). Similarly, peripheral injection of MK-801 produces a reversible reduction of responses to noxious stimuli in wide dynamic range cells in the spinal cord dorsal horn (Ushida et al., 1999). These spinal cord data lend further support to the hypothesis that peripheral glutamate may be critically involved in the generation of sensitization in central trigeminal neurons. Thus, it is reasonable to assume that blockade of peripheral glutamate receptors may be an effective way to prevent increases in central neuronal activity and the resulting plasticity that contributes to prolonged craniofacial muscle hypersensitivity.

Unresolved Issues

The presence of different subtypes of EAA receptors on peripheral terminals of muscle nociceptive afferents, as shown on cutaneous unmyelinated axons (Carlton et al., 1995; Coggeshall and Carlton, 1998; Bhave et al., 2001), has not been clearly demonstrated. In TG, mRNAs or proteins for NR1, NR2A, NR2B, GluR1, GluR21, and mGluR5 have been detected (Fig. 2; Sahara et al., 1997; Lee and Ro, 2007a). An unanticipated finding was that mGluR 1 is not reliably detected from TG or from the masseter nerve (Lee and Ro, 2007b). These data are consistent with the lack of effect of mGluR1 antagonists on DHPG-induced masseter hypersensitivity. However, it is possible that mGluR1 splice variants that are not detected by the antibodies used in this study exist in TG and the masseter nerve. Additional information on the distribution of functional EAA receptors on muscle nociceptive afferents and how the expression level of these receptors is modulated under inflammatory conditions will prove valuable in understanding relative contributions from each EAA receptor subtype in mediating muscle pain and hyperalgesia under normal and inflammatory conditions.

Finally, studies are needed to reveal the mechanisms of peripheral EAA receptor activation in pain transmission. Few studies to date have addressed the signaling mechanisms of glutaminergic transmission in the peripheral nerve endings following noxious stimulation (Hu et al., 2002; Lee and Ro, 2007b). Since glutamate receptors on peripheral terminals are not synaptically activated, the mechanisms of receptor activation in the periphery are likely to be different from those in the central nervous system. Furthermore, the physical linkage between mGluR and NMDA receptors demonstrated in the postsynaptic density in central neurons has not yet been determined in the peripheral endings of primary afferents (Naisbitt et al., 1999; Tu et al., 1999). The demonstration of intracellular signaling mechanisms specific to peripheral EAA receptor activation that eventually lead to sensitization of muscle nociceptors and of central trigeminal nociceptive neurons would have significant therapeutic implications.

Clinical Significance

The pathophysiology of pain and inflammation is a complex phenomenon that involves a large number of centrally and peripherally released chemical mediators, such as bradykinin, prostaglandin, serotonin, and histamine. In addition to these chemical mediators, recent studies clearly implicate peripheral glutamate and EAA receptors as important players in the development and maintenance of chronic pain. This chapter has summarized the evidence for the role of peripheral EAA receptors in mediating orofacial muscle pain and hyperalgesia. These results provide important new insights into pathophysiological mechanisms for the development of acute and persistent types of muscle pain. They provide a strong rationale for the development of pharmacological treatment alternatives that can be directed at the peripheral EAA receptors to ameliorate persistent craniofacial muscle pain.

Acknowledgments

I would like to thank Dr. JS Lee, Ms. Youping Zhang, and Mr. Gregory Haynes for their contribution to this project. I also thank Dr. Norman Capra for his valuable comments on this chapter. Research was supported by National Institute of Dental and Craniofacial Research Grants DE14549 and DE16062.

References

Aley KO, Messing RO, Mochly-Rosen D, Levine JD. Chronic hypersensitivity for inflammatory nociceptor sensitization mediated by the epsilon isozyme of protein kinase C. J Neurosci 2000;20:4680–4685.

Aley KO, Martin A, McMahon T, Mok J, Levine JD, Messing RO. Nociceptor sensitization by extracellular signal-regulated kinases. J Neurosci 2001;21:6933–6939.

Bhave G, Karim F, Carlton SM, Gereau RW IV. Peripheral group I metabotropic glutamate receptors modulate nociception in mice. Nat Neurosci 2001;4:417–423.

Bhave G, Gereau RW IV. Posttranslational mechanisms of peripheral sensitization. J Neurobiol 2004;61:88–106.

Cairns BE, Hu JW, Arendt-Nielsen L, Sessle BJ, Svensson P. Sex-related differences in human pain and rat afferent discharge evoked by injection of glutamate into the masseter muscle. J Neurophysiol 2001;86:782–791.

Cairns BE, Gambarota G, Svensson P, Arendt-Nielsen L, Berde CB. Glutamate-induced sensitization of rat masseter muscle fibers. Neuroscience 2002;109:389–399.

Cairns BE, Svensson P, Wang K, Hupfeld S, Graven-Nielsen T, Sessle BJ, Berde CB, Arendt-Nielsen L. Activation of peripheral NMDA receptors contributes to human pain and rat afferent discharges evoked by injection of glutamate into the masseter muscle. J Neurophysiol 2003;90:2098–2105.

Cairns BE, Svensson P, Wang K, Castrillon E, Hupfeld S, Sessle BJ, Arendt-Nielsen L. Ketamine attenuates glutamate-induced mechanical sensitization of the masseter muscle in human males. Exp Brain Res 2006;169:467–472.

Carlton SM, Hargett GL, Coggeshall RE. Localization and activation of glutamate receptors in unmyelinated axons of rat glabrous skin. Neurosci Lett 1995;197:25–28.

Cesare P, Dekker LV, Sardini A, Parker PJ. McNaughton PA. Specific involvement of PKC-epsilon in sensitization of the neuronal response to painful heat. Neuron 1999;23:617–624.

Chen J, Li H, Luo C, Li Z, Zheng J. Involvement of peripheral NMDA and non-NMDA receptors in development of persistent firing of spinal wide-dynamic-range neurons induced by subcutaneous bee venom injection in the cat. Brain Res 1999;844:98–105.

Coggeshall RE, Carlton SM. Ultra structural analysis of NMDA, AMPA, and kainate receptors on unmyelinated and myelinated axons in the periphery. J Comp Neurol 1998;391:78–86.

Conn PJ, Pin JP. Pharmacology and functions of metabotropic glutamate receptors. Annu Rev Pharmacol Toxicol 1997;37:205–237.

De Blasi A, Conn PJ, Pin J, Nicoletti F Molecular determinants of metabotropic glutamate receptor signaling. Trends Pharmacol Sci 2001;22:114–120.

Dogrul A, Ossipov MH, Lai J, Malan TP Jr, Porreca F. Peripheral and spinal antihyperalgesic activity of SIB-1757, a metabotropic glutamate receptor (mGLUR5) antagonist, in experimental neuropathic pain in rats. Neurosci Lett 2000;292:115–118.

Davidson EM, Coggeshall RE, Carlton SM. Peripheral NMDA and non-NMDA glutamate receptors contribute to nociceptive behaviors in the rat formalin test. Neuroreport 1997;8:941–946.

Dong XD, Mann MK, Sessle BJ, Arendt-Nielsen L, Svensson P, Cairns BE. Sensitivity of rat temporalis muscle afferent fibers to peripheral N-methyl-D-aspartate receptor activation. Neuroscience 2006;141:939–945.

Du J, Koltzenburg M, Carlton SM. Glutamate-induced excitation and sensitization of nociceptors in rat glabrous skin. Pain 2001;89:187–198.

Du J, Zhou S, Coggeshall RE, Carlton SM. N-methyl-D-aspartate-induced excitation and sensitization of normal and inflamed nociceptors. Neuroscience 2003;118:547–562.

Dubner R, Ruda MA. Activity-dependent neuronal plasticity following tissue injury and inflammation. Trends Neurosci 1992;15:96–103.

Ferreira J, Triches KM, Medeiros R, Calixto JB. Mechanisms involved in the nociception produced by peripheral protein kinase C activation in mice. Pain 2005;117:171–181.

Ge HY, Madeleine P, Arendt-Nielsen L. Gender differences in pain modulation evoked by repeated injections of glutamate into the human trapezius muscle. Pain 2005;113:134–140.

Gold MS, Flake NM. Inflammation-mediated hyperexcitability of sensory neurons. Neurosignals 2005;14:147–157.

Harper RP, Kerins CA, Talwar R, Spears R, Hutchins B, Carlson DS, McIntosh JE, Bellinger LL. Meal pattern analysis in response to temporomandibular joint inflammation in the rat. J Dent Res 2000;79:1704–1711.

Hu HJ, Bhave G, Gereau RW IV. Prostaglandin and protein kinase A-dependent modulation of vanilloid receptor function by metabotropic glutamate receptor 5: potential mechanism for thermal hyperalgesia. J Neurosci 2002;22:7444–7452.

Jackson DL, Graff CB, Richardson JD, Hargreaves KM. Glutamate participates in the peripheral modulation of thermal hyperalgesia in rats. Eur J Pharmacol 1995;284:321–325.

Ji RR, Woolf CJ. Neuronal plasticity and signal transduction in nociceptive neurons: implications for the initiation and maintenance of pathological pain. Neurobiol Dis 2001;8:1–10.

Lawand NB, McNearney T, Westlund KN. Amino acid release into the knee joint: key role in nociception and inflammation. Pain 2000;86:69–74.

Lee HJ, Choi HS, Ju JS, Bae YC, Kim SK, Yoon YW, Ahn DK. Peripheral mGluR5 antagonist attenuated craniofacial muscle pain and inflammation but not mGluR1 antagonist in lightly anesthetized rats. Brain Res Bull 2006;70:378–385.

Lee JS, Ro JY. Differential regulation of glutamate receptors in trigeminal ganglia following masseter inflammation. Neuroscience Lett 2007a;421:91–95.

Lee JS, Ro, JY. Peripheral metabotropic glutamate receptor 5 mediates mechanical hypersensitivity in craniofacial muscle via protein kinase C dependent mechanisms. Neuroscience 2007b;146:375–383.

Naisbitt S, Kim E, Tu JC, Xiao B, Sala C, Valtschanoff J, Weinberg RJ, Worley PF, Sheng, M. Shank, a novel family of postsynaptic density proteins that binds to the NMDA receptor/PSD-95/GKAP complex and cortactin. Neuron 1999;23:569–582.

Nies M, Ro JY. Bite force measurement in awake rats: revisited. Brain Res Protocol 2004;12:180–185.

Omote K, Kawamata T, Kawamata M, Namiki A. Formalin-induced release of excitatory amino acids in the skin of the rat hindpaw. Brain Res 1998;787:161–164.

Rees H, Sluka KA, Westlund KN, Willis WD. Do dorsal root reflexes augment peripheral inflammation? Neuroreport 1994;21:821–824.

Ren K. An improved method for assessing mechanical allodynia in the rat. Physiol Behav 1999;67:711–716.

Ro JY. Contribution of central and peripheral NMDA receptors in craniofacial muscle nociception and edema formation. Brain Res 2003;979:78–84.

Ro JY. Bite force measurement in awake rats: a behavioral model for persistent orofacial muscle pain and hyperalgesia. J Orofac Pain 2005;19:159–167.

Ro JY, Capra NF. Assessing mechanical sensitivity of masseter muscle in lightly anesthetized rats: a model for craniofacial muscle hyperalgesia. Neurosci Res 2006;56:119–123.

Ro JY, Capra NF, Lee JS, Masri R, Chun YH. Hypertonic saline-induced muscle nociception and c-fos activation are partially mediated by peripheral NMDA receptors. Eur J Pain 2007;11:398–405.

Ro JY, Capra NF, Masri R. Development of a behavioral assessment of craniofacial muscle pain in lightly anesthetized rats. Pain 2003;104:179–185.

Ro JY, Capra NF, Masri R. Contribution of central and peripheral *N*-methyl-D-aspartate receptors to *c-fos* expression in the trigeminal spinal nucleus following acute masseteric inflammation. Neuroscience 2004;123:213–219.

Ro JY, Nies M, Zhang Y. The role of peripheral N-methyl-D-aspartate receptors in muscle hyperalgesia. Neuroreport 2005;16:485–489.

Sahara Y, Noro N, Iida Y, Soma K, Nakamura Y. Glutamate receptor subunits GluR5 and KA-2 are coexpressed in rat trigeminal ganglion neurons. J Neurosci 1997;17:6611–6620.

Shigenaga Y, Sera M, Nishimori T, Suemune S, Nishimura M, Yoshida A, Tsuru K. The central projection of masticatory afferent fibers to the trigeminal sensory nuclear complex and upper cervical spinal cord. J Comp Neurol 1988;268:489–507.

Svensson P, Wang K, Arendt-Nielsen L, Cairns BE, Sessle BJ. Pain effects of glutamate injections into human jaw or neck muscles. J Orofac Pain 2005;19:109–118.

Thut PD, Hermanstyne TO, Flake NM, Gold MS. An operant conditioning model to assess changes in feeding behavior associated with temporomandibular joint inflammation in the rat. J Orofac Pain 2007;21:7–18.

Tu JC, Xiao B, Naisbitt S, Yuan JP, Petralia RS, Brakeman P, Doan A, Aakalu VK, Lanahan AA, Sheng M, Worley PF. Coupling of mGluR/Homer and PSD-95 complexes by the Shank family of postsynaptic density proteins. Neuron 1999;23:583–592.

Ushida T, Tani T, Kawasaki M, Iwatsu O, Yamamoto H. Peripheral administration of an *N*-methyl-D-aspartate receptor antagonist (MK-801) changes dorsal horn neuronal responses in rats. Neurosci Lett 1999;260:89–92.

Walker K, Reeve A, Bowes M, Winter J, Wotherspoon G, Davis A, Schmid P, Gasparini F, Kuhn R, Urban L. mGlu5 receptors and nociceptive function II. mGlu5 receptors functionally expressed on peripheral sensory neurones mediate inflammatory hyperalgesia. Neuropharmacology 2001;40:10–19.

Wong EHF, Kemp JA. Sites for antagonism on the *N*-methyl-D-aspartate receptor channel complex. Annu Rev Pharmacol Toxicol 1991;31:401–425.

Woolf CJ, Salter MW. Neuronal plasticity: increasing the gain in pain. Science 2000;288:1765–1769.

You HJ, Chen J, Morch CD, Arendt-Nielsen L. Differential effect of peripheral glutamate (NMDA, non-NMDA) receptor antagonists on bee venom-induced spontaneous nociception and sensitization. Brain Res Bull 2002;58:561–567.

Zhou S, Bonasera L, Carlton SM. Peripheral administration of NMDA, AMPA, or KA results in pain behaviors in rats. Neuroreport 1996;7:895–900.

Zhu CZ, Hsieh G, Ei-Kouhen O, Wilson SG, Mikusa JP, Hollingsworth PR, Chang R, Moreland RB, Brioni J, Decker MW, Honore P. Role of central and peripheral mGluR5 receptors in post-operative pain in rats. Pain 2005;114:195–202.

Correspondence to: Jin Y. Ro, PhD, Department of Biomedical Sciences, University of Maryland Baltimore School of Dentistry, 650 W. Baltimore Street, Baltimore, MD 21201, USA. Tel: 1-410-706-6027; fax: 1-410-706-0865; email: jro@umaryland.edu.

Facilitated Response of Muscle Thin-Fiber Receptors in Mechanical Hyperalgesia after Exercise

Kazue Mizumura and Toru Taguchi

Department of Neuroscience II, Research Institute of Environmental Medicine, Nagoya University, Nagoya, Japan

Delayed-onset muscle soreness (DOMS) is described as an unpleasant sensation or pain after unaccustomed strenuous exercise. Lengthening contraction (also termed *eccentric contraction*; an example is downhill running) can induce DOMS more easily than shortening (*concentric*) contraction (an example is uphill running) (Armstrong, 1984). DOMS is not apparent immediately after exercise, but emerges within 24 hours and reaches a peak within 24–48 hours. It disappears within 3 to 7 days (Armstrong, 1984; Graven-Nielsen and Arendt-Nielsen, 2003). There is usually no spontaneous pain (Graven-Nielsen and Arendt-Nielsen, 2003). To investigate the neural mechanism of mechanical hyperalgesia in DOMS, we developed an animal model by applying repetitive lengthening muscular contraction in rats. This model allowed us to examine changes in the sensitivity of muscle thin-fiber sensory afferents after exercise.

How is DOMS Generated?

Several mechanisms have been proposed for DOMS, but they are mainly related to its generation and do not explain the neural component of mechanical hyperalgesia. Lactic acid, found in increased levels in muscles and plasma shortly after exercise (Schwane et al., 1983), was once considered to be a cause of DOMS. However, this hypothesis has been strongly refuted by the fact that concentric (shortening) exercise, which involves higher metabolism, fails to produce DOMS (Schwane et al., 1983). In addition, lactic acid levels return to pre-exercise levels within an hour after exercise. Therefore, while lactic acid may contribute to the acute pain associated with fatigue during and shortly after intense exercise, it does not explain DOMS.

Spasm was considered to be a cause of DOMS based on the observation that resting muscle activity (EMG activity) increased after lengthening exercise (De Vries, 1966). The smaller elbow joint angle after lengthening exercises of the elbow flexors would support this hypothesis, but reports on EMG activity in exercised muscles have been inconclusive. Damage to the connective tissue that forms sheaths around bundles of muscle fibers has also been proposed as a cause of DOMS. The content and composition of connective tissue differ between muscle fiber types; type I (slow-twitch) fibers display a more robust structure than type II (fast-twitch) fibers. Moreover, fast-twitch fibers are selectively recruited during eccentric exercise and are thus more likely to be damaged, possibly resulting in muscle soreness (Lieber and Friden, 1988).

Histological studies (Armstrong et al., 1983) and ultrastructural investigations (Newham et al., 1983) in humans and animals have revealed micro-injuries in exercised muscles, including broadening and streaming of Z-bands that mechanically bind neighboring sarcomeres, focal disruption of the striated band pattern, and disorganized sarcomeres. Biochemical studies have shown leakage of enzymes such as creatine kinase and lactic dehydrogenase from the exercised muscle (Armstrong et al., 1983). These observations have led to the hypothesis that muscle damage is the cause of DOMS. Observation of invading inflammatory cells (macrophages) into the muscle has led to the inflammation theory (see Smith, 1991, for review). A recent intensive, comprehensive study (Malm et al., 2004) in humans found no difference in the markers for inflammation between subjects who underwent lengthening versus shortening contraction. The involvement of inflammation was also examined by using anti-inflammatory drugs. However, the effects of the drugs differed among laboratories, and there were more reports of effective results when a drug was administered prophylactically (before exercise) than when it was given therapeutically (after exercise) (Cheung et al., 2003).

None of the hypothetical mechanisms described above is sufficient to explain DOMS. A combination of tissue damage and inflammation mechanisms is often accepted, but further experimental results are needed using other approaches.

To date, no reports have directly addressed the neural component of mechanical hyperalgesia. Investigation of the neural mechanism of DOMS will require an animal model, but virtually no studies have demonstrated the existence of muscular mechanical hyperalgesia (tenderness and movement-related pain) in animals.

Mechanical Hyperalgesia in an Animal Model of DOMS

Many studies have used downhill running to induce DOMS in humans and animals. In our study, however, we electrically contracted the hindpaw extensors, mainly the extensor digitorum longus (EDL), while mechanically stretching the muscles (Taguchi et al., 2005a) so that we could compare the unexercised and exercised sides and also study the central processing of afferent information in the spinal cord. The gastrocnemius muscle has also been used for this purpose (Itoh and Kawakita, 2002).

The extensor muscles of the hindpaw, including the EDL, were contracted for 1 second by electrically stimulating the common peroneal nerve through a pair of needles inserted near the nerve. The ankle joint was plantarflexed to stretch the EDL synchronously with muscle contraction for 1 second. The contraction was repeated every 4 seconds for a

total of 500 repetitions. A control group of rats underwent needle inser-
tion, but no current was applied to their nerves, and the ankle joint was
repetitively plantarflexed as for rats in the exercise group.

Mechanical hyperalgesia was demonstrated by two methods:
measurement of withdrawal threshold and recording of c-Fos expression
in the superficial dorsal horn of the spinal cord. The mechanical withdrawal threshold of the exercised muscle was measured by applying a
probe (tip diameter 2.6 mm) to the EDL muscle through the skin with
a Randall-Selitto analgesiometer, which is considered to transmit force
to deeper muscles better than von Frey hairs (Takahashi et al., 2005).
Fig. 1A shows the change in withdrawal threshold after exercise. The
threshold significantly decreased 1 day after lengthening contraction in
7-week-old rats. It reached its lowest point on the second day and remained decreased until the third day after exercise (Taguchi et al., 2005a,

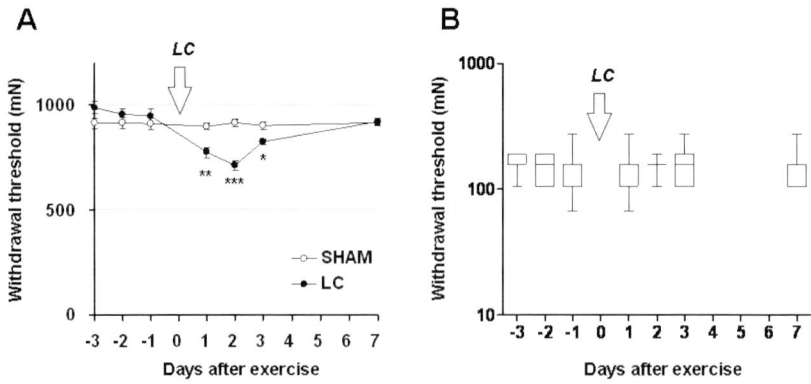

Fig. 1. Mechanical hyperalgesia in muscles of rats after lengthening contraction (LC). (A)
Mechanical withdrawal threshold measured with Randall-Selitto apparatus decreased after
LC. Solid circles: LC group ($n = 6$), open circles: sham exercise group ($n = 6$). Arrow: day
of lengthening contraction or sham exercise. Data are presented as means ± SEM. *$P < 0.05$,
** $P < 0.01$, ***$P < 0.001$ compared with 1 day before exercise (one-way ANOVA followed
by Bonferroni's multiple comparison test) and compared between the sham and LC groups
(unpaired t test). Modified from Taguchi et al. (2005a), with permission. (B) Withdrawal
threshold for the skin over the exercised muscle of the LC group ($n = 7$) measured by von
Frey hairs. Data are represented as box (median ± interquartile range [IQR]) and whiskers
(10 and 90 percentile values). Other presentation as in panel A. No significant differences
were found between 1 day before LC and each day after LC (nonparametric Friedman test
followed by Dunn's multiple comparison test). Modified from Taguchi et al. (2005a).

2007). On day four the threshold completely returned to baseline levels (Taguchi et al., 2007). The withdrawal threshold of the contralateral side (without exercise) remained unchanged throughout the entire period of observation. There was no change in mechanical withdrawal threshold of the skin over the EDL or the sole of the hindpaw as measured with von Frey hairs (Fig. 1B). With a diameter of 2.6 mm at the tip, our probe was larger than commercially available probes, and we confirmed that withdrawal threshold, as measured with the Randall-Selitto apparatus equipped with this probe, was not influenced by surface anesthesia of the skin over the EDL (Nasu et al., 2007). Considering all these results, we concluded that the deep tissues (probably the exercised muscle) of the exercised side were hyperalgesic to mechanical stimulation.

Itoh and Kawakita (2002) used another method to detect mechanical hyperalgesia in exercised muscles in rabbits. They applied repeated lengthening contractions of the gastrocnemius muscle in lightly anesthetized rabbits by manually extending the muscle during contractions induced by electrical stimulation of the tibial nerve. The investigators then measured reflex EMG activity of the biceps femoris muscle in response to electrical stimulation or manual extension of the gastrocnemius muscle. Under normal conditions, electrical stimulation or extension of the gastrocnemius muscle induced very little EMG activity in the biceps femoris muscle, whereas 1 day after exercise these manipulations induced considerable EMG activity, which reached a peak 2 days after exercise. The investigators also detected a sensitive point at the musculotendinous attachment area located on the ropy band (a palpable taut band of hardened tissue). They assumed that this point was an experimentally induced trigger point. In our rat model, it was impossible to detect a taut band because the muscle is too small.

c-Fos Study

To be sure that the decreased mechanical withdrawal threshold, as measured with Randall-Selitto equipment, reflects mechanical hyperalgesia in the exercised muscles, we examined c-Fos expression in the dorsal horn.

This protein has been used as a neural marker of pain since Hunt et al. (1987) reported that various kinds of noxious stimuli induce its expression in the superficial dorsal horn, which contains secondary neurons receiving nociceptive C-fiber inputs (Ling et al., 2003). Characteristics of DOMS are hyperalgesia to compression and movement-induced pain with almost no spontaneous pain. We thus examined c-Fos expression after the animals received compression of the exercised muscles. Pressure stimulation (160 g with a Randall-Selitto apparatus for 10 seconds followed by a 20-second rest period) was applied to the exercised muscle through the skin on day 2, when mechanical hyperalgesia was at its peak (as shown in Fig. 1A). Stimulation was repeated for 30 minutes under anesthesia with pentobarbital (50 mg/kg, i.p.). Two hours later (or 2 days after the exercise session in control groups without compression), the animals were deeply anesthetized and perfused with fixative, and then the tissue was processed for immunohistochemistry.

The number of c-Fos-immunoreactive neurons in the dorsal horn was small in the sham group (which had undergone stretching without muscle contraction), in the lengthening contraction only (LC only) group, and in the sham + compression group, and was no different from the contralateral side (Taguchi et al., 2005a). Thus, the compression used in this experiment did not activate the nociceptive pathway in anesthetized animals, nor did lengthening contraction itself activate the nociceptive pathway 2 days later. This observation agrees with the finding that there is usually no spontaneous pain in DOMS. In the group that received muscle compression 2 days after lengthening contraction (LC + compression), however, c-Fos immunoreactivity clearly increased, especially in the superficial dorsal horn corresponding to laminae I/II. The most prominent change was found in L4 (Taguchi et al., 2005a). This observation is consistent with a previous report that the great majority of sensory neurons innervating the EDL muscle are located in the L4 dorsal root ganglia. The increased expression of c-Fos in the superficial dorsal horn in the LC + compression group was completely suppressed with morphine (10 mg/kg i.p., given 20 minutes before compression 2 days after lengthening contraction) (Taguchi et al., 2005a); morphine is known to suppress transmission of nociceptive information at the spinal level.

These observations provide further evidence that the muscle was hyper-algesic 2 days after lengthening contraction.

Facilitated Response of Muscle Thin-Fiber Afferents in DOMS

To examine whether the activity of muscle thin-fiber afferents, which transmit noxious information to the central nervous system, changes during mechanical hyperalgesia after lengthening contraction, we recorded the activity of single nerve fibers from in vitro preparations of EDL muscle and common peroneal nerve. We compared the mechanical sensitivity of thin fibers (conduction velocity < 2.0 m/s) in control animals and those that had received lengthening contraction 2 days earlier (Taguchi et al., 2005b).

Some thin fibers were spontaneously active, but there was no difference between the control and LC groups, with a median of 0.12 impulses/s (range = 0–0.52 impulses/s) in the control group (n = 33) and a median of 0 impulses/s (range = 0–0.42 impulses/s) in the LC group (n = 25). These values were consistent with those reported previously from experiments in vivo (Franz and Mense, 1975; Kumazawa and Mizumura, 1977) and indicate that the recorded receptors were in good condition. In addition, the observation that the spontaneous activity of fibers recorded in the LC group was low and did not differ from the control group conforms with the observation that DOMS does not usually involve spontaneous pain. The receptive fields of the thin-fiber sensory receptors were distributed all over the muscle, with a tendency to be concentrated near musculotendinous junctions. The receptive fields seemed to be more densely located near the musculotendinous junction in the LC group than in controls (Taguchi et al., 2005b).

A ramp-shaped mechanical stimulation, linearly increasing from 0 to 196 mN in 10 seconds (shown in the inset of Fig. 2) was applied by a mechanical stimulator with a flat circular tip (with a diameter of about 1.7 mm) to the point identified as being most sensitive. Mechanical stimulation excited all fibers identified (33 fibers in control preparations, and 25 fibers in LC preparations). A sample response of a fiber recorded from the control preparations is shown in Fig. 2A. The control preparations with no treatment showed, on average, an intensity-dependent increase of discharge rate during a ramp-shaped mechanical stimulation (open triangle in Fig. 3). On the other hand, the build-up of the response in the LC preparations was steeper than that in the control preparations (solid circle in Fig. 3). Thus, the mechanical threshold in the LC preparation (median = 38.2 mN, interquartile range [IQR] = 26.8–55.8 mN, n = 25) was lower than in the control preparations (median = 65.4 mN, IQR = 46.6–122.0 mN, n = 33, P < 0.001) (Taguchi et al., 2005b). In addition, the

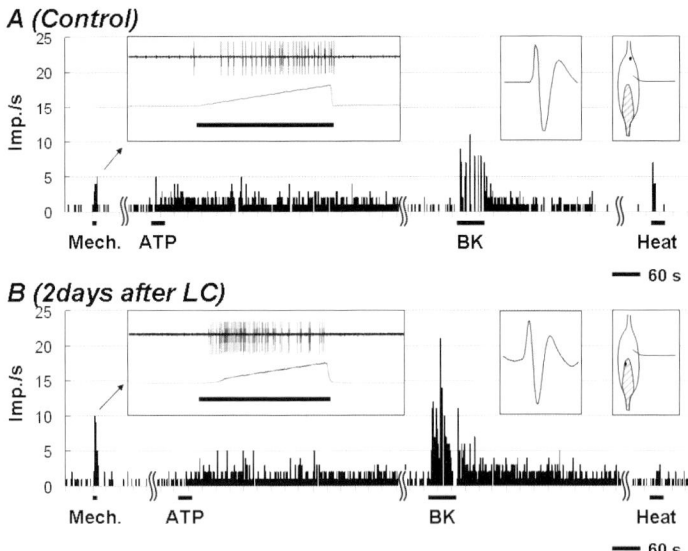

Fig. 2. Responses of C-fiber sensory afferent fibers to noxious stimuli. (A) A sensory receptor recorded in the control preparation. Conduction velocity = 0.50 m/s. The receptive field (marked with a dot in the schema of the extensor digitorum longus [EDL]) is at the right side of the EDL muscle near the proximal end on the front surface. (B) Receptor recorded in the lengthening contraction (LC) preparation. Conduction velocity = 0.34 m/s. The receptive field is at the right side of the EDL muscle at the muscle-tendon junction on the front surface. Black bars under the abscissa show the period of the stimuli. Mech.: ramp mechanical stimulation (196 mN in 10 s); raw recordings of the discharges and applied force are shown in the insets. ATP = application of 10 mM adenosine triphosphate for 30 s; BK = application of 10 μM bradykinin for 60 s; Heat = application of hot Krebs solution for 30 s (from 34 to 50°C).

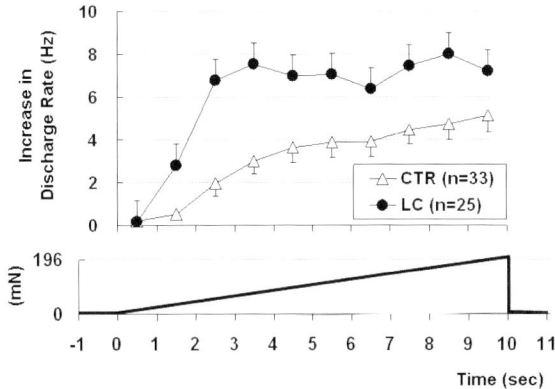

Fig. 3. Time course of the mechanical responses of thin-fiber receptors in lengthening contraction (LC) and control (CTR) preparations. Response to ramp mechanical stimulation (from 0 to 196 mN) was counted every second, and the net increase was calculated by subtracting the discharge rate during the control period. Averages of 25 (LC) and 33 (CTR) receptors are shown along the time after the start of stimulation. A schema of mechanical stimulation is shown beneath the abscissa.

total number of evoked discharges during a ramp mechanical stimulation as an index of the magnitude of the mechanical response was significantly larger in the LC than in the control preparations (Fig. 3). This increased sensitivity of thin fibers to mechanical stimulation is considered to be responsible for mechanical hyperalgesia after lengthening contraction.

Except for the increased sensitivity to mechanical stimulation, no difference was found in responses to any other stimuli, algesic substances, acid, heat, or cold (Taguchi et al., 2005b). For example, application of adenosine triphosphate (ATP) 10 mM activated 34.5% of fibers (10/29) in the control preparation and 50.0% (10/20) of fibers in the lengthening contraction preparation (a sample response in Fig. 2). These percentages were not statistically different. The magnitude of the response to ATP was no different between control and LC preparations. Application of 10 μM bradykinin activated 65.5% (19/29) of control fibers and in 70.0% (14/20) of LC fibers (a sample response in Fig. 2). These percentages are not significantly different. The response to bradykinin was the same in the two preparations. The fibers that were sensitive to ATP (n = 10 in controls, n = 10 in the LC group) all responded to bradykinin.

These findings clearly demonstrated that mechanical sensitivity of thin-fiber receptors was facilitated 2 days after lengthening contraction, and this increased sensitivity is considered to be responsible for mechanical hyperalgesia after lengthening contraction. Sensitization to mechanical stimulation of muscle thin-fiber receptors has been reported in inflammatory conditions (Diehl et al., 1993), but only qualitatively. Ours is the first observation of clear sensitization to mechanical stimuli after lengthening contraction with quantitative data to show the threshold and magnitude of the response. In cutaneous tissues, mechanical sensitization in inflammatory conditions has rarely been observed.

The mechanism for the facilitated mechanical sensitivity in muscle afferents after lengthening contraction has yet to be studied, and there are several possibilities to investigate. First, mechanical sensitivity could be facilitated by chemical mediators in the muscle after lengthening contraction. ATP (Mork et al., 2003) and nerve growth factor (Svensson et al., 2003) induced mechanical hyperalgesia when injected into human muscle, but bradykinin, serotonin, and substance P did not (Babenko et al., 1999). Treatment with low pH caused a significant and lasting decrease in the mechanical thresholds of almost all C-fibers in rat skin-nerve preparations in vitro (Steen et al., 1992). Bradykinin also lowered the mechanical threshold of muscle nociceptors in vivo (Mense and Meyer, 1988) and sensitized visceral nociceptors to mechanical stimuli in vitro (Koda and Mizumura, 2002). In addition, prostaglandin E_2 (Koda and Mizumura, 2002), histamine (Koda and Mizumura, 2002), and ATP (Page et al., 2000) are known to sensitize visceral nociceptor responses to mechanical stimulus. All these substances also sensitize cutaneous and visceral nociceptors to heat (Mizumura and Kumazawa, 1996; Yajima et al., 2005), although the concentration needed to sensitize sensory receptors to mechanical stimulation is higher than that needed to sensitize them to heat (Koda and Mizumura, 2002). These substances, however, are unlikely to be responsible for the sensitization to mechanical stimulus in the LC group in our experiment described above, because heat sensitivity was not altered. Nerve growth factor also facilitates the mechanical response of muscle nociceptors (Mann et al., 2006), but it also facilitates the response of nociceptors to heat (Rueff and Mendell, 1996), although with a different time course and in the skin. A second possibility is that since DOMS involves muscle edema (Crenshaw et al., 1994), edema-induced changes in the mechanical properties of the exercised muscle might contribute to the mechanical hyperalgesia after lengthening contraction. Another possibility is that the augmented mechanical response might result from an increased number of putative mechanotransducer or ion channels at the terminals of muscle thin-fiber receptors after eccentric exercise. Clarification of this point must await the identification of such mechanotransduction channels.

DOMS provides a good model of mechanical hyperalgesia (tenderness and movement-related pain). We observed that mechanical hyperalgesia after lengthening contraction lasted for up to 5 weeks in a stressed condition (Mizumura et al., 2007), suggesting that DOMS can develop into a clinically important chronic muscle pain condition. Demonstration of the peripheral and possibly central neural mechanisms of DOMS will shed light on clinically important muscle pain.

Acknowledgment

This work was supported in part by a Health and Labour Sciences Research Grant from the Ministry of Health, Labour and Welfare, Japan (H14-Choju-29), and by a Grant-in-Aid for Exploratory Research from the Ministry of Education, Culture, Sports, Science and Technology (No. 14657014).

References

Armstrong RB. Mechanisms of exercise-induced delayed onset muscular soreness: a brief review. Med Sci Sports Exerc 1984;16:529–538.

Armstrong RB, Oglive RW, Schwane JA. Eccentric exercise-induced injury to rat skeletal muscle. J Appl Physiol 1983;54:80–93.

Babenko V, Graven-Nielsen VT, Svensson P, Drewes AM, Jensen TS, Arendt-Nielsen L. Experimental human muscle pain induced by intramuscular injections of bradykinin, serotonin, and substance P. Eur J Pain 1999;3:93–102.

Cheung K, Hume P, Maxwell L. Delayed onset muscle soreness: treatment strategies and performance factors. Sports Med 2003;33:145–164.

Crenshaw AG, Thornell LE, Friden J. Intramuscular pressure, torque and swelling for the exercise-induced sore vastus lateralis muscle. Acta Physiol Scand 1994;152:265–277.

De Vries HA. Quantitative electromyographic investigation of the spasm theory of muscle pain. Am J Phys Med 1966;45:119–134.

Diehl B, Hoheisel U, Mense S. The influence of mechanical stimuli and of acetylsalicylic acid on the discharges of slowly conducting afferent units from normal and inflamed muscle in the rat. Exp Brain Res 1993;92:431–440.

Franz M, Mense S. Muscle receptors with group IV afferent fibres responding to application of bradykinin. Brain Res 1975;92:369–383.

Graven-Nielsen T, Arendt-Nielsen L. Induction and assessment of muscle pain, referred pain, and muscular hyperalgesia. Curr Pain Headache Rep 2003;7:443–451.

Hunt SP, Pini A, Evan G. Induction of c-*fos*-like protein in spinal cord neurons following sensory stimulation. Nature 1987;328:632–634.

Itoh K, Kawakita K. Effect of indomethacin on the development of eccentric exercise-induced localized sensitive region in the fascia of the rabbit. Jpn J Physiol 2002;52:173–180.

Koda H, Mizumura K. Sensitization to mechanical stimulation by inflammatory mediators, by second messengers possibly mediating these sensitizing effects, and by mild burn in canine visceral nociceptors in vitro. J Neurophysiol 2002;87:2043–2051.

Kumazawa T, Mizumura K. Thin-fibre receptors responding to mechanical, chemical, and thermal stimulation in the skeletal muscle of the dog. J Physiol (Lond) 1977;273:179–194.

Lieber RL, Friden J. Selective damage of fast glycolytic muscle fibres with eccentric contraction of the rabbit tibialis anterior. Acta Physiol Scand 1988;133:587–588.

Ling LJ, Honda T, Shimada Y, Ozaki N, Shiraishi Y, Sugiura Y. Central projection of unmyelinated (C) primary afferent fibers from gastrocnemius muscle in the guinea pig. J Comp Neurol 2003;461:140–150.

Malm C, Sjodin TL, Sjoberg B, Lenkei R, Renstrom P, Lundberg IE, Ekblom B. Leukocytes, cytokines, growth factors and hormones in human skeletal muscle and blood after uphill or downhill running. J Physiol (Lond) 2004;556:983–1000.

Mann MK, Dong XD, Svensson P, Cairns BE. Influence of intramuscular nerve growth factor injection on the response properties of rat masseter muscle afferent fibers. J Orofac Pain 2006;20:325–336.

Mense S, Meyer H. Bradykinin-induced modulation of the response behaviour of different types of feline group III and IV muscle receptors. J Physiol (Lond) 1988;398:49–63.

Mizumura K, Kumazawa T. Modification of nociceptor responses by inflammatory mediators and second messengers implicated in their action- a study in canine testicular polymodal receptors. In: Kumazawa T, Kruger L, Mizumura K, editors. The polymodal receptor—a gateway to pathological pain, Vol. 113. Amsterdam: Elsevier;1996. p 115–141.

Mizumura K, Taguchi T, Nasu T. Persistent muscular mechanical hyperalgesia induced by lengthening contraction followed by repetitive cold stress. J Musculoskeletal Pain 2007;15(Suppl):64.

Mork H, Ashina M, Bendtsen L, Olesen J, Jensen R. Experimental muscle pain and tenderness following infusion of endogenous substances in humans. Eur J Pain 2003;7:145–153.

Nasu T, Terazawa E, Sato J, Mizumura K. Randall-Selitto device measures the mechanical withdrawal thresholds of different tissues in rats depending on its probe diameter. J Physiol Sci 2007;57(Suppl):S112.

Newham DJ, McPhail G, Mills KR, Edwards RHT. Ultrastructural changes after concentric and eccentric contractions of human muscle. J Neurol Sci 1983;61:109–122.

Page AJ, O'Donnell TA, Blackshaw LA. P2X purinoceptor-induced sensitization of ferret vagal mechanoreceptors in oesophageal inflammation. J Physiol (Lond) 2000;523:403–411.

Rueff A, Mendell LM. Nerve growth factor and NT-5 induce increased thermal sensitivity of cutaneous nociceptors in vitro. J Neurophysiol 1996;76:3593–3596.

Schwane JA, Watrous BG, Johnson SR, Armstrong RB. Is lactic acid related to delayed-onset muscle soreness? Phys Sports Med 1983;11:124–131.

Smith LL. Acute inflammation—the underlying mechanism in delayed onset muscle soreness. Med Sci Sports Exerc 1991;23:542–551.

Steen KH, Reeh PW, Anton F, Handwerker HO. Protons selectively induce lasting excitation and sensitization to mechanical stimulation of nociceptors in rat skin, in vitro. J Neurosci 1992;12:86–95.

Svensson P, Cairns BE, Wang K, Arendt-Nielsen L. Injection of nerve growth factor into human masseter muscle evokes long-lasting mechanical allodynia and hyperalgesia. Pain 2003;104:241–247.

Taguchi T, Matsuda T, Mizumura K. Change with age in muscular mechanical hyperalgesia after lengthening contraction in rats. Neurosci Res 2007;57:331–338.

Taguchi T, Matsuda T, Tamura R, Sato J, Mizumura K. Muscular mechanical hyperalgesia revealed by behavioural pain test and c-Fos expression in the spinal dorsal horn after eccentric contraction in rats. J Physiol (Lond) 2005a;564:259–268.

Taguchi T, Sato J, Mizumura K. Augmented mechanical response of muscle thin-fiber sensory receptors recorded from rat muscle-nerve preparations *in vitro* after eccentric contraction. J Neurophysiol 2005b;94:2822–2831.

Takahashi K, Taguchi T, Itoh K, Okada K, Kawakita K, Mizumura K. Influence of surface anesthesia on the pressure pain threshold measured with different-sized probes. Somatosens Mot Res 2005;22:299–305.

Yajima H, Sato J, Giron R, Nakamura R, Mizumura K. Inhibitory, facilitatory, and excitatory effects of ATP and purinergic receptor agonists on the activity of rat cutaneous nociceptors in vitro. Neurosci Res 2005;51:405–416.

Correspondence to: Kazue Mizumura, MD, PhD, Department of Neuroscience II, Research Institute of Environmental Medicine, Nagoya University, Furo-cho, Chikusa-ku, Nagoya 464-8601, Japan. Tel: 81-52-789-3861; fax: 81-52-789-3889; email: mizu@riem.nagoya-u.ac.jp.

Mechanisms of Central Nervous Hyperexcitability Due to Activation of Muscle Nociceptors

Siegfried Mense[a] and Ulrich Hoheisel[b]

[a]Institute of Anatomy and Cell Biology, University Heidelberg, Heidelberg, Germany; [b]Institute of Pharmacology and Toxicology, Charité, Humboldt University, Berlin, Germany

Patients with muscle pain often show signs of sensitization such as muscle allodynia, hyperalgesia, and pain referral. In the clinical setting, it is often difficult to distinguish between sensitization of peripheral muscle nociceptors (peripheral sensitization) and that of central neurons (central sensitization). Basically, every long-lasting input from muscle nociceptors to the spinal cord or brainstem is likely to lead to changes in the excitability of central neurons. The main acute and chronic changes found in dorsal horn neurons in animal models of muscle pain are: (1) Increased background activity, i.e., higher discharge frequency in the absence of intentional stimulation. (2) Increased responsiveness to electrical stimulation of the nerve of the damaged muscle. (3) The appearance (within minutes) of new receptive fields following intramuscular (i.m.) injection of a pain-producing substance (Hoheisel et al., 1993). (4) The spread of excitation to spinal segments that do not normally receive input from the damaged muscle.

The hyperexcitability of central neurons—an expression of central sensitization—is just the first step, followed in chronic cases by changes in the connectivity, and finally the structure, of dorsal horn neurons and glial cells. Input from muscle nociceptors is more effective in inducing increased central excitability than is input from cutaneous nociceptors (Wall and Woolf, 1984). Central sensitization is an important prerequisite for the transition from acute to chronic pain and is therefore of major importance for both basic research and clinical treatment.

Various animal models have been developed to study central nervous system hyperexcitability. The focus of the present chapter is on two of these models, the first using experimental muscle inflammation and the second based on i.m. injection of nerve growth factor (NGF).

Myositis-Induced Excitability Changes in the Spinal Dorsal Horn

In experiments we conducted in anesthetized rats, changes in spinal neuronal excitability and connectivity occurred within a few hours after induction of experimental muscle inflammation. At the spinal level, three effects were induced by inflammation of the gastrocnemius-soleus (GS) muscle: (1) an increase in the background (or spontaneous) activity of dorsal horn neurons, (2) an increase in response to mechanical stimulation in the main target segments of the GS muscle (L4 and L5), and (3) expansion of the input region of the muscle nerve to adjacent lumbar segments and regions that do not normally receive strong input from the electrically stimulated GS muscle nerve (Hoheisel et al., 1994). The last effect is the most interesting, because the electrical stimulation of the muscle nerve circumvents the sensitized peripheral nociceptors, and thus the observed change must be due to central sensitization.

The most likely explanation for the expansion of the myositis-induced excitation to adjacent segments is that existing—but ineffective—synaptic connections between muscle afferents and neurons in these segments became more effective (Li and Zhuo, 1998). The opening of ineffective synapses leads to hyperexcitability of the neurons, which then respond to an input that does not normally excite them. In patients, hyperexcitability is likely to elicit pain during movements (allodynia) and hyperalgesia during noxious stimulation, whereas the expansion of the myositis-induced excitation in the dorsal horn may be the reason for the spread and referral of muscle pain.

One out of many possible mechanisms of central sensitization is that nociceptive afferent activity releases glutamate together with substance P from presynaptic boutons of the muscle afferent fibers. The postsynaptic cell is equipped with a multitude of receptor molecules, including two types of ionotropic glutamate receptor: N-methyl-D-aspartate (NMDA) receptors and AMPA (α-amino-3-hydroxy-5 methyl-4-isoxazole propionic acid), also known as "non-NMDA," receptors. Activation of these receptors results in the opening of ion channels that are permeable to cations, the NMDA channels mainly to Ca^{2+}, and the AMPA channels mainly to Na^+.

Under normal circumstances, many of the AMPA channels are ineffective, i.e., few ions pass through them per given unit of time. However, during a longer-lasting nociceptive input, the number of Na^+ ions entering the postsynaptic cell is large enough to depolarize the cell. The depolarization removes the Mg^{2+} ion that normally blocks the NMDA channel. Ca^{2+} ions can now enter the cell and activate intracellular enzymes such as protein kinases A and C. The enzymes phosphorylate the AMPA and NMDA channels, i.e., they couple a phosphate residue to the channel proteins. Phosphorylated ion channels are more permeable to ions and create larger ion currents. Eventually, gene expression changes in the nucleus of the postsynaptic neuron, so that a novel synthesis of ion channel proteins occurs. The result of these processes is a neuron that has a higher density of more effective ion channels in its membrane. These structural changes lead to a long-lasting hyperexcitability of the neuron to noxious and innocuous stimuli. A further factor involved in the sensitizing process is the action of substance P on postsynaptic G-protein-coupled neurokinin-1 (NK1) receptors (Liu and Sandkühler, 1998; Millan, 1999; Usunoff et al., 2006; Fig. 1).

Neurotransmitters and Neuropeptides Involved in Myositis-Induced Central Sensitization

The activation of NMDA and NK1 receptors contributes to myositis-induced central sensitization. In experiments on rats, intrathecal administration of antagonists to NK1 and NMDA receptors prevented the

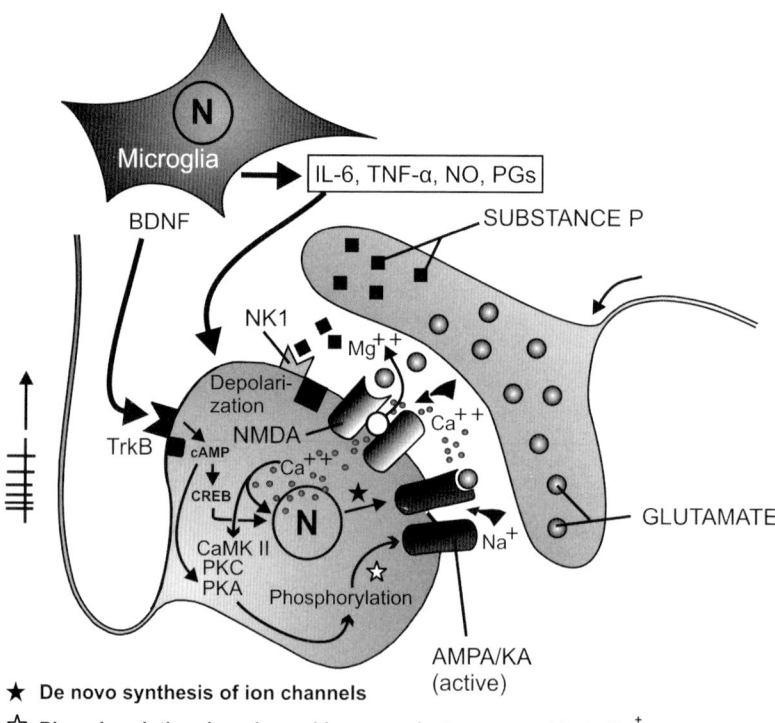

★ **De novo synthesis of ion channels**

☆ **Phosphorylation: ion channel becomes better permeable to Na$^+$**

Fig. 1. Some of the mechanisms involved in central sensitization. To the right, a presynaptic terminal of a nociceptive muscle afferent fiber is shown that contacts a postsynaptic neuron. The upper part depicts a microglial cell as it releases cytokines and brain-derived neurotrophic factor (BDNF). AMPA/KA = α-amino-3-hydroxy-5 methyl-4-isoxazole propionic acid/kainate, CaMK II = calcium/calmodulin protein kinase II, cAMP = cyclic adenosine monophosphate, IL-6 = interleukin-6, NO = nitric oxide, NK1 = neurokinin 1, NMDA = N-methyl-D-aspartate, PGs = prostaglandins, PKA = protein kinase A, PKC = protein kinase C, TNF-α = tumor necrosis factor alpha, TrkB = tyrosine kinase B (BDNF receptor).

expansion of the spinal target area to the L3 segment in animals with inflammation of the GS muscle (Hoheisel et al., 1997). On the other hand, blocking the AMPA receptors had no significant influence on the expansion. There may be a difference between muscle and joint hyperalgesia in this regard, because the latter may be reduced by administration of an AMPA-receptor antagonist (Sluka et al., 1994). Chronic central sensitization may become independent of the muscle input soon after its induction. In a model of acid-induced muscle hyperalgesia, an interruption of the muscle input by local anesthesia or dorsal rhizotomy 24 hours after induction of sensitization did not abolish the hyperalgesia (Sluka et al., 2001).

The increased background activity of dorsal horn neurons in animals with experimental myositis depends strongly on the release of nitric oxide (NO) in the spinal cord (Hoheisel et al., 2000). A lumbar spinal block of the enzyme nitric oxide synthase (NOS) with L-NAME significantly increased background activity only in nociceptive neurons. This finding indicates that NO is released tonically in the dorsal horn and inhibits the background discharge of the neurons. In contrast to the increased background activity induced by L-NAME, the mechanical responsiveness of the neurons was decreased by intrathecal (i.t.) injection of L-NAME. Thus, in dorsal horn neurons, background activity and responsiveness can change independently from each other (Hoheisel et al., 1995). Background activity is of clinical importance because it is assumed to be responsible for spontaneous pain and dysesthesia in patients with myositis.

The effects of NO in nociception and pain are controversial in the literature, with some groups regarding it as a pronociceptive and some as an antinociceptive agent. A recent report showed that NO and cyclic guanosine monophosphate (cGMP, a second messenger that requires NO for synthesis) have different actions at the spinal and supraspinal level. At the supraspinal level, NO and cGMP were found to be pronociceptive, and at the spinal level, antinociceptive (Hoheisel et al., 2005). If blockers of NO synthesis such as L-NAME are administered systemically, the supraspinal antinociceptive action prevails. Therefore, NOS-blocking drugs could be used to alleviate hyperalgesia.

The Role of Glial Cells in Central Sensitization

It is only recently that the involvement of glial cells in pain mechanisms has been appreciated. Microglia (immunocompetent brain macrophages) and astrocytes have been shown to be activated by peripheral pathological changes, including inflammation (Dong and Benveniste, 2001; Watkins and Maier, 2002). The process of glial activation together with the release of cytokines such as proinflammatory interleukins, tumor necrosis factor-α (TNF-α), and brain-derived neurotrophic factor (BDNF) in the central nervous system (neuroinflammation) are considered important factors leading to central sensitization (Hunt et al., 2001; Marchand et al., 2005; Fig. 1).

Few data are available on the involvement of glia in muscle pain. Results from our group show that astrocytes were activated after chronic inflammation (lasting 12 days) was induced by i.m. injection of complete Freund's adjuvant (CFA) into the rat GS muscle. The astrocytes exhibited morphological changes and increased expression of glial fibrillary acidic protein and fibroblast growth factor 2 (Tenschert et al., 2004). Activated astrocytes are known to be capable of releasing proinflammatory cytokines such as interleukin-6 and TNF-α, and thus they may contribute to the myositis-induced sensitization of nociceptive dorsal horn neurons (Dong and Benveniste, 2001; Kostrzewa and Segura-Aguilar, 2003). More recent data from our group indicate that chronic CFA-induced myositis also activates microglial cells. The myositis-induced pain-related behavior of the rats can be attenuated by blocking the microglia with intrathecal administration of minocycline (U. Hoheisel, D. Lambertz, and S. Mense, unpublished data).

Interestingly, other groups reported that inflammation induced in the rat paw by a subcutaneous injection of CFA did not activate microglial cells, whereas a neuropathic lesion did (Zhang et al., 2003). Apparently, microglial activation requires input from a particular set of peripheral receptors or a special pattern of discharge. The latter assumption is supported by the finding that zymosan-induced, but not CFA-induced, paw inflammation is associated with activation of microglia (Clark et al.,

2007). Likewise, the allodynia evoked by repeated i.m. injections of acidic saline in rats cannot depend on glial activation, because it was not reversed by blocking microglia and astrocytes (Ledeboer et al., 2006). Thus, it appears that not all muscle lesions that elicit chronic hypersensitivity in animal models are associated with an activation of glial cells.

Central Sensitization Induced by Nerve Growth Factor

Among the substances released in inflamed muscle, NGF is of particular interest, because it is synthesized in muscle and represents a major sensitizing substance for nociceptors in pathologically altered tissue (Pezet and McMahon, 2006). A special feature of NGF is that when injected intramuscularly in humans it induces sensitization without causing acute pain during the injection. The sensitization is expressed as long-lasting muscle allodynia and hyperalgesia (Svensson et al., 2003).

Although injection of NGF does not cause immediate pain, it excites a large proportion of group IV muscle afferents, as shown in recent rat experiments by our group. The activated receptors had a high mechanical stimulation threshold and presumably were nociceptors (Hoheisel et al., 2005). Despite the strong excitation of muscle nociceptors, awake rats did not exhibit signs of pain during NGF injection into the GS muscle. One possible explanation for the lack of pain is that the NGF-induced input excited just a few spinal neurons at a low frequency or evoked mainly subthreshold synaptic potentials. Intracellular recordings from dorsal horn neurons in rats showed that NGF injections into the GS muscle caused mainly subthreshold synaptic potentials at the spinal level (Graven-Nielsen et al., 2006; Hoheisel et al., 2007). Only a few neurons fired action potentials at a low frequency.

The long-lasting allodynia and hyperalgesia observed in humans after i.m. NGF injection raises the question as to whether low-frequency activation or even subthreshold potentials in dorsal horn neurons are sufficient to sensitize the cells. In the past, many groups studying sensitization of central neurons have used high-frequency stimulation to induce long-term potentiation (LTP), whereas low-frequency stimulation was reported to induce mainly long-term depression (LTD) or depotentiation (Froc and Racine, 2005; Ikeda et al., 2006). Recently, the sensitizing action of low-frequency stimulation has attracted more interest. In rat hippocampal slices, stimulation at 1 Hz induced a novel form of LTP characterized by slow onset and independence from activation of NMDA receptors (Lante et al., 2006).

The sensitizing action of low-frequency input to the spinal cord may be of particular importance for the development of chronic muscle pain, because pathological changes of muscle tissue are typically associated with low-frequency (and not high-frequency) activation of nociceptors. For instance, muscle receptors with group IV afferent fibers—most of which are nociceptive—exhibit an average discharge of less than 1 Hz in inflamed muscle (Diehl et al., 1993).

In contrast to NGF, a 5% solution of hypertonic saline (HS) causes immediate pain when injected intramuscularly in humans (Capra and Ro, 2004; Graven-Nielsen, 2006). For rat group IV receptors from muscle, HS is likewise a strong stimulus, but it differs from NGF in that it excites both low- and high-threshold unmyelinated muscle afferent units (Hoheisel et al., 2004). Thus, the spectrum of afferent fibers excited by NGF and HS is different.

The working hypothesis derived from these data was that although i.m. injection of NGF elicits only low-frequency action potentials or subthreshold effects (excitatory postsynaptic potentials; EPSPs) in dorsal horn neurons, it sensitizes the cells. To test the hypothesis, we made intracellular recordings from dorsal horn neurons in anesthetized rats.

Because NGF is known to sensitize peripheral nociceptors, in most experiments we used electrical stimulation of the muscle nerve, which circumvents the sensitized muscle nociceptors. In dorsal horn neurons, the first signs of sensitization were seen a few minutes after NGF injection into the GS muscle. The neuron shown in Fig. 2 reacted to electrical stimulation only with EPSPs, prior to NGF injection. Thirty minutes after injection, the neuron responded with action potentials to the stimulation (Hoheisel et al., 2007). In recent studies on NGF-induced sensitization in rats and mice, similar allodynia/hyperalgesia has been reported (Malik-Hall et al., 2005; Hathway and Fitzgerald, 2006).

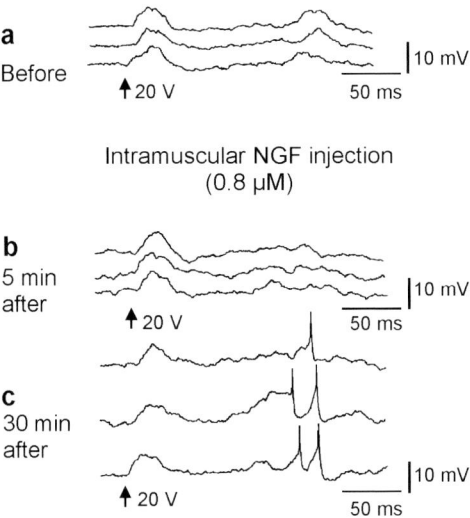

Fig. 2. Short-latency effects of nerve growth factor (NGF) on the responses of dorsal horn neurons to electrical nerve stimulation. Original registrations of excitatory postsynaptic potentials (EPSPs) and action potentials elicited by electrical stimulation of rat gastrocnemius-soleus (GS) muscle nerves are shown before (a) and a few minutes after i.m. injection of NGF (b, c). Upward arrows indicate the time of electrical stimulation. The neuron was not excited by the NGF injection (modified from Hoheisel et al. 2007).

By the day after NGF injection, the proportion of dorsal horn neurons responding with action potentials to electrical stimulation of the GS muscle nerve had increased significantly. In contrast, in rats that had been treated with an injection of HS one day prior to testing, the dorsal horn neurons showed no significant increase in the mechanically induced responses. The lack of a sensitizing effect of HS was surprising, because this treatment elicited responses of much higher discharge frequency in the dorsal horn neurons (Hoheisel et al., 2007). The strong sensitizing action of NGF—which induced mainly EPSPs in dorsal horn neurons—may indicate that conscious sensations are not required for a sensitizing effect of peripheral stimulation. Indeed, studies in humans have shown that nonpainful irritation of the skin with ultraviolet B light causes secondary hyperalgesia (Gustorff et al., 2004). This effect may be based on the same mechanisms that induce hyperalgesia after a painless i.m. injection of NGF.

Results from a study on crayfish giant fibers point in the same direction by showing that subthreshold input was sufficient for inducing potentiation of signaling in the synapses onto the giant fibers (Tsai et al., 2005). In superficial dorsal horn neurons of rats, low-frequency stimulation of afferent C fibers has also been reported to induce LTP (Ikeda et al., 2006). Evidence indicates that in these cells, Ca^{2+} is mobilized from intracellular stores during low-level presynaptic activation, which in turn could amplify pain-related information (Ikeda et al., 2006).

At the level of primary afferent unit, NGF has unique actions in that it excites exclusively nociceptive group IV receptors in muscle (Hoheisel et al., 2005). Nociceptive afferent fibers from muscle and other tissues have been shown to possess tetrodotoxin-resistant (TTX-r) Na^+ channels (Akopian et al., 1999; Steffens et al., 2003), which appear to carry particularly effective information to the spinal cord. In contrast, HS excited every group IV ending tested, irrespective of its mechanical threshold (Hoheisel et al., 2004). Therefore, the overall input to the spinal cord evoked by HS is greater and includes fibers that were excited by NGF.

Possible explanations for the greater sensitizing action of NGF on central neurons in comparison to HS are: (1) The NGF-driven nociceptive muscle afferents release BDNF in the spinal cord, which sensitizes dorsal horn neurons (Zhao et al., 2006; Fig. 1). The NGF-sensitive muscle afferent units are equipped with tyrosine kinase A (TrkA) receptor molecules, and these units are assumed to be nociceptive (Mannion et al., 1999). (2) The simultaneous input in non-nociceptive group IV units elicited by HS inhibits the sensitizing effects of the NGF-induced input.

We also conducted behavioral experiments in which mechanical stimulation of the GS muscle was used to test for allodynic and hyperalgesic effects of NGF vs. HS. In these experiments, the sensitizing action of NGF was also much stronger than that of HS (Fig. 3). We showed that the NGF-induced sensitization involved the activation of NMDA ion channels by simultaneously injecting NGF and ketamine into the GS muscle. Injection of ketamine (100 mg/kg i.p.) completely abolished the NGF-induced allodynia and hyperalgesia to mechanical stimulation of the GS muscle.

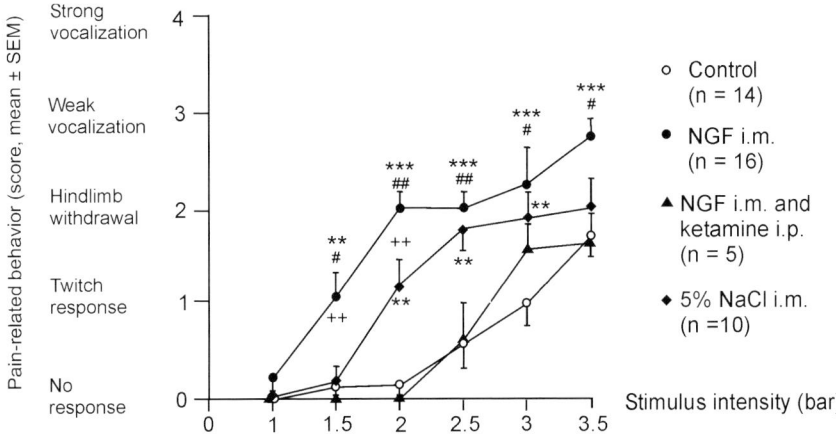

Fig. 3. Sensitizing effects of nerve growth factor (NGF) vs. 5% hypertonic saline (HS) on the responses of awake rats to pressure stimulation of the gastrocnemius-soleus (GS) muscle. Pressure stimuli were applied with a pneumatic forceps; the stimulus intensity is given in bar (abscissa). Pain-related behavior was scored as follows: 0 = no response, 1 = twitching of hindlimb muscles but no withdrawal. 2 = hindlimb withdrawal, 3 = weak vocalization, 4 = strong vocalization. Open circles, control animals without prior i.m. injection; filled circles, 1 day after NGF i.m.; diamonds, 1 day after i.m. HS; triangles, 1 day after NGF plus ketamine. Asterisks (*) indicate significant differences compared to control animals, plus signs (+) show significant differences between NGF and HS, and pound signs (#) show significant differences between NGF and NGF plus ketamine. #, $P < 0.05$; **, ##, ++, $P < 0.01$; *** $P < 0.001$. There were no significant differences between the control and the NGF plus ketamine group (modified from Hoheisel et al. 2007).

The sensitizing action of NGF-induced subthreshold or low-frequency spinal activity offers an intriguing explanation for some chronic muscle pain syndromes that are not well understood at present, such as work-related musculoskeletal disorders (Novak, 2004; Sbriccoli et al., 2004). It is conceivable that individuals who repeatedly perform tonic muscle contractions at low force (e.g., musicians) may sustain microtraumas (followed by sterile inflammation; Barr et al., 2004). These microtraumas might elicit subthreshold potentials or low-frequency discharges at the spinal level that might not evoke subjective sensations but could sensitize central neurons. In the long run, the central sensitization may develop into a chronic muscle pain syndrome.

References

Akopian AN, Souslova V, England S, Okuse K, Ogata N, Ure J, Smith A, Kerr BJ, McMahon SB, Boyce S, Hill R, Stanfa LC, Dickenson AH, Wood JN. The tetrodotoxin-resistant sodium channel SNS has a specialized function in pain pathways. Nat Neurosci 1999;2:541–548.

Barr AE, Barbe MF, Clark BD. Systemic inflammatory mediators contribute to widespread effects in work-related musculoskeletal disorders. Exerc Sport Sci Rev 2004;32:135–142.

Capra NF, Ro JY. Human and animal experimental models of acute and chronic muscle pain: intramuscular algesic injection. Pain 2004;110:3–7.

Clark AK, Gentry C, Bradbury EJ, McMahon SB, Malcangio M. Role of spinal microglia in rat models of peripheral nerve injury and inflammation. Eur J Pain 2007;11:223–230.

Diehl B, Hoheisel U, Mense S. The influence of mechanical stimuli and of acetylsalicylic acid on the discharges of slowly conducting afferent units from normal and inflamed muscle in the rat. Exp Brain Res 1993;92:431–440.

Dong Y, Benveniste EN. Immune functions of astrocytes. Glia 2001;36:180–190.

Froc DJ, Racine RJ. Interactions between LTP- and LTD-inducing stimulation in the sensorimotor cortex of the awake freely moving rat. J Neurophysiol 2005;93:548–556.

Graven-Nielsen T. Fundamentals of muscle pain, referred pain and deep tissue hyperalgesia. Scan J Rheum 2006;(Suppl 122):1–43.

Graven-Nielsen T, Curatolo M, Mense S. Central sensitization, referred pain, and deep tissue hyperalgesia in musculoskeletal pain. In: Flor H, Kalso E, Dostrovsky JO, editors. Proceedings of the 11th World Congress on Pain. Seattle: IASP Press; 2006. p 217–230.

Gustorff B, Hoechtl K, Sycha T, Felouzis E, Lehrs S, Kress HG. The effects of remifentanil and gabapentin on hyperalgesia in a new extended inflammatory skin pain model in healthy volunteers. Anesth Analg 2004;98:401–407.

Hathway GJ, Fitzgerald M. Time course and dose-dependence of nerve growth factor-induced secondary hyperalgesia in the mouse. J Pain 2006;7:57–61.

Hoheisel U, Mense S, Simons DG, Yu XM. Appearance of new receptive fields in rat dorsal horn neurons following noxious stimulation of skeletal muscle: a model for referral of muscle pain? Neurosci Lett 1993;153:9–12.

Hoheisel U, Koch K, Mense S. Functional reorganization in the rat dorsal horn during an experimental myositis. Pain 1994;59:111–118.

Hoheisel U, Reinert A, Mense S. The excitability and background activity of rat dorsal horn neurons is differentially influenced by an experimental myositis. Pain Clinic 1995;9:209–215.

Hoheisel U, Sander B, Mense S. Myositis-induced functional reorganization of the rat dorsal horn: effects of spinal superfusion with antagonists to neurokinin and glutamate receptors. Pain 1997;69:219–230.

Hoheisel U, Unger T, Mense S. A block of the nitric oxide synthesis leads to increased background activity predominantly in nociceptive dorsal horn neurons in the rat. Pain 2000;88:249–257.

Hoheisel U, Reinöhl J, Unger T, Mense S. Acidic pH and capsaicin activate mechanosensitive group IV muscle receptors in the rat. Pain 2004;110:149–157.

Hoheisel U, Unger T, Mense S. The possible role of the NO-cGMP pathway in nociception: different spinal and supraspinal action of enzyme blockers on rat dorsal horn neurones. Pain 2005;117:358–367.

Hoheisel U, Unger T, Mense S. Sensitization of rat dorsal horn neurones by NGF-induced subthreshold potentials and low-frequency activation. A study employing intracellular recordings in vivo. Brain Res 2007;1169:34–43.

Hunt SP, Mantyh PW. The molecular dynamics of pain control. Nature Rev Neurosci 2001;2:83–91.

Ikeda H, Stark J, Fischer H, Wagner M, Drdla R, Jäger T, Sandkühler J. Synaptic amplifier of inflammatory pain in the spinal dorsal horn. Science 2006;312:1659–1662.

Kostrzewa RM, Segura-Aguilar J. Novel mechanisms and approaches in the study of neurodegeneration and neuroprotection. A review. Neurotox Res 2003;5:375–383.

Lante F, Cavalier M, Cohen-Solal C, Guiramand J, Vignes M. Developmental switch from LTD to LTP in low frequency-induced plasticity. Hippocampus 2006;16:981–989.

Ledeboer A, Mahoney JH, Milligan ED, Martin D, Maier SF, Watkins LR. Spinal cord glia and inter-leukin-1 do not appear to mediate persistent allodynia induced by intramuscular acidic saline in rats. J Pain 2006;7:757–767.

Li P, Zhuo M. Silent glutamatergic synapses and nociception in mammalian spinal cord. Nature 1998;393:695–698.

Liu XG, Sandkühler J. Activation of spinal N-methyl-D-aspartate or neurokinin receptors induces long-term potentiation of spinal C-fibre-evoked potentials. Neuroscience 1998;86:1209–1216.

Malik-Hall M, Dina OA, Levine JD. Primary afferent nociceptor mechanisms mediating NGF-induced mechanical hyperalgesia. Eur J Neurosci 2005;21:3387–3394.

Mannion RJ, Costigan M, Decosterd I, Amaya F, Ma QP, Holstege J, Ji RR, Acheson A, Lindsay RM, Wilkinson GA, Woolf CJ. Neurotrophins: peripherally and centrally acting modulators of tactile stimulus-induced inflammatory pain hypersensitivity. Proc Natl Acad Sci USA 1999;96:9385–9390.

Marchand F, Perretti M, McMahon SB. Role of the immune system in chronic pain. Nature Rev Neurosci 2005;6:521–532.

Millan MJ. The induction of pain: an integrative review. Prog Neurobiol 1999;57:1–164.

Novak CB. Upper extremity work-related musculoskeletal disorders: a treatment perspective. J Orthop Sports Phys Ther 2004;34:628–637.

Pezet S, McMahon SB. Neurotrophins: mediators and modulators of pain. Annu Rev Neurosci 2006;29:507–538.

Sbriccoli P, Yousuf K, Kupershtein I, Solomonow M, Zhou H, Zhu MP, Lu Y. Static load repetition is a risk factor in the development of lumbar cumulative musculoskeletal disorder. Spine 2004;29:2643–2653.

Sluka KA, Jordan HH, Westlund KN. Reduction in joint swelling and hyperalgesia following post-treatment with a non-NMDA glutamate receptor antagonist. Pain 1994;59:95–100.

Sluka KA, Kalra A, Moore SA. Unilateral intramuscular injections of acidic saline produce a bilateral long-lasting hyperalgesia. Muscle Nerve 2001;24:37–46.

Steffens H, Eek B, Trudrung P, Mense S. Tetrodotoxin block of A-fibre afferents from skin and muscle—a tool to study pure C-fibre effects in the spinal cord. Eur J Physiol 2003;445:607–613.

Svensson P, Cairns BE, Wang K, Arendt-Nielsen L. Injection of nerve growth factor into human masseter muscle evokes long-lasting mechanical allodynia and hyperalgesia. Pain 2003;104:241–247.

Tenschert S, Reinert A, Hoheisel U, Mense S. Effects of a chronic myositis on structural and functional features of spinal astrocytes in the rat. Neurosci Lett 2004;361:196–199.

Tsai LY, Tseng SH, Yeh SR. Long-lasting potentiation of excitatory synaptic signalling of the crayfish lateral giant neuron. J Comp Physiol A Neuroethol Sens Neural Behav Physiol 2005;191:347–354.

Usunoff KG, Popratiloff A, Schmitt O, Wree A. Functional anatomy of pain. Adv Anat Embryol Cell Biol 2006;184:1–115.

Wall PD, Woolf CJ. Muscle but not cutaneous C-afferent input produces prolonged increases in the excitability of the flexion reflex in the rat. J Physiol 1984;356:443–458.

Watkins LR, Maier SF. Glia: A novel drug discovery target for clinical pain. Nat Rev Drug Discov 2002;2:973–985.

Zhang J, Hoffert C, Vu HK, Groblewski T, Ahmad S, O'Donnell D. Induction of CB2 receptor expression in the rat spinal cord of neuropathic but not inflammatory chronic pain models. Eur J Neurosci 2003;17:2750–2754.

Zhao J, Seereeram A, Nassar MA, Levato A, Pezet S, Hathaway G, Morenilla-Palao C, Stirling C, Fitzgerald M, McMahon SB, Rios M, Wood JN. Nociceptor-derived brain-derived neurotrophic factor regulates acute and inflammatory but not neuropathic pain. Mol Cell Neurosci 2006;31:539–548.

Correspondence to: Prof. Dr. med. S. Mense, Institut für Anatomie und Zellbiologie III, Universität Heidelberg, Im Neuenheimer Feld 307, 69120 Heidelberg, Germany. Tel: 49-6221-544193; fax: 49-6221-546071; email: mense@urz.uni-heidelberg.de.

Bilateral, Long-Lasting Hyperalgesia Due to Repeated Excitation of Muscle Nociceptors: A Role for ASIC3

Roxanne Y. Walder and Kathleen A. Sluka

Physical Therapy and Rehabilitation Science Graduate Program, Pain Research Program, University of Iowa, Iowa City, Iowa, USA

Clinically, musculoskeletal pain can arise in a variety of disorders including myofascial pain, fibromyalgia syndrome, myositis, temporomandibular joint disorder, low back pain, neck pain, or joint pain (Barr and Barbe, 2002; Chen et al., 2002; Fricton, 2002; Clauw and Crofford, 2003; Barr et al., 2004; Clauw, 2007). The etiology and pathogenesis of these musculoskeletal pain conditions are poorly understood, and current therapeutic approaches have a limited scientific basis, largely due to incomplete knowledge of the peripheral and central mechanisms underlying musculoskeletal pain.

Chronic Muscle Pain

Chronic pain is a major economic problem costing billions of dollars in health care and lost wages. Population-based studies indicate that among types of chronic pain, musculoskeletal pain is the most prevalent (Gran, 2003). In spite of its prevalence, the biological mechanisms that generate and maintain chronic muscle pain are poorly understood. Whereas numerous animal models for cutaneous pain exist, few models of chronic muscle pain have been established. Importantly, muscle pain is distinctly different from cutaneous pain because it results in longer lasting, more diffuse, poorly localized pain.

Chronic musculoskeletal pain syndromes include both inflammatory and non-inflammatory components. Conditions such as repetitive strain injury and tendonitis are clearly associated with peripheral tissue damage that includes inflammation of the muscle (Barr and Barbe, 2002; Barr et al., 2004; Stauber, 2004). These conditions are common, accounting for 2–15% of work-related musculoskeletal disorders and resulting in a significant loss of productivity and disability.

Approximately 10–15% of the population in the United States and England have chronic widespread pain (CWP), and 20–25% of the population have chronic regional muscle pain (Clauw and Crofford, 2003; Gran, 2003). These widespread and regional chronic pain conditions are non-inflammatory, with minimal peripheral tissue damage. One form of CWP is fibromyalgia syndrome (FMS), which is classified as a chronic generalized muscle pain with hyperalgesia to pressure over multiple tender points (Wolfe et al., 1990). It is commonly accepted that there is a generalized decrease in mechanical pain threshold in patients with CWP (Quimby et al., 1988; Tunks et al., 1988; Granges and Littlejohn, 1993). Still, there is no consensus as to the etiology and pathology of CWP. For FMS, it is generally accepted that pain is maintained by central neuronal changes. Nonsteroidal anti-inflammatory drugs (NSAIDs) are ineffective as analgesic agents in FMS, whereas opioids, gabapentin, and exercise can reverse some of the pain (Busch et al., 2002; Rao and Bennett, 2003; Arnold et al., 2007; Clauw, 2007). While central sensitization plays a role in the maintenance of FMS, the peripheral initiators of these central changes are unknown. We propose that ASIC3 (one of the acid-sensing ion channels) in the dorsal root ganglia (DRG) innervating muscle is key to the development of CWP associated with peripheral muscle inflammation, as well as that maintained by central neuronal changes.

Animal Models of Muscle Pain

Inflammatory model. To directly address both inflammatory and non-inflammatory musculoskeletal pain conditions, we developed and characterized several animal models. All these models are associated with long-lasting, widespread hyperalgesia after insult to deep somatic tissue, i.e., muscle or joint. For example, injection of carrageenan or capsaicin into the muscle or joint of rats produces bilateral hyperalgesia that lasts for weeks and results in a local inflammatory response (Sluka, 2002; Radhakrishnan et al., 2003). The finding that hyperalgesia spreads to the contralateral side when the inflammation becomes chronic suggests that chronic inflammation of deep tissues is associated with widespread hyperalgesia. Inflammation of muscle sensitizes neurons in both the peripheral and central nervous systems (Mense, 1993). Muscle nociceptors increase their resting activity and responses to mechanical stimuli following intramuscular injection of carrageenan (Berberich et al., 1988; Diehl et al., 1988). Similar changes occur in dorsal horn neurons in response to carrageenan-induced muscle inflammation, i.e., increases in background activity and decreases in the threshold to noxious stimulation (Hoheisel et al., 1994, 1997). Further, muscle inflammation induces development of receptive fields within the gastrocnemius muscle for dorsal horn neurons located in L3; these receptive fields are completely absent in control animals (Hoheisel et al., 1994). Thus, injection of carrageenan into muscle produces inflammation resulting in sensitization of peripheral and central neurons that is manifested as long-lasting widespread hyperalgesia.

Non-inflammatory model. Recently, we developed and characterized a model of chronic non-inflammatory musculoskeletal pain induced by two intramuscular injections of acidic (pH 4.0) saline spaced 5 days apart (Sluka et al., 2001).

Acidic saline (20 or 100 μL for mice or rats, respectively) is injected into the left gastrocnemius muscle, and hyperalgesia is assessed by measuring the paw withdrawal latency to mechanical stimuli (von Frey filaments) and to radiant heat (Sluka et al., 2001, 2003). Although the acidity of the injected solution is pH 4.0, pH in the muscle decreases only to pH 6.0 for approximately 6 minutes. Histological analysis of the injected muscle tissue shows little or no muscle tissue injury, even at the site of injection (Sluka et al., 2001). This model is characterized by long-lasting *bilateral* mechanical hyperalgesia of the paw without associated muscle tissue damage. Unique to this model, the *contralateral* hyperalgesia is not dependent on continued primary afferent input once developed (Sluka et al., 2001). Rather, central mechanisms appear to maintain the hyperalgesia. Blockade of NMDA or non-NMDA glutamate receptors spinally reverses the hyperalgesia once developed (Skyba et al., 2002), suggesting that continued activation of ionotropic glutamate receptors occurs during the development of widespread hyperalgesia. Release of glutamate increases in the spinal dorsal horn in response to the second intramuscular injection of acidic saline, and increased basal concentrations of glutamate in the spinal cord are detected at 1 week after the second acidic saline injection (Skyba et al., 2005). Wide-dynamic-range neurons in the dorsal horn sensitize with the expansion of receptive fields to include the contralateral limb and increase their responses to mechanical stimuli bilaterally (Sluka et al., 2003). Bilateral increases in phosphorylation of CREB (cAMP responsive element binding protein) occur in the dorsal horn of the spinal cord. Blockade of the cAMP pathway reverses the mechanical hyperalgesia as well as the increases in phosphorylated CREB (Hoeger-Bement and Sluka, 2003). However, while these studies show that the maintenance of hyperalgesia involves changes in the central nervous system, the factors involved in initiating the bilateral hyperalgesia have yet to be determined. We propose that activation of ASIC3 in DRG innervating muscle is responsible for initiating the bilateral mechanical hyperalgesia induced by muscle insult, both inflammatory and non-inflammatory in origin.

Muscle Pain versus Cutaneous Pain

The quality of pain associated with injury to a muscle differs from that associated with injury to the skin. Injury to deep structures results in diffuse, difficult to localize, aching pain (Kellgren, 1938; Simone et al.,

1994). In contrast, injury to the skin usually produces well-localized, sharp, stabbing or burning pain (Ochoa and Torebjork, 1983). For muscle pain, the size of the area of referred pain correlates with the intensity and duration of the primary muscle pain (Marchettini et al., 1996). In human subjects, painful intramuscular stimulation is rated as more unpleasant than painful cutaneous stimulation (Svensson et al., 1997). Capsaicin-induced intramuscular pain is longer lasting than capsaicin-induced skin pain, and referred pain is more frequent with intramuscular pain (Witting et al., 2000). Thus, pain associated with injury to muscle differs in quality from pain associated with injury to skin.

Different central anatomical pathways or different biochemical mediators could result in a different pattern of response. DRG neurons innervating muscle have less isolectin B4 and somatostatin, and more calcitonin gene-related peptide and substance P than do DRG neurons innervating cutaneous tissue (O'Brien et al., 1989; Plenderleith and Snow, 1993). Injection of neuropeptides into skin or muscle results in different responses. Substance P produces spontaneous pain when injected into skin but causes a decrease in the pressure pain threshold, without spontaneous pain, when injected into muscle (Jensen et al., 1991). Calcitonin gene-related peptide does not produce pain when injected alone into either skin or muscle, but it does cause pain when injected with substance P into muscle (Pedersen-Bjergaard et al., 1991). Interestingly, McCleskey and colleagues recently showed that small-diameter primary afferent neurons innervating muscle (~50%) are more likely to express ASIC3 than those innervating skin (~10–20%) (Molliver et al., 2005). This finding supports our hypothesis that ASIC3 is critical to the development of hyperalgesia associated with muscle insult.

The central projections from neurons innervating muscle are predominantly to lamina I and the deeper dorsal horn, whereas those from cutaneous tissue have a dense projection to lamina II (Mense and Craig, 1988; Mense, 1993). Formalin injected into the skin of the lower back increases c-fos expression throughout laminae I–V, but when it is injected into the muscles of the lower back there is no labeling in lamina II (Ohtori et al., 2000). Further, C-fiber stimulation of a muscle nerve produces a longer-lasting increase in the flexion reflex when compared to

C-fiber stimulation of a cutaneous nerve (Wall and Woolf, 1984). Thus, the biochemical, anatomical, and physiological differences support the hypothesis that injury to muscle results in distinctly different behavioral responses when compared to injury to the skin. These differences are observed in both the peripheral and central nervous systems.

Acid-Sensing Ion Channels and Pain

Effects of tissue acidosis on nociception. A decrease in pH is observed following inflammation, hematomas, and isometric exercise (Revici et al., 1949; Hood et al., 1988; Pan et al., 1988; Issberner et al., 1996). Tissue acidosis occurs in several physiological and disease states, including arthritis, inflammation, ischemia, myofascial pain, and cancer (Pan et al., 1988; Issberner et al., 1996; Reeh and Steen, 1996; Shah et al., 2005). In fact, there is a positive correlation between the pain experienced and local acidity (Issberner et al., 1996). Acidosis can be mimicked by infusing acidic solutions into muscle and joints. Constant infusion of pH 5.2 phosphate buffer into the flexor carpi radialis muscle in human subjects produces pain with a rating of 20% on the visual analogue scale that shows no adaptation during infusion (Issberner et al., 1996). Thus, acid infusion into muscle results in pain and can play a role in the development of referred pain and mechanical hyperalgesia.

ASIC3 and pain. Low pH activates acid-sensing ion channels (ASICs), which are encoded by four different genes. Three of the ASICs—ASIC1, ASIC2, and ASIC3—are found on primary afferent neurons (Waldmann and Lazdunski, 1998; Waldmann, 2001). Of these, ASIC3 plays a key role in mechanical hyperalgesia induced by muscle insult. ASIC3 is found in large- and small-diameter primary afferents and in free nerve endings of the skin and colocalizes with substance P receptors in small DRG neurons (Price et al., 2001). Further ASIC3 is found in DRG innervating muscle (Sluka et al., 2003; Molliver et al., 2005). In knockout mice lacking ASIC3 (ASIC3−/−) and without tissue injury, the behavioral response to mechanical and heat stimuli is similar to that of wild-type littermates (Price et al., 2001), indicating that ASIC3 does not play a role in normal sensory processing.

Cutaneous mechanical hyperalgesia that results after cutaneous inflammation is enhanced in ASIC3−/− mice (Price et al., 2001; Chen et al., 2002). Similarly, ASIC3−/− mice show increased sensitivity to mechanical stimuli in response to carrageenan of the paw (Mogil et al., 2005). Thermal hyperalgesia, produced by carrageenan paw inflammation, develops similarly in ASIC3−/− mice when compared to their wild-type littermates (Price et al., 2001; Chen et al., 2002). Taken together, these data argue against a role for ASIC3 in cutaneous inflammatory pain. However, ASIC3 mRNA is upregulated after complete Freund's adjuvant inflammation of the paw (Voilley et al., 2001), suggesting an increase in ASIC3 protein after inflammation. Application of pro-inflammatory cytokines to DRG neurons (nerve growth factor, serotonin, interleukin-1β, prostaglandin E_2, and bradykinin) mimics this increased expression of ASIC3 mRNA after inflammation (Mamet et al., 2002; Hou et al., 2003; Lin et al., 2006; Ma et al., 2006; Ozaktay et al., 2006). Further, application of these inflammatory mediators to DRG neurons results in a greater number of neurons expressing ASIC currents, including ASIC3-like currents, and increased coexpression of ASIC3 and TRPV1, another ion channel that plays an essential role in the development of acid-induced inflammation and hyperalgesia (Caterina et al., 1997; Liu et al., 2004; Leffler et al., 2006). For the ASIC3-like currents, there is an increase in current density and a greater number of neurons expressing ASIC3 (Mamet et al., 2002). These changes in ASIC3 current should increase acid-induced excitation of ASIC3 neurons and increase the number of neurons responding to acid. Thus, muscle inflammation should result in the release of inflammatory mediators that would sensitize primary afferent fibers, increasing expression of ASIC3 in muscle. The decreased pH that occurs after inflammation would activate ASIC3 on primary afferent fibers innervating muscle, increasing the input to the spinal cord and resulting in central sensitization manifested behaviorally in this model as secondary hyperalgesia of the paw.

In ASIC3−/− mice with muscle tissue injury, however, mechanical hyperalgesia is significantly reduced. Specifically, the mechanical hyperalgesia that occurs after repeated intramuscular acid injection (Sluka et al., 2003), or after muscle inflammation (Sluka et al., 2007), is significantly reduced in ASIC−/− mice when compared to wild-type controls.

Intramuscular injection of amiloride, a nonselective ASIC blocker, into C57BL/6 (ASIC3+/+) mice also prevents the mechanical hyperalgesia produced by the two intramuscular acid injections in mice (Sluka et al., 2003). Further, dorsal horn neurons in ASIC3−/− mice do not become sensitized after the second intramuscular injection of acid when compared to ASIC3+/+ mice. Infection of mouse DRG neurons innervating muscle of ASIC3−/− mice with an ASIC3-encoding virus results in functional expression of ASIC3 in muscle and DRG, completely restoring the mechanical hyperalgesia induced by carrageenan inflammation (Sluka et al., 2007). In contrast, infection of mouse DRG neurons innervating skin with an ASIC3-encoding virus results in functional expression of ASIC3 in skin and DRG, but does not restore the mechanical hyperalgesia induced by carrageenan inflammation. We therefore conclude that activation of ASIC3 in the primary afferent fibers innervating muscle is critical for the development of central sensitization after muscle insult and for the consequent mechanical hyperalgesia (Sluka et al., 2003, 2007).

Summary

Musculoskeletal pain is a major medical problem and is currently difficult to treat. Chronic widespread musculoskeletal pain is the result of numerous intracellular molecular reactions that act in concert to cause hyperalgesia, allodynia, and referred pain. Mechanisms of cutaneous pain are different than those which cause muscle pain. At present, we do not know what converts an acute pain to a chronic pain condition. The use of animal models of both inflammatory and non-inflammatory musculoskeletal pain can help us further understand the important proteins and pathways involved in the development and maintenance of CWP. Although central sensitization plays a critical role in the maintenance of widespread bilateral hyperalgesia, it is becoming clear that peripheral ion channels are critical to the development of muscle-induced hyperalgesia. We propose that peripheral ion channels such as ASIC3 and TRPV1 play a critical role in the development of both acute and chronic musculoskeletal pain. Further scientific understanding of the peripheral and central physiological mechanisms resulting in CWP could lead to new pharmacological treatments for clinical pain.

Acknowledgments

Supported by the National Institutes of Health NS39734, AR053509, and AR052316.

References

Arnold LM, Goldenberg DL, Stanford SB, et al. Gabapentin in the treatment of fibromyalgia: a randomized, double-blind, placebo-controlled, multicenter trial. Arthritis Rheum 2007;56:1336–1344.

Barr AE, Barbe MF. Pathophysiological tissue changes associated with repetitive movement: a review of the evidence. Phys Ther 2002;82:173–187.

Barr AE, Barbe MF, Clark BD. Work-related musculoskeletal disorders of the hand and wrist: epidemiology, pathophysiology, and sensorimotor changes. J Orthop Sports Phys Ther 2004;34:610–627.

Berberich P, Hoheisel U, Mense S. Effects of a carrageenan-induced myositis on the discharge properties of group III and IV muscle receptors in the cat. J Neurophysiol 1988;59:1395–1409.

Busch A, Schachter CL, Peloso PM, Bombardier C. Exercise for treating fibromyalgia syndrome. Cochrane Database Syst Rev 2002;3:CD003786.

Caterina MJ, Schumacher MA, Tominaga M, Rosen TA, Levine JD, Julius D. The capsaicin receptor: a heat-activated ion channel in the pain pathway. Nature 1997;389:816–824.

Chen CC, Zimmer A, Sun WH, Hall J, Brownstein MJ, Zimmer A. A role for ASIC3 in the modulation of high-intensity pain stimuli. Proc Natl Acad Sci USA 2002;99:8992–8997.

Clauw DJ. Fibromyalgia: update on mechanisms and management. J Clin Rheumatol 2007;13:102–109.

Clauw DJ, Crofford LJ. Chronic widespread pain and fibromyalgia: what we know, and what we need to know. Best Pract Res Clin Rheumatol 2003;17:685–701.

Diehl B, Hoheisel U, Mense S. Histological and neurophysiological changes induced by carrageenan in skeletal muscle of cat and rat. Agents Actions 1988;25:210–213.

Fricton JR. Masticatory myofascial pain: an explanatory model of regional muscle pain syndromes. J Musculoskel Pain 2002;10:131–150.

Gran JT. The epidemiology of chronic generalized musculoskeletal pain. Best Pract Res Clin Rheumatol 2003;17:547–561.

Granges G, Littlejohn G. Pressure pain threshold in pain-free subjects, in patients with chronic regional pain syndromes, and in patients with fibromyalgia syndrome. Arthritis Rheum 1993;36:642–646.

Hoeger-Bement MK, Sluka KA. Phosphorylation of CREB and mechanical hyperalgesia is reversed by blockade of the cAMP pathway in a time-dependent manner after repeated intramuscular acid injections. J Neurosci 2003;23:5437–5445.

Hoheisel U, Koch K, Mense S. Functional reorganization in the rat dorsal horn during an experimental myositis. Pain 1994;59:111–118.

Hoheisel U, Sander B, Mense S. Myositis-induced functional reorganization of the rat dorsal horn: effects of spinal superfusion with antagonists to neurokinin and glutamate receptors. Pain 1997;69:219–230.

Hood VL, Schubert C, Keller U, Muller S. Effect of systemic pH on pHi and lactic acid generation in exhaustive forearm exercise. Am J Physiol 1988;255:F479–85.

Hou L, Li W, Wang X. Mechanism of interleukin-1 beta-induced calcitonin gene-related peptide production from dorsal root ganglion neurons of neonatal rats. J Neurosci Res 2003;73:188–197.

Issberner U, Reeh PW, Steen KH. Pain due to tissue acidosis: a mechanism for inflammatory and ischemic myalgia? Neurosci Lett 1996;208:191–194.

Jensen K, Tuxen C, Pedersen-Bjergaard U, Jansen I. Pain, tenderness, wheal and flare induced by substance-P, bradykinin and 5-hydroxytryptamine in humans. Cephalalgia 1991;11:175–182.

Kellgren JH. Observations on referred pain arising from muscle. Clin Sci 1938;3:175–190.

Leffler A, Monter B, Koltzenburg M. The role of the capsaicin receptor TRPV1 and acid-sensing ion channels (ASICS) in proton sensitivity of subpopulations of primary nociceptive neurons in rats and mice. Neuroscience 2006;139:699–709.

Lin CR, Amaya F, Barrett L, Wang H, Takada J, Samad TA, Woolf CJ. Prostaglandin E2 receptor EP4 contributes to inflammatory pain hypersensitivity. J Pharmacol Exp Ther 2006;319:1096–1103.

Liu M, Willmott NJ, Michael GJ, Priestley JV. Differential pH and capsaicin responses of Griffonia simplicifolia IB4 (IB4)-positive and IB4-negative small sensory neurons. Neuroscience 2004;127:659–672.

Ma C, Greenquist KW, Lamotte RH. Inflammatory mediators enhance the excitability of chronically compressed dorsal root ganglion neurons. J Neurophysiol 2006;95:2098–2107.

Mamet J, Baron A, Lazdunski M, Voilley N. Proinflammatory mediators, stimulators of sensory neuron excitability via the expression of acid-sensing ion channels. J Neurosci 2002;22:10662–10670.

Marchettini P, Simone DA, Caputi G, Ochoa JL. Pain from excitation of identified muscle nociceptors in humans. Brain Res 1996;740:109–116.

Mense S. Nociception from skeletal muscle in relation to clinical muscle pain. Pain 1993;54:241–289.

Mense S, Craig AD Jr. Spinal and supraspinal terminations of primary afferent fibers from the gastrocnemius-soleus muscle in the cat. Neuroscience 1988;26:1023–1035.

Mogil JS, Breese NM, Witty MF, Ritchie J, Rainville ML, Ase A, Abbadi N, Stucky CL, Seguela P. Transgenic expression of a dominant-negative ASIC3 subunit leads to increased sensitivity to mechanical and inflammatory stimuli. J Neurosci 2005;25:9893–9901.

Molliver DC, Immke DC, Fierro L, Pare M, Rice FL, McCleskey EW. ASIC3, an acid-sensing ion channel, is expressed in metaboreceptive sensory neurons. Mol Pain 2005;1:35.

O'Brien C, Woolf CJ, Fitzgerald M, Lindsay RM, Molander C. Differences in the chemical expression of rat primary afferent neurons which innervate skin, muscle or joint. Neuroscience 1989;32:493–502.

Ochoa J, Torebjork E. Sensations evoked by intraneural microstimulation of single mechanoreceptor units innervating the human hand. J Physiol 1983;342:633–654.

Ohtori S, Takahashi K, Chiba T, Takahashi Y, Yamagata M, Sameda H, Moriya H. Fos expression in the rat brain and spinal cord evoked by noxious stimulation to low back muscle and skin. Spine 2000;25:2425–2430.

Ozaktay AC, Kallakuri S, Takebayashi T, Cavanaugh JM, Asik I, DeLeo JA, Weinstein JN. Effects of interleukin-1 beta, interleukin-6, and tumor necrosis factor on sensitivity of dorsal root ganglion and peripheral receptive fields in rats. Eur Spine J 2006;15:1529–1537.

Pan JW, Hamm JR, Rothman DL, Shulman RG. Intracellular pH in human skeletal muscle by 1H NMR. Proc Natl Acad Sci USA 1988;85:7836–7839.

Pedersen-Bjergaard U, Nielsen LB, Jensen K, Edvinsson L, Jansen I, Olesen J. Calcitonin gene-related peptide, neurokinin A and substance P: effects on nociception and neurogenic inflammation in human skin and temporal muscle. Peptides 1991;12:333–337.

Plenderleith MB, Snow PJ. The plant lectin *Bandeiraea simplicifolia* I-B4 identifies a subpopulation of small diameter primary sensory neurones which innervate the skin in the rat. Neurosci Lett 1993;159:17–20.

Price MP, McIlwrath SL, Xie J, Cheng C, Qiao J, Tarr DE, Sluka KA, Brennan TJ, Lewin GR, Welsh MJ. The DRASIC cation channel contributes to the detection of cutaneous touch and acid stimuli in mice. Neuron 2001;32:1071–1083.

Quimby LG, Block SR, Gratwick GM. Fibromyalgia: generalized pain intolerance and manifold symptom reporting. J Rheumatol 1988;15:1264–1270.

Radhakrishnan R, Moore SA, Sluka KA. Unilateral carrageenan injection into muscle or joint induces chronic bilateral hyperalgesia in rats. Pain 2003;104:567–577.

Rao SG, Bennett RM. Pharmacological therapies in fibromyalgia. Best Pract Res Clin Rheumatol 2003;17:611–627.

Reeh PW, Steen KH. Tissue acidosis in nociception and pain. Prog Brain Res 1996;113:143–151.

Revici E, Stoopen E, Frenk E, Ravich RA. The painful focus. II. The relation of pain to local physiochemical changes. Bull Inst Appl Biol 1949;1:21–38.

Shah JP, Phillips TM, Danoff JV, Gerber LH. An in vivo microanalytical technique for measuring the local biochemical milieu of human skeletal muscle. J Appl Physiol 2005;99:1977–1984.

Simone DA, Marchettini P, Caputi G, Ochoa JL. Identification of muscle afferents subserving sensation of deep pain in humans. J Neurophysiol 1994;72:883–889.

Skyba DA, King EW, Sluka KA. Effects of NMDA and non-NMDA ionotropic glutamate receptor antagonists on the development and maintenance of hyperalgesia induced by repeated intramuscular injection of acidic saline. Pain 2002;98:69–78.

Skyba DA, Lisi TL, Sluka KA. Excitatory amino acid concentrations increase in the spinal cord dorsal horn after repeated intramuscular injection of acidic saline. Pain 2005;119:142–149.

Sluka KA. Stimulation of deep somatic tissue with capsaicin produces long-lasting mechanical allodynia and heat hypoalgesia that depends on early activation of the cAMP pathway. J Neurosci 2002;22:5687–5693.

Sluka KA, Kalra A, Moore SA. Unilateral intramuscular injections of acidic saline produce a bilateral, long-lasting hyperalgesia. Muscle Nerve 2001;24:37–46.

Sluka KA, Price MP, Breese NM, Stucky CL, Wemmie JA, Welsh MJ. Chronic hyperalgesia induced by repeated acid injections in muscle is abolished by the loss of ASIC3, but not ASIC1. Pain 2003;106:229–239.

Sluka KA, Radhakrishnan R, Benson CJ, Eshcol JO, Price MP, Babinski K, Audette KM, Yeomans DC, Wilson SP. ASIC3 in muscle mediates mechanical, but not heat, hyperalgesia associated with muscle inflammation. Pain 2007;129,102–112.

Stauber WT. Factors involved in strain-induced injury in skeletal muscles and outcomes of prolonged exposures. J Electromyogr Kinesiol 2004;14:61–70.

Svensson P, Beydoun A, Morrow TJ, Casey KL. Human intramuscular and cutaneous pain: psychophysical comparisons. Exp Brain Res 1997;114:390–392.

Tunks E, Crook J, Norman G, Kalaher S. Tender points in fibromyalgia. Pain 1988;34:11–19.

Voilley N, de Weille J, Mamet J, Lazdunski M. Nonsteroid anti-inflammatory drugs inhibit both the activity and the inflammation-induced expression of acid-sensing ion channels in nociceptors. J Neurosci 2001;21:8026–8033.

Waldmann R. Proton-gated cation channels—neuronal acid sensors in the central and peripheral nervous system. Adv Exp Med Biol 2001;502:293–304.

Waldmann R, Lazdunski M. H^+-gated cation channels: neuronal acid sensors in the NaC/DEG family of ion channels. Curr Opin Neurobiol 1998;8:418–424.

Wall PD, Woolf CJ. Muscle but not cutaneous C-afferent input produces prolonged increases in the excitability of the flexion reflex in the rat. J Physiol 1984;356:443–458.

Witting N, Svensson P, Gottrup H, Arendt-Nielsen L, Jensen TS. Intramuscular and intradermal injection of capsaicin: a comparison of local and referred pain. Pain 2000;84:407–412.

Wolfe F, Smythe HA, Yunus MB, et al. The American College of Rheumatology 1990 criteria for the classification of fibromyalgia. Report of the Multicenter Criteria Committee. Arthritis Rheum 1990;33:160–172.

Correspondence to: Prof. Kathleen A. Sluka, PT, PhD, University of Iowa, Physical Therapy and Rehabilitation Science Graduate Program, Pain Research Program, 1-242 MEB, Iowa City, IA 52242, USA. Tel: 1-319-335-9799 (office); fax: 1-319-335-9707; email: kathleen-sluka@uiowa.edu.

Central Mechanisms of Craniofacial Musculoskeletal Pain: A Review

Barry J. Sessle

Faculty of Dentistry and Centre for the Study of Pain,
University of Toronto, Toronto, Ontario, Canada

Most acute and chronic pain conditions in the craniofacial region affect musculoskeletal craniofacial tissues such as the temporomandibular joint (TMJ), masticatory muscles, and teeth. These pain conditions are very common, and chronic pain states affecting these deep tissues are frequently difficult to diagnose and manage, largely because their etiology and pathogenesis are not clear. Moreover, the craniofacial sensory system has many differences from the spinal sensory system (see Table I), and so findings in one system cannot automatically be extrapolated to the other. Thus, this chapter reviews recent advances in understanding of the neural mechanisms underlying deep craniofacial pain, with a special focus on the brainstem processes underlying pain in the TMJ, masticatory muscles, and tooth pulp.

Table I
Trigeminal sensory systems: differences from spinal sensory systems

---

A. *Peripheral Tissues and Innervation*
1. Tissues that are unique to the craniofacial region (e.g., tooth pulp, cornea)
2. Higher innervation density in many craniofacial tissues than in most spinally innervated tissues
3. Shorter conduction distances of peripheral nerve pathways
4. Slower conduction velocities of peripheral nerve fibers
5. Higher ratio of myelinated : unmyelinated fibers
6. Lower proportion of sympathetic efferents
7. Certain craniofacial receptors (e.g., some periodontal mechanoreceptors, jaw muscle spindles) have their primary afferent cell bodies *within* the CNS

B. *Central Nervous System*
1. Face and mouth are represented completely at most rostrocaudal levels of VBSNC, and a dual representation of some tissues occurs in Vc
2. Distinctive brainstem termination patterns of some nociceptive afferents
3. Transitional regions between Vc and Vi, and between Vc and CDH, with distinctive properties (e.g., bilateral afferent inputs to Vc/Vi)
4. "Deep bundle" fiber system is especially prominent in Vc (connects caudal and rostral levels of VBSNC), whereas Lissauer's tract is absent
5. Significant ipsilateral and contralateral projections from VBSNC to the thalamus

C. *Pain Conditions Specific to the Craniofacial Region*
1. Headaches (e.g., migraine, cluster headache)
2. Toothaches (e.g., pulpitis pain)
3. Trigeminal neuralgia
4. Miscellaneous (e.g., atypical facial pain, burning mouth syndrome, atypical odontalgia)

Source: From Sessle (2005a).
Abbreviations: VBSNC = trigeminal brainstem sensory nuclear complex, CDH = upper cervical dorsal horn, Vc = subnucleus caudalis, Vi = subnucleus interpolaris.

Overview of Trigeminal Brainstem and Thalamocortical Mechanisms

Brainstem Nociceptive Processes

The small-diameter primary afferents that innervate the TMJ, masticatory muscles, and tooth pulp have their cell bodies in the trigeminal ganglion and project to the brainstem, where they mainly terminate in the trigeminal brainstem sensory nuclear complex (VBSNC). Here, they release excitatory neurochemicals such as excitatory amino acids (e.g., glutamate) and neuropeptides (e.g., substance P) that are involved in the activation of second-order neurons in the VBSNC (see Dubner et al., 1978; Capra and Dessem, 1992; Sessle, 2000, 2005a). The VBSNC can be subdivided into the principal or main sensory nucleus and the spinal tract nucleus, which comprises three subnuclei: oralis, interpolaris, and caudalis. While some nociceptive afferents may access rostral components of the VBSNC (e.g., subnuclei interpolaris and oralis) and play some role in craniofacial pain (see below), there is considerable evidence that subnucleus caudalis is the principal brainstem relay site of trigeminal nociceptive information from neurons responsive to nociceptive afferent inputs, including those from the TMJ, masticatory muscles and tooth pulp (see Dubner et al., 1978; Capra and Dessem, 1992; Bereiter et al., 2000; Sessle, 2000, 2005a; Woda, 2003).

This evidence is summarized as follows: (i) The subnucleus caudalis is a laminated structure, and it has cell types that morphologically resemble those of the spinal dorsal horn, which is the essential spinal cord region of the spinal nociceptive system. (ii) Nearly all the small-diameter (Aδ and C-fiber) primary afferents carrying nociceptive information from the craniofacial tissues terminate in the subnucleus caudalis, in its laminae I, II, V, and VI, whereas the larger A-fiber primary afferents conducting low-threshold mechanosensitive (e.g., tactile) information terminate mainly in its laminae III–VI (as well as in the more rostral components of the VBSNC). The termination sites of TMJ, muscle, and tooth pulp afferents include in particular the superficial laminae of the caudalis as well as its deeper laminae, i.e., superficial and deep laminar sites where nociceptive neurons responsive to stimulation of craniofacial deep tissues are located. (iii) Immunocytochemical markers of neuronal activity, such as c-Fos protein, are increased in caudalis neurons following noxious stimulation of craniofacial tissues, including the TMJ, muscles, or tooth pulp. (iv) The endings in caudalis of trigeminal primary afferents, as well as inputs emanating from intrinsic central nervous system (CNS) circuits, release excitatory or inhibitory neurotransmitters and neuromodulators that act upon receptors and ion channels in caudalis neurons and regulate trigeminal nociceptive transmission. (v) Transection of the trigeminal spinal tract at the rostral pole of the caudalis in humans relieves the excruciating pain of trigeminal neuralgia and markedly reduces the patient's ability to perceive noxious stimuli (especially those applied to the face). Analogous lesions or pharmacologically induced disruption of the caudalis in experimental animals reduce behavioral, autonomic, and muscle reflex responses to noxious facial stimuli. These findings suggest that the functional integrity of the subnucleus caudalis is necessary for the relay of nociceptive signals from the brainstem terminals of the small-diameter nociceptive primary afferents to second-order neurons in the subnucleus caudalis. Consistent with this view are more recent findings (see below) that the subnucleus caudalis plays an integral role in central sensitization in trigeminal nociceptive pathways. (vi) The output of caudalis neurons includes regions of the brain involved in the processing or modulation of pain. (vii) Electrophysiological recordings in the VBSNC have revealed that many neurons in the subnucleus caudalis can be activated by noxious stimulation of cutaneous or deep tissues. Most neurons in the superficial and deep laminae of the subnucleus caudalis can be activated by cutaneous (or mucosal) noxious stimuli, and have been categorized as either nociceptive-specific (NS) neurons or wide-dynamic-range (WDR) neurons. These neurons typically have a localized mechanoreceptive field (RF), and many have only a cutaneous (or mucosal) RF and respond with a progressively increasing discharge as the intensity of a cutaneous or mucosal noxious stimulus applied to the RF is gradually increased or as more of the neuronal RF is stimulated. Their RF and response properties are consistent with a role for many NS and WDR neurons in the detection, localization, intensity coding, and discrimination of superficial pain (Dubner et al., 1978; Dubner, 1985; Sessle, 2000). Each NS neuron receives small-diameter afferent inputs from $A\delta$ and/or C fibers and responds only to noxious stimuli (e.g., pinch, heat) applied to its RF in the face or mouth. The WDR neuron, in contrast, may receive large-diameter and small-diameter A-fiber inputs as well as C-fiber inputs, and can be excited by non-noxious (e.g., tactile) stimuli as well as by noxious stimuli applied to its craniofacial RF. As noted below, most NS and WDR caudalis neurons also receive musculoskeletal afferent inputs.

Many of these features of the subnucleus caudalis are similar to those of the spinal dorsal horn. Because of its structural and functional similarity with the spinal dorsal horn, the subnucleus caudalis is now often termed the *medullary dorsal horn*. However, there are some important differences that bring into question whether the subnucleus caudalis and spinal dorsal horn have a complete structural and functional homology; for example, the rostral and caudal parts of the subnucleus caudalis have different functions (see below).

Projections from the VBSNC

Many neurons in all components of the VBSNC are relay neurons that project to the thalamus, either directly, or indirectly via polysynaptic pathways that may involve the reticular formation (see Dubner et al., 1978; Sessle and Hu, 1991; Dostrovsky and Craig, 2006; Shigenaga and Yoshida, 2006). Some of the projections involving the reticular formation are components of circuits whereby craniofacial noxious stimuli may influence autonomic functions (e.g., respiration, cardiovascular function, salivation, and lacrimation). In addition, some VBSNC neurons project directly or indirectly to cranial nerve motor nuclei and thus serve as interneurons in muscle reflex circuits. Other neurons may have only intrinsic projections, i.e., their axons do not leave the VBSNC but instead terminate within it. One example is the intrinsic projections from the subnucleus caudalis that influence the activity of nociceptive neurons in the subnucleus oralis. Of particular note are the neurons in the superficial laminae of the subnucleus caudalis that include the substantia gelatinosa (SG). This caudalis zone represents one of the main sites by which peripheral afferents and brain centers modulate somatosensory transmission.

Thalamus and Cortex

The projections from the VBSNC to the thalamus can activate neurons in parts of the thalamus, mainly the lateral thalamus (e.g., the ventrobasal complex), the posterior nuclear group, and the medial thalamus. Both the lateral thalamus and the medial thalamus contain NS and WDR neurons that receive craniofacial nociceptive information relayed through the VBSNC (Sessle and Hu, 1991; Chiang et al., 2005a; Dostrovsky and Craig, 2006). The RF and response properties of the ventrobasal NS and WDR neurons and their connections with the overlying somatosensory cerebral cortex indicate that their role is principally in the sensory-discriminative dimension of pain. Nociceptive neurons also occur in the somatosensory cerebral cortex with properties similar to those of caudalis or ventrobasal NS or WDR neurons, indicating their potential role in pain localization and intensity coding. In contrast, the properties of most NS and WDR neurons in the medial thalamus suggest that their role is mainly in the affective dimension of pain, similar to the nociceptive neurons that occur in cortical regions such as the anterior cingulate cortex. However, no detailed information is available on how nociceptive information from the TMJ and masticatory muscles is processed in the thalamus or cortex. Nonetheless, in the case of the tooth pulp, several studies have shown that many neurons in these thalamic and cortical regions can be activated by tooth pulp stimulation; nearly all of these neurons also have a cutaneous nociceptive RF in the craniofacial region and may be either NS or WDR on the basis of their cutaneous RF properties (e.g., Iwata et al., 1999; Chiang et al., 2005a).

Modulation of Nociceptive Transmission

Modification of somatosensory transmission can occur at the brainstem, thalamus, and cerebral cortex. The intricate organization of each subdivision of the VBSNC and the variety of inputs to each of them from peripheral tissues or from different parts of the CNS provide a particularly important substrate for numerous interactions between the various inputs, and this modulation of VBSNC activity can then be reflected in changes in neuronal properties at the higher CNS levels (see Dubner et al., 1978; Sessle and Hu, 1991; Sessle, 2000, 2005a; Woda, 2003; see also Maixner, this volume). For example, the responses of caudalis nociceptive neurons to noxious stimulation of musculoskeletal tissues can be suppressed by influences derived from structures within the VBSNC itself (e.g., the SG of the subnucleus caudalis), as well as from other parts of the brainstem and higher centers (e.g., the periaqueductal gray and somatosensory cortex). These modulatory influences act by releasing one or more endogenous neurochemicals such as opioids, serotonin (5-HT), or gamma-aminobutyric acid (GABA), and through such inhibitory actions they may contribute to the analgesic efficacy of a number of therapeutic procedures such as narcotic analgesics and acupuncture. Some modulatory influences on nociceptive transmission in the VBSNC may instead have facilitatory effects, and thus contribute to processes such as central sensitization in the VBSNC and at higher CNS levels.

Special Features of Brainstem Processing and Modulation of Deep Craniofacial Nociceptive Inputs

Convergence of Afferent Inputs

As noted earlier, many NS and WDR caudalis neurons have spatiotemporal properties indicative of an important role in superficial pain. While the vast majority of caudalis NS and WDR neurons have a superficial RF, many also have a deep tissue RF (e.g., in TMJ or muscle). Indeed, most can be excited by one or more other afferent inputs as well as by cutaneous or mucosal afferent inputs. For example, in the cat and rat, electrical or noxious mechanical stimuli that activate small-diameter primary afferents supplying jaw or tongue muscles, TMJ, or tooth pulp may activate 60% or more of the NS and WDR caudalis neurons having a cutaneous RF (see Sessle and Hu, 1991; Sessle, 2000; Hu et al., 2005; Morch et al., 2007). Moreover, algesic chemicals (e.g., mustard oil, capsaicin, or glutamate) can also activate a substantial proportion of NS and WDR neurons

A

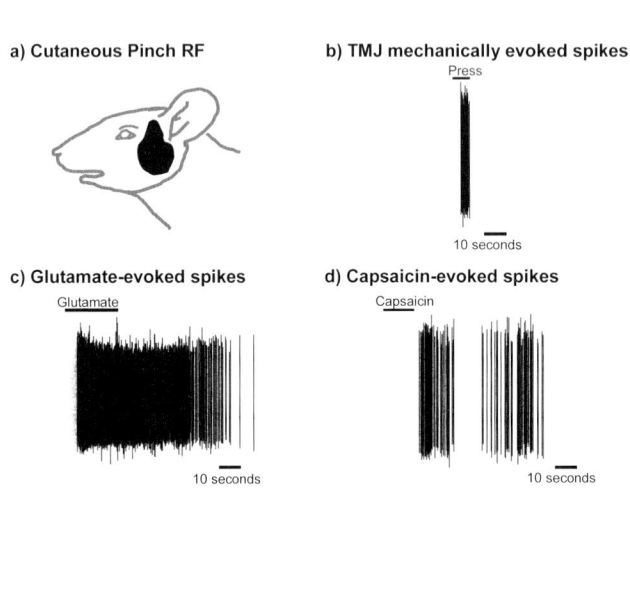

B

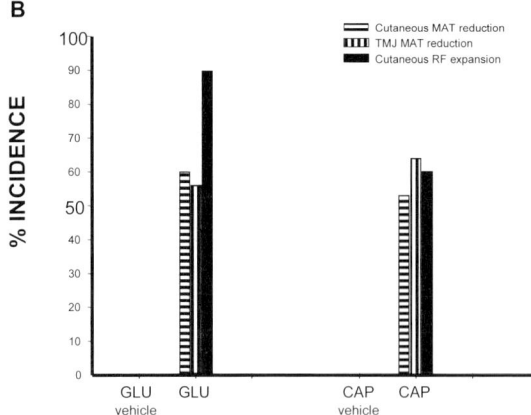

Fig. 1. Panel A shows an example of a TMJ responsive nociceptive specific (NS) neuron recorded in the junctional region of caudalis and Cl. Panels a and b show the neuron's cutaneous mechanoreceptive field (RF) and its response to mechanical probing of the TMJ, and panels c and d show its responses to injection of glutamate or capsaicin into the TMJ. Panel B shows that in TMJ-responsive nociceptive neurons ($n = 49$), injection of glutamate (GLU) or capsaicin (CAP) into the TMJ significantly increased the incidence of cutaneous mechanical activation threshold (MAT) reduction, TMJ MAT reduction, and cutaneous RF expansion compared with control injections of vehicle for GLU or CAP ($P < 0.05$, Fisher exact test). (From D. Lam, J. Hu, and B. Sessle, unpublished data.)

with a cutaneous RF when the chemical is applied to the TMJ, masticatory muscle, or tooth pulp (Sessle and Hu, 1991; Sessle, 2000; Okamoto et al., 2003; see also Chapter 3 by Ro, this volume). An example is shown in Fig. 1. In contrast, very few neurons that respond only to low-threshold (e.g., tactile) afferent inputs receive these convergent excitatory inputs from deep as well as superficial tissues. In addition, very few caudalis NS and WDR neurons are activated exclusively by deep noxious stimuli. Rather, the vast majority of the caudalis neurons transmitting deep nociceptive information receive additional inputs from afferents supplying other tissues, including skin, suggesting that many of these neurons are the brainstem neural elements crucial for the appreciation of deep pain in the craniofacial region. Furthermore, their features of extensive afferent convergence and susceptibility to central sensitization induced by deep nociceptive afferent inputs appear also to be integral mechanisms underlying pain spread and referral, which are common in craniofacial musculoskeletal pain conditions. Sex differences in caudalis nociceptive neuronal responses to deep noxious stimuli (e.g., Okamoto et al., 2003), along with the sex differences in responsivity of TMJ and jaw muscle primary afferents to some noxious or pain-modulatory chemicals (see Chapter 14 by Cairns and Dong), may be factors contributing to sex differences in many clinical chronic musculoskeletal pain conditions such as temporomandibular disorders.

Regional Differences

There is evidence that different parts of the subnucleus caudalis may have different functional roles. The rostral and caudal portions of the caudalis have some different neuronal RF and response properties, including differences in their receipt of bilateral versus ipsilateral deep craniofacial afferent inputs, and they appear to be differentially involved in the autonomic, endocrine, and muscle reflex responses to noxious stimulation of deep craniofacial tissues (Ren and Dubner, 1999; Bereiter et al., 2000; Dubner and Ren, 2004). Furthermore, more rostral components of the VBSNC (e.g., subnuclei interpolaris and oralis) also contribute to trigeminal nociceptive processes, especially those related to intraoral pain (e.g., in the tooth pulp) and perioral pain (for review, see Sessle, 2000, 2005a; Woda, 2003).

Neurochemical Processes

As in the spinal dorsal horn, several neurochemicals including excitatory amino acids (e.g., glutamate and aspartate), adenosine triphosphate (ATP), and neuropeptides (e.g., substance P, calcitonin gene-related peptide [CGRP], and neurokinin A) are released from the central endings of trigeminal nociceptive primary afferents in the VBSNC, where they normally act via receptors and ion channels in second-order neurons to exert excitatory effects on the neurons. In the case of nociceptive transmission related to craniofacial musculoskeletal tissues, most of the limited attention has focused on glutamatergic transmission involving glutamate receptor subtypes AMPA (α-amino-3-hydroxy-5-methyl-4-isoxazole propionate) and NMDA (N-methyl-D-aspartate) in the subnucleus caudalis. For example, glutamate-evoked deep inputs can excite caudalis nociceptive neurons; glutamate is released in the subnucleus caudalis by TMJ noxious stimulation; and application to the subnucleus caudalis of AMPA-receptor antagonists (such as CNQX) and NMDA-receptor antagonists (such as MK-801 and APV) can attenuate nociceptive transmission in the subnucleus caudalis from TMJ, masticatory muscle, or tooth pulp afferents (e.g., Cairns et al., 1998; Chiang et al., 1998; Ro et al., 2004; see also Sessle, 2000; Woda, 2003; Chapter 3 by Ro). There is also evidence suggesting that substance P acting through neurokinin receptors and ATP acting via purinergic (P2X) receptors may facilitate caudalis nociceptive transmission from these deep afferents.

Inhibitory neurochemical processes also modulate caudalis nociceptive transmission, as in the spinal dorsal horn, and there is evidence for such inhibitory influences on caudalis nociceptive neurons transmitting deep craniofacial information (e.g., Sessle et al., 1981; Chiang et al., 1995; see Chapter 17 by Maixner). Some of the descending pathways influence nociceptive transmission by the release from their endings of certain of the chemicals mentioned above (e.g., 5-HT), whereas other pathways may cause the release of chemicals such as the enkephalins and

GABA from the endings of interneurons intrinsic to the VBSNC (e.g., in the SG of the subnucleus caudalis) that act respectively on opioid or GABA receptors within the subnucleus caudalis. Nociceptive transmission in the subnucleus caudalis from craniofacial musculoskeletal tissues can also be modulated by so-called segmental or afferent influences initiated by stimulation of peripheral afferents and involving the interneuronal circuitry existing within the subnucleus caudalis.

Central Sensitization

As noted above, some of the descending influences on nociceptive transmission can produce facilitatory influences, thereby contributing to the augmentation of pain that can occur in certain situations, e.g., anxiety and some forms of stress. Peripheral afferent inputs into the CNS operating through segmental mechanisms or through activation of descending influences may also facilitate nociceptive transmission under some conditions; this process involves the extensive convergence of afferent inputs onto nociceptive neurons. For example, inflammation or injury of craniofacial musculoskeletal tissues or nerve fibers may produce a barrage of nociceptive primary afferent inputs into the CNS, which in turn releases neurochemicals from the afferent endings onto NS and WDR neurons, leading to a cascade of intracellular events in the neurons manifesting as increased neuronal excitability. The prolonged augmentation of nociceptive neuronal properties in the subnucleus caudalis (and spinal dorsal horn) has been termed "central sensitization." Inputs from deep tissues (e.g., TMJ, muscle, and tooth pulp) are especially effective in inducing central sensitization in caudalis nociceptive neurons (see Ren and Dubner, 1999; Sessle, 2000, 2005a,b; Dubner and Ren, 2004; Salter, 2004; Woolf and Salter, 2006; see also Chapter 3 by Ro). Caudalis central sensitization has been documented in both acute and chronic models of inflammatory musculoskeletal craniofacial pain. This central sensitization reflects neuroplastic changes that can be manifested as an increase in spontaneous activity, expansion of the neuronal cutaneous and/or deep RF, lowering of activation threshold, and augmentation of the responses of both NS and WDR caudalis neurons to craniofacial stimuli (e.g., Figs. 1 and 2).

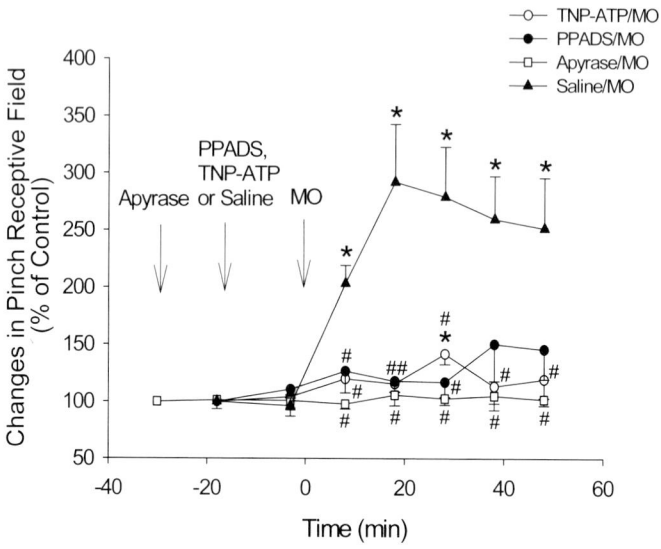

Fig. 2. Changes in neuronal pinch/pressure receptive field (RF) induced by mustard oil (MO) application to the tooth pulp after continuous i.t. superfusion of P2X antagonists (TNP-ATP, PPADS), apyrase, or isotonic saline. Note that after saline superfusion, MO application to the pulp (at 0 minutes) produced significant increases in pinch/pressure RF size throughout the 50-minute observation period ($P < 0.001$, repeated-measures analysis of variance [RM ANOVA]; * $P < 0.05$, Dunnett's test), whereas after TNP-ATP (5 µg/mL), PPADS (33 µg/mL) or apyrase (30 U/mL) superfusion, MO application no longer produced increases in pinch RF size. There were significant differences between the three drug groups and the saline/MO group (all $P < 0.001$, two-way RM ANOVA) in the values at most post-MO test time points (# $P < 0.05$, Bonferroni t-test). Each group consisted of six NS neurons located in deep laminae of Vc, and each value reflects mean ± SE. Arrows indicate the application time of drugs or saline. (From Chiang et al., 2005b.)

It is thought that these central nociceptive neuronal changes contribute, respectively, to the spontaneous pain, spread or referral of pain, allodynia, and hyperalgesia that characterize many pain states arising from peripheral tissue injury or inflammation. In addition, the occurrence of central sensitization indicates that the central nociceptive mechanisms and circuits are not "hard-wired" but rather are plastic. Moreover, central sensitization is usually reversible after a transient, uncomplicated trauma or inflammation, but depending on the type of injury or inflammation and other factors, it can be associated with pain behavior that can last for hours, days, or even weeks.

Several neuropeptides (e.g., substance P and CGRP) and excitatory amino acids (e.g., glutamate) appear to be crucial for the production of central sensitization. For example, centrally acting NMDA-receptor antagonists are particularly effective in preventing the caudalis central sensitization and accompanying increased jaw muscle activity and other nociceptive behaviors induced by afferent inputs from TMJ, masticatory muscle, or tooth pulp (e.g., Cairns et al., 1998; Chiang et al., 1998; Ro et al., 2004; see also Chapter 3 by Ro). The importance of the subnucleus caudalis in trigeminal central sensitization is evidenced by recent findings that central sensitization induced in other components of the trigeminal somatosensory system (e.g., ventrobasal thalamus or subnucleus oralis) and the associated prolonged increase in jaw muscle activity can be abolished by disruption of caudalis activity (Cairns et al., 1998; Hu et al., 2002; Woda, 2003; Park et al., 2006; Zhang et al., 2006).

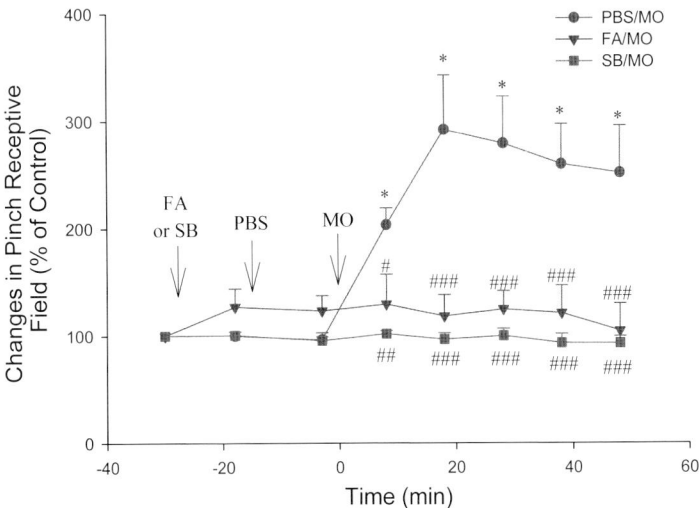

Fig. 3. Changes in neuronal pinch/pressure receptive field (RF) induced by mustard oil (MO) application to the tooth pulp after i.t. application of phosphate-buffered saline (PBS, as control) or glial cell inhibitors fluoroacetate (FA, an inhibitor of the astroglial metabolic enzyme aconitase) and SB203580 (SB, an inhibitor of p38 MAP kinase). Mean (± SE) values are shown for each group at the different time points. *$P < 0.05$ compared to the baseline within the group (RM ANOVA on Ranks followed by Dunnett's test); # $P < 0.05$, ## $P < 0.01$, ### $P < 0.001$ compared to the PBS/MO group at different time points tested (two-way ANOVA followed by Tukey t-test). Arrows indicate the application time of drugs or PBS. (From Xie et al., 2007.)

Several other neurochemicals that are released from central neurons (e.g., in SG of the subnucleus caudalis) may modulate these central effects; these include 5-HT, opioids, and GABA. Indeed, there are complex receptor and intracellular mechanisms underlying the induction and maintenance of central sensitization (Salter, 2004; Woolf and Salter, 2006). For example, the release of glutamate may be influenced by the action of ATP on purinergic receptors on the central endings of deep nociceptive afferents within the subnucleus caudalis, given that trigeminal central sensitization can be induced by ATP agonists and attenuated by ATP antagonists acting through P2X receptors in the caudalis (Chiang et al., 2005b; Jennings et al., 2006) (e.g., Fig. 2). The source of the ATP is unclear but may include non-neural cells in the caudalis.

Evidence is emerging of an important role of glial cells (astrocytes and microglia) in chronic pain states (see Tsuda et al., 2005; Watkins and Maier, 2005). Recent studies in craniofacial pain models are consistent with this role, given that the application of glial inhibitors to the subnucleus caudalis can block the induction of caudalis central sensitization (e.g., Fig. 3) and prevent nociceptive behavior in inflammatory craniofacial pain models (Piao et al., 2006; Chiang et al., 2007; Guo et al., 2007; Xie et al., 2007). In the case of craniofacial musculoskeletal pain, Xie et al. (2007) and Chiang et al. (2007) have recently provided the first documentation in either the spinal or trigeminal nociceptive system that central sensitization (induced in this case by inflammatory irritant application to the rat molar pulp) in functionally identified dorsal horn nociceptive neurons can be effectively abolished by application to the caudal brainstem of inhibitors that suppress astrocytic metabolic processes or release of modulatory substances from astrocytes. Interestingly, these investigators found that the normal nociceptive responses in the neurons were unaffected, supporting the spinal literature that glia play an important role in exaggerated pain states but not in normal pain processing. Furthermore, Guo et al. (2007) have shown in their rat model of chronic masseter muscle inflammatory hyperalgesia that the nociceptive afferent input to the CNS leads to the induction of cytokines and other chemical mediators in caudalis glia that enhance central sensitization and cause increased craniofacial pain. These neurochemical processes as well as non-neural cells may be important targets for the development of new therapeutic approaches to manage musculoskeletal pain.

Conclusions

This chapter has provided a brief overview of the neural pathways and mechanisms involved in craniofacial musculoskeletal pain, with a particular focus on processes in the VBSNC. The subnucleus caudalis is the integral brainstem relay of craniofacial nociceptive signals, and the majority of its nociceptive neurons receive convergent afferent inputs from deep tissues as well as other craniofacial tissues. Of particular note is evidence from acute and chronic craniofacial musculoskeletal pain models that these inputs can induce caudalis neuroplastic changes that reflect a central sensitization that most likely contributes to the clinical features of TMJ pain, masticatory muscle pain, and dental pain. Further definition of these sensitization phenomena, including their underlying neurochemical basis and the role that non-neural cells in the CNS may play, holds the promise of new or more effective therapeutic approaches to manage craniofacial musculoskeletal pain.

Acknowledgments

The secretarial assistance of Fong Yuen and Dorothy Tsang is gratefully acknowledged. The cited studies of the author were supported by Canadian MRC Grant MT-4918 and NIH Grants DE04786 and DE015420.

References

Bereiter DA, Hiraba H, Hu JW. Trigeminal subnucleus caudalis: beyond homologies with the spinal dorsal horn. Pain 2000;88:221–224.

Cairns BE, Sessle BJ, Hu JW. Evidence that excitatory amino acid receptors within the temporomandibular joint region are involved in the reflex activation of the jaw muscles. J Neurosci 1998;18:8056–8064.

Capra NF, Dessem D. Central connections of trigeminal primary afferent neurons: topographical and functional considerations. Crit Rev Oral Biol Med 1992;4:1–52.

Chiang CY, Sessle BJ, Hu JW. Parabrachial area and nucleus raphe magnus-induced modulation of electrically evoked trigeminal subnucleus caudalis neuronal responses to cutaneous or deep A-fiber and C-fiber inputs in rats. Pain 1995;62:61–68.

Chiang C.Y, Park SJ, Kwan CL, Hu JW, Sessle BJ. NMDA receptor mechanisms contribute to neuroplasticity induced in caudalis nociceptive neurons by tooth pulp stimulation. J Neurophysiol 1998;80:2621–2631.

Chiang CY, Wang J, Xie YF, Zhang S, Hu JW, Dostrovsky JO, Sessle BJ. Astroglial glutamate-glutamine shuttle is involved in central sensitization of nociceptive neurons in rat medullary dorsal horn. J Neurosci 2007;27:9068–9076.

Chiang CY, Zhang S, Park SJ, Hu JW, Dostrovsky JO, Sessle BJ. Mechanoreceptive field and response properties of nociceptive neurons in ventral posteromedial thalamic nucleus of the rat. In: Willis WD, Jones EG, editors. Thalamus and related systems. Cambridge: Cambridge University Press; 2005a. p 41–51.

Chiang CY, Zhang S, Xie YF, Hu JW, Dostrovsky JO, Salter MW, Sessle BJ. Endogenous ATP involvement in mustard oil-induced central sensitization in trigeminal subnucleus caudalis (medullary dorsal horn). J Neurophysiol 2005b;94:1751–1760.

Dostrovsky JO, Craig AD. Ascending projection systems. In: McMahon SB, Koltzenburg M, editors. Wall and Melzack's textbook of pain. London: Churchill Livingstone; 2006. p 187–203.

Dubner R. Recent advances in our understanding of pain. In: Klineberg I, Sessle BJ, editors. Orofacial pain and neuromuscular dysfunction: mechanisms and clinical correlates. Oxford: Pergamon; 1985. p 3–19.

Dubner R, Ren K. Brainstem mechanisms of persistent pain following injury. J Orofac Pain 2004;18:299–305.

Dubner, R, Sessle BJ, Storey AT. The neural basis of oral and facial function. New York: Plenum; 1978.

Guo W, Wang H, Watanabe M, Shimizu K, Zou S, LaGraize SC, Wei F, Dubner R, Ren K. Glial-cytokine-neuronal interactions underlying the mechanisms of persistent pain. J Neurosci 2007;27:6006–6018.

Hu B, Chiang CY, Hu JW, Dostrovsky JO, Sessle BJ. P2X receptors in trigeminal subnucleus caudalis modulate central sensitization in trigeminal subnucleus oralis. J Neurophysiol 2002;88:1614–1624.

Hu JW, Sun KQ, Vernon H, Sessle BJ. Craniofacial inputs to upper cervical dorsal horn: implications for somatosensory information processing. Brain Res 2005;1044:93–106.

Iwata K, Yoshiyuki T, Akimasa T, Sakamoto M, Sumino R. Integration of tooth-pulp pain at the level of cerebral cortex. In: Nakamura Y, Sessle BJ, editors. Neurobiology of mastication: from molecular to systems approach. Amsterdam: Elsevier; 1999. p 471–481.

Jennings EA, Christie MJ, Sessle BJ. ATP potentiates neurotransmission in the rat trigeminal subnucleus caudalis. Neuroreport 2006;17:1507–1510.

Morch CD, Hu JW, Arendt-Nielsen L, Sessle BJ. Convergence of cutaneous, musculoskeletal, dural and visceral afferents onto nociceptive neurons in the first cervical dorsal horn. Eur J Neurosci 2007;26:142–154.

Okamoto K, Hirata H, Takeshita S, Bereiter DA. Response properties of TMJ neurons in superficial laminae at the spinomedullary junction of female rats vary over the estrous cycle. J Neurophysiol 2003;89:1467–1477.

Park SJ, Zhang S, Chiang CY, Hu JW, Dostrovsky JO, Sessle BJ. Central sensitization induced in thalamic nociceptive neurons by tooth pulp stimulation is dependent on the functional integrity of trigeminal brainstem subnucleus caudalis but not subnucleus oralis. Brain Res 2006;1112:134–145.

Piao ZG, Cho IH, Park CK, Hong JP, Choi SY, Lee SJ, Lee S, Park K, Kim JS, Oh SB. Activation of glia and microglia p38MAPK in medullary dorsal horn contributes to tactile hypersensitivity following trigeminal sensory nerve injury. Pain 2006;121:219–231.

Ren K, Dubner R. Central nervous system plasticity and persistent pain. J Orofac Pain 1999;13:155–163.

Ro JY, Capra NF, Masri R. Contribution of peripheral N-methyl-D-aspartate receptors to c-fos expression in the trigeminal spinal nucleus following acute masseteric inflammation. Neuroscience 2004;123:213–219.

Salter MW. Cellular neuroplasticity mechanisms mediating pain persistence. J Orofac Pain 2004;18:218–324.

Sessle BJ. Acute and chronic craniofacial pain: brainstem mechanisms of nociceptive transmission and neuroplasticity, and their clinical correlates. Crit Rev Oral Biol Med 2000;11:57–91.

Sessle BJ. Orofacial pain. In: Merskey H, Loeser D, Dubner R (Eds). The paths of pain 1975–2005. Seattle: IASP Press, 2005a, pp 131–150.

Sessle BJ. Trigeminal central sensitization. Rev Analg 2005b;8:85–102.

Sessle BJ, Hu JW. Mechanisms of pain arising from articular tissues. Can J Physiol Pharmacol 1991;69:617–626.

Sessle BJ, Hu JW, Dubner R, Lucier GE. Functional properties of neurons in trigeminal subnucleus caudalis of the cat. II. Modulation of responses to noxious and non-noxious stimuli by periaqueductal gray, nucleus raphe magnus, cerebral cortex and afferent influences, and effect of naloxone. J Neurophysiol 1981;45:193–207.

Shigenaga Y, Yoshida A. Trigeminal brainstem nuclear complex, anatomy. In: Schmidt RF, Willis WD, editors. Encyclopedia of pain. Berlin: Springer; 2006. p 2536–2541.

Tsuda M, Inoue K, Salter MW. Neuropathic pain and spinal microglia: a big problem from molecules in "small" glia. Trends Neurosci 2005;28:101–107.

Watkins LR, Maier SF. Glia and pain: past, present, and future. In: Merskey H, Loeser D, Dubner R, editors. The paths of pain 1975–2005. Seattle: IASP Press; 2005. p 165–175.

Woda A. Pain in the trigeminal system: from orofacial nociception to neural network modeling. J Dent Res 2003;82:764–768.

Woolf C, Salter MW. Plasticity and pain: role of the dorsal horn. In: McMahon SB, Koltzenburg M (Eds). Wall and Melzack's textbook of pain. London: Churchill Livingstone, 2006, pp 91–106.

Xie YF, Zhang S, Chiang CY, Hu JW, Dostrovsky JO, Sessle BJ. Involvement of glia in central sensitization in trigeminal subnucleus caudalis (medullary dorsal horn). Brain Behav Immun 2007;21:634–641.

Zhang S, Chiang CY, Xie YF, Lu Y, Hu JW, Dostrovsky JO, Sessle BJ. Central sensitization in thalamic nociceptive neurons induced by mustard oil application to rat molar tooth pulp. Neuroscience 2006;142:833–842.

Correspondence to: Barry J. Sessle, MDS, PhD, DSc (hc), FRSC, Faculty of Dentistry and Centre for the Study of Pain, University of Toronto, 124 Edward Street, Toronto, ON, Canada M5G 1G6. Tel: 1-416-979-4921; fax: 1-416-979-4936; email: barry.sessle@dentistry.utoronto.ca.

New Perspectives on Descending Pain-Modulating Systems in Musculoskeletal Pain

Wahida Rahman and Anthony H. Dickenson

Department of Pharmacology, University College London, London, United Kingdom

Pain is a series of neuronal processes that involve the peripheral nerves, spinal cord, and brain. In 1965, the gate control theory of pain proposed that in addition to spinal mechanisms, descending controls from the brain could modulate pain transmission. Thus, both "bottom-up" and "top-down" processes interact to generate the final perception of the stimulus.

Musculoskeletal pains, such as pain arising from traumas such as whiplash injury and from musculoskeletal disorders such as fibromyalgia and osteoarthritis, are often chronic and widespread (see references in Bergman 2007). The ability of the nervous system, at many levels, to change in response to dysfunction evoked by injury or disease is considerable and leads to changes that can be observed throughout the pathways involved in the perception of pain. This plasticity can lead to an unreliable relationship between the impact of the original insult, the magnitude of transmission of peripheral stimuli, and the perception of pain. For instance, despite an apparent lack of tissue damage in fibromyalgia patients, abnormal sensitivity to digital pressure (hyperalgesia) and widespread allodynia (hypersensitive behavioral responses to normally innocuous stimuli) suggest the abnormal central processing of otherwise normal peripheral sensory stimuli (Brady and Schneider, 2001). In contrast, a number of causes for pathological joint changes have been put forward as driving the pain seen in osteoarthritis, yet despite this disparity in the originating factors, similar changes in the central nervous system are likely to be driving the pain in both fibromyalgia and osteoarthritis. Evidence to date points toward a key role for mechanisms of central sensitization in these pain states, including increasing evidence supporting abnormal temporal summation and central sensitization in fibromyalgia patients (Morris et al., 1998; Staud et al., 2001, 2003b; Price et al., 2002).

Novel and developing pharmacological, anatomical, molecular, and genomic techniques have allowed researchers to describe a myriad of cellular and molecular mechanisms that contribute to the initiation and maintenance of central hyperexcitability. Thus, in addition to peripheral and central spinal mechanisms, it is well documented that descending pain modulation from midbrain brainstem areas such as the periaqueductal gray (PAG) and rostral ventromedial medulla (RVM) onto the spinal cord plays a major role in the modulation of nociception in ascending pathways (Urban and Gebhart, 1999; Millan, 2002).

The role of descending inhibitory control of pain and the actions of the neurotransmitters norepinephrine and serotonin in mediating this inhibitory modulatory influence are most extensively described, although a number of other neurotransmitters are implicated (Millan, 2002). Earlier animal studies reported an increase in spinal neuronal activity and an increase in pain behaviors in animals following interruption of descending pathways arising from the brainstem. A recent study investigating the analgesic mechanism of Neurotropin in rats with adjuvant-induced arthritis suggests that enhanced activation of descending monoaminergic pathways reduces arthritic hyperalgesia (Miura et al., 2005). Furthermore, there is evidence showing stronger tonic descending inhibition of neurons that mediate deep tissue pain as compared to inhibitory control of cutaneous pain (Yu et al., 1991). Agents that increase levels of norepinephrine and serotonin, such as antidepressants, have proven useful therapy in patients with fibromyalgia, although the evidence supporting the use of antidepressants in other musculoskeletal pains is not convincing (Curatolo and Bogduk, 2001).

Some reports suggest impaired diffuse noxious inhibitory control (DNIC) in patients with osteoarthritis (Kosek and Ordeberg, 2000), fibromyalgia (Kosek et al., 1996, Kosek and Hansson, 1997; Lautenbacher and Rollman, 1997) and in patients with temporomandibular disorder (Maixner et al., 1995; Kashima et al., 1999). However others have reported normal inhibitory controls in fibromyalgia patients (Staud et al., 2003a, 2004). Nonetheless, reduced function within descending inhibitory pathways is still a possible mechanism underlying the pathology of pain associated with musculoskeletal disorders.

Reduced activity within descending inhibitory pathways is only one mechanism by which nociceptive inputs can be increased. More recently, attention has turned toward the contribution of descending facilitation arising from within the midbrain and brainstem that can further enhance the spinal mechanisms of pain, independent of, but in concert with, direct peripheral and spinal events, which may have a role in the development and maintenance of persistent pain states (Calejesan et al., 1998; Urban and Gebhart, 1999; Burgess et al., 2002; Porreca et al., 2002).

This chapter outlines recent findings regarding the role of descending pain modulatory pathways on mechanisms of spinal hyperexcitability, focusing in particular on a spinobulbospinal loop that engages a descending facilitatory drive back onto spinal neurons to amplify nociceptive transmission in ascending pathways. Activity within this pathway in nonpathological conditions is important for regulating the baseline level of spinal neuronal activity. Moreover, plasticity within the spinobulbospinal loop plays a role in determining the level of nociceptive transmission in other models of chronic pain such as neuropathy and cancer-induced bone pain. This pathway accesses areas of the brain involved in the integration and regulation of the affective component of the pain response. Given that patients with chronic pain often experience a number of comorbid conditions including anxiety, depression, fear, fatigue, and sleep disturbance, plasticity within this pathway could be important in the development and maintenance of chronic musculoskeletal pain. Disorders such as fibromyalgia might even be a consequence of abnormal neuronal processes in these affective parts of the brain that not only produce the mood and sleep problems but also inappropriately activate descending facilitations that amplify otherwise normal inputs into the spinal cord. Importantly, monoamine systems have been implicated in sleep and mood disorders, anxiety, and sensory abnormalities (Millan, 2002, 2003).

Descending Facilitation and Spinal Neuronal Hyperexcitability

The RVM is a critical center for effecting descending modulation of spinal transmission of pain. The neurons within this area are classified into three types based on their firing patterns in response to noxious thermal stimuli. ON-cells increase their firing immediately before a nocifensive response and are thought to facilitate nociception, whereas OFF-cells, considered to mediate inhibition, pause in their firing just prior to a nociceptive withdrawal reflex. Neutral cells do not appear to play a role in physiological pain, although a role in neuropathic pain has been reported (Fields et al., 1983; Fields and Heinricher, 1985; Pertovaara et al., 2001). The differential activation of these neurons may form the basis of the bidirectional output from this brainstem area, and a shift toward a more dominant role for descending facilitation could increase nociception. In a model of nerve injury, inactivation of the RVM with lidocaine attenuated tactile and thermal hyperalgesia (Porreca et al., 2001; Burgess et al., 2002) and significantly reduced noxious evoked neuronal responses (Bee and Dickenson, 2007). These findings suggest an inappropriate activation of descending facilitatory influences mediating some of the neuropathy-induced plasticity observed at the spinal level. In addition, administration of a cholecystokinin B (CCKB) antagonist into the RVM reversed neuropathic pain behaviors, suggesting that tonic activity of CCK may have a role in modulating abnormal pain (Kovelowski et al., 2000) in addition to its potential role in anxiety.

Recent evidence suggests that one such descending excitatory pathway requires serotonin (5-HT), released into the spinal cord from pathways that originate in the RVM, to exert powerful excitatory effects via activation of spinal 5-HT$_3$ receptors (Suzuki et al., 2002). Pharmacological and genetic knockout studies have revealed a pronociceptive role for these receptors, which are predominantly localized in the superficial dorsal horn, where they are expressed on the nerve terminals of small-diameter afferents (Ali et al., 1996; Green et al., 2000; Zeitz et al., 2002; Maxwell et al., 2003; Conte et al., 2005). We will return to this receptor later in the chapter.

Superficial NK1-Expressing Lamina I Neurons are at the Origin of a Descending Excitatory Pathway

Lamina I neurons that express the neurokinin-1 (NK1) receptor for substance P are predominantly (approximately 80%) projection neurons (Todd et al., 2000). A primary target is the parabrachial (PB) area, which receives a dense afferent projection from these cells and comprises a major link between the spinal cord and the brainstem through pathways that arrive at the RVM. Anatomical and pharmacological data implicate a role for PB neurons in the integration of sensory nociceptive processing with autonomic and homeostatic regulation to generate affective-emotional responses (e.g., fear or memory of aggression), motivational-behavioral responses (e.g., flight or freezing), and autonomic neuroendocrine reactions (Bernard et al., 1996). The two main forebrain targets of PB neurons are the nucleus centralis of the amygdala and the ventrolateral medial hypothalamus. Less dense, but still significant, projections are seen from the PB to the midbrain and brainstem ventromedial periaqueductal gray (PAG) and the ventrolateral medulla (RVM) (Gauriau and Bernard, 2002; Todd, 2002). These latter areas modulate descending monoaminergic pathways from the brainstem, which in turn project back to the spinal cord, forming complex loops, such as the facilitatory RVM projection onto spinal 5-HT$_3$ receptors, that allow the brain to further regulate spinal activity. A recent neuroimaging study demonstrated that arthritic pain was associated with increased activity in the cingulate cortex, the thalamus, and the amygdala; these areas are involved in the processing of fear, in emotional responses, and in aversive conditioning (Kulkarni et al., 2007).

NK1 receptor-expressing lamina I neurons play an important role in the central sensitization, allodynia, and hyperalgesia that underlie abnormal pain states (Hunt and Mantyh, 2001). In rat models, selective ablation of superficial NK1-receptor-expressing neurons is achieved via intrathecal injection of the neurotoxin saporin conjugated to SP (SP-SAP) (Mantyh et al., 1997). This treatment markedly attenuates pain behavior after intraplantar capsaicin injection, in various models of inflammatory pain induced by carrageenan, formalin, or complete Freund's adjuvant (Mantyh et al., 1997), and in models of neuropathic pain induced by nerve damage and spinal cord injury (Nichols et al., 1999; Oatway et al., 2004; Suzuki et al., 2005). The behavioral consequences of SP-SAP treatment fits well with observed alterations in the neuronal response characteristics of neurons of laminae V–VI of the dorsal horn in these animals. Changes include clear and marked reduction in receptive field size, in the second phase of the formalin response, and in wind-up and long term potentiation (LTP)—all indicative of reduced central sensitization. Deficits in mechanical and thermal evoked responses are also seen (Suzuki et al., 2002, 2005; Rygh et al., 2006).

Given that these superficial (laminae I/III) NK1 receptor-bearing neurons form part of an important ascending pathway to the brainstem (Todd et al., 2000), loss of the ascending lamina I–PB pathway was proposed to underlie these reduced pain responses, seen both behaviorally and in deep spinal neurons. Importantly, most of the effects of ablating these lamina I/III neurons were reproduced by blocking spinal $5HT_3$ receptors in unlesioned animals, further providing pharmacological evidence for a serotonergic descending facilitatory influence from the brainstem. Interestingly, wind-up is unaffected by ondansetron, although it was highly sensitive to SP-SAP treatment. Thus, wind-up is an intrinsic spinal phenomenon relying on lamina I/III-lamina V circuitry but not on descending excitations. Furthermore, spinal LTP—another measure of central sensitization—is also dependent on these NK1 receptor expressing lamina I/III neurons, but its full expression depends only minimally on descending facilitation via spinal $5\text{-}HT_3$ receptors.

Taken together, these results provide evidence that NK1-receptor-expressing lamina I/III projection neurons, which project to the PB and to other areas implicated in emotional responses, are at the origin of a spinobulbospinal loop that engages the RVM to control spinal excitability pain sensitivity through the activation of a descending serotonergic pathway (Fig. 1). In parallel with descending drives, indicators of central sensitization, such as wind-up, temporal summation, and LTP, are intrinsic spinal events, but the two systems will interact to produce the final onward transmission of pain messages.

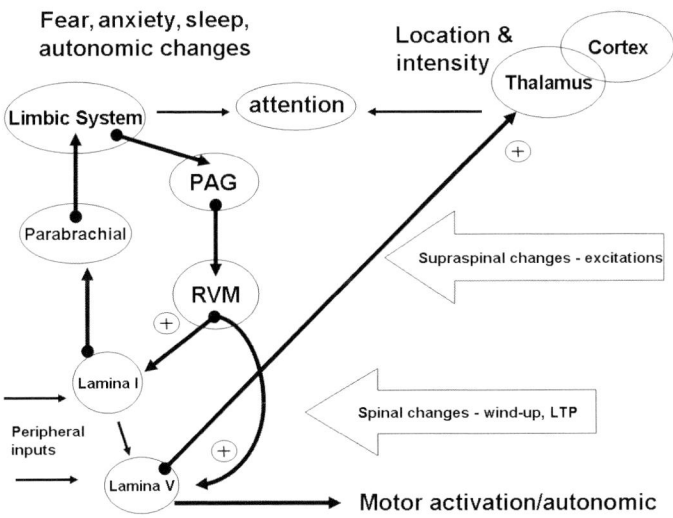

Fig. 1. A diagram showing the projections of lamina I neurokinin-1 (NK1)-expressing neurons that relay to limbic regions and the lamina V pathways to the thalamus and cortex that generate the affective and sensory components of pain. Wind-up and long-term potentiation (LTP), intrinsic spinal mechanisms, can potentiate the output of lamina V neurons, as can activation of lamina I NK1-expressing neurons. These cells are at the origin of the spinobulbospinal loop. Loss of these lamina I neurons disrupts descending projections to the spinal cord, affecting in particular a 5-HT$_3$-receptor-mediated excitatory pathway. Thus, activation of lamina I NK1-expressing neurons and subsequent engagement of the spinobulbospinal loop, culminating with 5-HT acting at spinal 5-HT$_3$ receptors, can further enhance ascending activity from the dorsal horn. Areas of the brainstem and limbic regions, which are accessed by lamina I NK1-expressing cells, are involved in anxiety, fear, and depression. Thus, this pathway may represent one way in which mood can affect the level of pain experienced.

Descending Excitatory Serotonergic Pathways and Chronic Pain

Serotonergic modulation of spinal nociceptive transmission is bidirectional; thus, in addition to well-documented inhibitory effects, the brain can amplify spinal pain processes through a serotonergic circuit (Oyama et al., 1996; Dubner and Ren, 1999; Ossipov et al., 2001; Millan, 2002). Evidence from studies in neuropathic rats suggests an overdrive or inappropriate activation of descending facilitation onto mechanically evoked spinal neuronal responses mediated by serotonin acting on spinal 5-HT$_3$ receptors (Suzuki et al., 2004). Depletion of endogenous spinal 5-HT reduced mechanical allodynia in neuropathic rats and also in a model of spinal cord injury (Oatway et al., 2004; Rahman et al., 2004).

Further evidence for the involvement of 5-HT$_3$ receptor systems in pain behavior has emerged from a recently developed model of cancer-induced bone pain in rats (Donovan-Rodriguez et al., 2006). Antagonism of spinal 5-HT$_3$ receptors produced much greater reductions in mechanical- and thermal-evoked neuronal responses compared with the effects of the drug in sham controls, again suggesting an enhanced descending excitatory drive onto spinal neurons in this model of chronic pain. In contrast, in a model of acute inflammation, although descending facilitation was demonstrated in both sham and inflamed rats, no difference was seen between the animal groups. These findings suggest that the pattern of descending facilitatory influences may vary with time and may depend on particular pathophysiological states. A recent clinical study demonstrated a significant, albeit small, reduction in pain scores in neuropathic pain patients given an i.v. injection of the selective 5-HT$_3$-receptor antagonist ondansetron, compared with a placebo control (McCleane et al., 2003). Similar evidence exists for patients with fibromyalgia that exhibit diffuse widespread pain, where oral and i.v. administration of the 5-HT$_3$ antagonist tropisetron significantly reduced pain scores (Papadopoulos et al., 2000; Stratz et al., 2001). Whether models of longer-term joint inflammation such as osteoarthritis and other deep tissue pains also exhibit enhanced descending facilitation remains to be determined, although preliminary data from our laboratory suggests that this may indeed be the case. A significantly greater role for descending facilitation, mediated by spinal 5-HT$_3$ receptors, on brush-evoked and low-intensity mechanical punctate-evoked neuronal responses was seen in osteoarthritic rats compared with sham controls (unpublished results) (Fig. 2).

Thus, descending facilitation, mediated by activation of spinal 5-HT$_3$ receptors, not only is crucial for the full coding of polymodal peripheral inputs by spinal neurons under normal conditions, but also suggests increased participation of supraspinal sites in driving sustained facilitatory influences on the spinal cord in chronic pain states (Kovelowski et al., 2000; Ossipov et al., 2000; Burgess et al., 2002; Porreca et al., 2002; Suzuki et al., 2004). Interestingly, ondansetron produced a significantly greater effect on the mechanical punctate-evoked neuronal responses compared with its effects on thermal evoked neuronal responses in neuropathic animals (Suzuki et al., 2004). This evidence, together with the finding that spinal transection (severing supraspinal

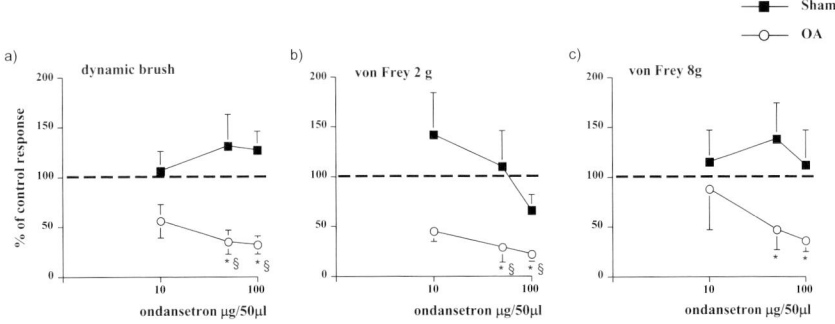

Fig. 2. Effects of spinal administration of the 5-HT$_3$-receptor antagonist ondansetron on low-intensity, mechanically evoked dorsal horn wide-dynamic-range neuronal responses in rats with experimental osteoarthritis (OA) and sham-operated animals: (a) dynamic brush, (b) von Frey 2 g, and (c) von Frey 8 g. Ondansetron produced significant dose-related inhibitions of the evoked responses to brush and von Frey 2 g and 8 g in the OA rats only. The neuronal responses in the OA animals were reduced significantly by the drug. No significant effects of ondansetron were seen on the same neuronal measures in the sham-operated group, and indeed, the increased responses after the drug compared to prior to the drug suggests a tendency to facilitation. The results demonstrate an important role for descending facilitation after onset of osteoarthritis. Data are expressed as maximal mean percentage of predrug control values ± SEM. * Significance ($P < 0.05$) from predrug control values (one-way analysis of variance followed by Dunnet's post-test comparison on raw data). § Significance ($P < 0.05$) compared with the sham-operated group (unpaired t test on normalized data).

circuits) blocks nerve-injury-induced tactile allodynia but not thermal nocifensive responses (Bian et al., 1998), may indicate strong descending facilitatory influences on allodynia.

Descending monoamine systems, and in particular 5-HT projections, innervate most segments of the spinal cord in a diffuse and often nonsynaptic manner. Thus, increases in activity in these pronociceptive pathways would be expected to cause widespread changes in sensitivity over many dermatomes, myotomes, and sclerotomes rather than any discrete focal change.

With regard to musculoskeletal pain, the clear evidence for abnormal temporal summation and central sensitization seen in fibromyalgia patients (Morris et al., 1998; Staud et al., 2001, 2003, 2005; Price et al., 2002) could arise from increased descending facilitations from the midbrain and brainstem, areas also responsible for the sleep and mood changes in these patients. Indeed, the data from Staud et al. (2001, 2004) suggest considerably higher baseline responses in fibromyalgia patients compared to controls so that temporal summation produces even greater pain. This difference is reminiscent of the influence of descending $5HT_3$-mediated facilitations on the process of LTP in the spinal cord of animals (Rygh et al., 2006).

Conclusions

This chapter has reviewed the involvement of descending modulatory pathways in pain processing. In particular, we have reviewed the evidence for the role of $5\text{-}HT_3$-mediated descending facilitation in the enhancement of central spinal pain processing. Not only does this system determine how spinal neurons respond to peripheral inputs, but plasticity within this system, resulting in an enhanced facilitatory drive, may be one of the underlying mechanisms for chronic pain states, as evidenced in models of nerve injury and cancer-induced bone pain, and may well have an important role in chronic musculoskeletal pain although direct evidence is currently minimal. Given that serotonin and the brainstem areas involved in these sensory controls are also implicated in emotions, sleep, and autonomic responses, the well-established links between these states and pain may well involve these same pathways and provide a basis for alterations in the degree of pain experienced as a result of affective changes.

The anatomy and pharmacology of descending facilitation are not yet fully understood, nor do we understand the extent to which this mechanism underpins pain states, such as chronic musculoskeletal pain. There is, however, evidence supporting the therapeutic effectiveness of 5-HT$_3$ antagonists in patients with fibromyalgia, rheumatoid arthritis, tendinopathies, and myofascial pain (Farber et al., 2004). Therefore, further research into the role of descending facilitation as a potential target for pain therapy is necessary.

Acknowledgments

Funded by the Wellcome Trust.

References

Ali Z, Wu G, Kozlov A, Barasi S. The role of 5HT$_3$ in nociceptive processing in the rat spinal cord: results from behavioural and electrophysiological studies. Neurosci Lett 1996;208:203–207.

Bee LA, Dickenson AH. Rostral ventromedial medulla control of spinal sensory processing in normal and pathophysiological states. Neuroscience 2007;147:786–793.

Bergman S. Management of musculoskeletal pain. Best Pract Res Clin Rheumatol 2007;21:153–166.

Bernard J, Bester H, Besson J. Involvement of the spino-parabrachio -amygdaloid and -hypothalamic pathways in the autonomic and affective emotional aspects of pain. Prog Brain Res 1996;107:243–255.

Bian D, Ossipov MH, Zhong C, Malan TPJ, Porreca F. Tactile allodynia, but not thermal hyperalgesia, of the hindlimbs is blocked by spinal transection in rats with nerve injury. Neurosci Lett 1998;241:79–82.

Brady DM, Schneider MJ. Fibromyalgia syndrome: a new paradigm for differential diagnosis and treatment. J Manipulative Physiol Ther 2001;24:529–541.

Burgess SE, Gardell LR, Ossipov MH, Malan TP, Jr., Vanderah TW, Lai J, Porreca F. Time-dependent descending facilitation from the rostral ventromedial medulla maintains, but does not initiate, neuropathic pain. J Neurosci 2002;22:5129–5136.

Calejesan A, Ch'ang M, Zhuo M. Spinal serotonergic receptors mediate facilitation of a nociceptive reflex by subcutaneous formalin injection into the hindpaw in rats. Brain Res 1998;798:46–54.

Conte D, Legg ED, McCourt AC, Silajdzic E, Nagy GG, Maxwell DJ. Transmitter content, origins and connections of axons in the spinal cord that possess the serotonin (5-hydroxytryptamine) 3 receptor. Neuroscience 2005;134:165–173.

Curatolo M, Bogduk N. Pharmacologic pain treatment of musculoskeletal disorders: current perspectives and future prospects. Clin J Pain 2001,17.25–32.

Donovan-Rodriguez T, Urch CE, Dickenson AH. Evidence of a role for descending serotonergic facilitation in a rat model of cancer-induced bone pain. Neurosci Lett 2006;393:237–242.

Dubner R, Ren K. Endogenous mechanisms of sensory modulation. Pain Suppl 1999;6:S27–S35.

Farber L, Haus U, Spath M, Drechsler S. Physiology and pathophysiology of the 5-HT$_3$ receptor. Scand J Rheumatol 2004;119:2–8.

Fields HL, Heinricher MM. Anatomy and physiology of a nociceptive modulatory system. Philos Trans R Soc Lond B Biol Sci 1985;308:361–374.

Fields H, Bry J, Hentall I, Zorman G. The activity of neurones in the rostral medulla of the rat during withdrawal from noxious heat. J Neurosci 1983;3:2545–2552.

Gauriau C, Bernard JF. Pain pathways and parabrachial circuits in the rat. Exp Physiol 2002;87:251–258.

Green GM, Scarth J, Dickenson A. An excitatory role for 5-HT in spinal inflammatory nociceptive transmission: state-dependent actions via dorsal horn 5-HT(3) receptors in the anaesthetized rat. Pain 2000;89:81–88.

Hunt SP, Mantyh PW. The molecular dynamics of pain control. Nat Rev Neurosci 2001;2:83–91.

Kashima K, Rahman OI, Sakoda S, Shiba R. Increased pain sensitivity of the upper extremities of TMD patients with myalgia to experimentally-evoked noxious stimulation: possibility of worsened endogenous opioid systems. Cranio 1999;17:241–246.

Kosek E, Hansson P. Modulatory influence on somatosensory perception from vibration and heterotopic noxious conditioning stimulation (HNCS) in fibromyalgia patients and healthy subjects. Pain 1997;70:41–51.

Kosek E, Ekhol J, Hansson P. Sensory dysfunction in fibromyalgia patients with implications for pathogenic mechanisms. Pain 1996;68:375–383.

Kovelowlowski CJ, Ossipov MH, Sun H, Lai J, Malan TP, Porreca F. Supraspinal cholecystokinin may drive tonic descending facilitation mechanisms to maintain neuropathic pain in the rat. Pain 2000;87:265–273.

Kulkarni B, Bentley DE, Elliott R, Julyan PJ, Boger E, Watson A, Boyle Y, El-Deredy W, Jones AK. Arthritic pain is processed in brain areas concerned with emotions and fear. Arthritis Rheum 2007;56:1345–1354.

Lautenbacher S, Rollman GB. Possible deficiencies of pain modulation in fibromyalgia. Clin J Pain 1997;13:189–196.

Maixner W, Fillingim R, Booker D, Sigurdsson A. Sensitivity of patients with painful temporomandibular disorders to experimentally evoked pain. Pain 1995;63:341–351.

Mantyh P, Rogers S, Honore P, Allen B, Ghilardi J, Li J, Daughters R, Lappi D, Wiley R, Simone D. Inhibition of hyperalgesia by ablation of lamina I spinal neurons expressing the substance P receptor. Science 1997;278:275–279.

Maxwell DJ, Kerr R, Rashid S, Anderson E. Characterisation of axon terminals in the rat dorsal horn that are immunoreactive for serotonin 5-HT3A receptor subunits. Exp Brain Res 2003;149:114–124.

McCleane GJ, Suzuki R, Dickenson AH. Does a single intravenous injection of the 5HT$_3$ receptor antagonist ondansetron have an analgesic effect in neuropathic pain? A double-blinded, placebo-controlled cross-over study. Anesth Analg 2003;97:1474–1478.

Millan MJ. Descending control of pain. Prog Neurobiol 2002;66:355–474.

Millan MJ. The neurobiology and control of anxious states. Prog Neurobiol 2003;70:83–244.

Miura T, Okazaki R, Yoshida H, Namba H, Okai H, Kawamura M. Mechanisms of analgesic action of Neurotropin on chronic pain in adjuvant-induced arthritic rat: roles of descending noradrenergic and serotonergic systems. J Pharmacol Sci 2005;97:429–436.

Morris V, Cruwys S, Kidd B. Increased capsaicin-induced secondary hyperalgesia as a marker of abnormal sensory activity in patients with fibromyalgia. Neurosci Lett 1998;250:205–207.

Nichols M, Allen B, Rogers S, Ghilardi J, Honore P, Luger N, Finke M, Li J, Lappi D, Simone D, Mantyh P. Transmission of chronic nociception by spinal neurons expressing the substance P receptor. Science 1999;286:1558–1561.

Oatway MA, Chen Y, Weaver LC. The 5-HT$_3$ receptor facilitates at-level mechanical allodynia following spinal cord injury. Pain 2004;110:259–268.

Ossipov M, Lai J, Malan TJ, Porreca F. Spinal and supraspinal mechanisms of neuropathic pain. Ann NY Acad Sci 2000;909:12–24.

Ossipov M, Lai J, Malan Jr T, Vanderah T, Porreca F. Tonic descending facilitation as a mechanism of neuropathic pain. In: Hansson P, Fields H, Hill R, Marchettini P, editors. Neuropathic pain: pathophysiology and treatment. Progress in Pain Research and Management, Vol. 21. Seattle: IASP Press; 2001. p 107–124.

Oyama T, Ueda M, Kuraishi Y, Akaike A, Satoh M. Dual effect of serotonin on formalin-induced nociception in the rat spinal cord. Neurosci Res 1996;25:129–135.

Papadopoulos IA, Georgiou PE, Katsimbri PP, Drosos AA. Treatment of fibromyalgia with tropisetron, a 5HT$_3$ serotonin antagonist: a pilot study. Clin Rheumatol 2000;19:6–8.

Pertovaara A, Keski-Vakkuri U, Kalmari J, Wei H, Panula P. Response properties of neurons in the rostroventromedial medulla of neuropathic rats: attempted modulation of responses by [1DMe]NPYF, a neuropeptide FF analogue. Neuroscience 2001;105:457–468.

Porreca F, Burgess SE, Gardell LR, Vanderah TW, Malan TP, Jr., Ossipov MH, Lappi DA, Lai J. Inhibition of neuropathic pain by selective ablation of brainstem medullary cells expressing the mu-opioid receptor. J Neurosci 2001;21:5281–5288.

Porreca F, Ossipov MH, Gebhart GF. Chronic pain and medullary descending facilitation. Trends Neurosci 2002;25:319–325.

Price DD, Staud R, Robinson ME, Mauderli AP, Cannon R, Vierck CJ. Enhanced temporal summation of second pain and its central modulation in fibromyalgia patients. Pain 2002;99:49–59.

Rahman W, Suzuki R, Rygh LJ, Dickenson AH. Descending serotonergic facilitation mediated through rat spinal 5HT$_3$ receptors is unaltered following carrageenan inflammation. Neurosci Lett 2004;361:229–231.

Rygh LJ, Suzuki R, Rahman W, Wong Y, Vonsy JL, Sandhu H, Webber M, Hunt S, Dickenson AH. Local and descending circuits regulate long-term potentiation and zif268 expression in spinal neurons. Eur J Neurosci 2006;24:761–772.

Staud R, Vierck C, Cannon R, Mauderli A, Price D. Abnormal sensitization and temporal summation of second pain (wind-up) in patients with fibromyalgia syndrome. Pain 2001;91:165–175.

Staud R, Robinson ME, Vierck CJ, Price DD. Diffuse noxious inhibitory controls (DNIC) attenuate temporal summation of second pain in normal males but not in normal females or fibromyalgia patients, Pain 2003a;101:167–174.

Staud R, Robinson M, Vierck C, Cannon R, Mauderli A, Price D. Ratings of experimental pain and pain-related negative affect predict clinical pain in patients with fibromyalgia syndrome. Pain 2003b;105:215–222.

Staud R, Vierck CJ, Robinson ME, Price DD. Spatial summation of heat pain within and across dermatomes in fibromyalgia patients and pain-free subjects. Pain 2004;111:342–350.

Stratz T, Farber L, Varga B, Baumgartner C, Haus U, Muller W. Fibromyalgia treatment with intravenous tropisetron administration. Drugs Exp Clin Res 2001;27:112–118.

Suzuki R, Morcuende S, Webber M, Hunt SP, Dickenson AH. Superficial NK1-expressing neurons control spinal excitability through activation of descending pathways. Nat Neurosci 2002;5:1319–1326.

Suzuki R, Rahman W, Hunt SP, Dickenson AH. Descending facilitatory control of mechanically evoked responses is enhanced in deep dorsal horn neurones following peripheral nerve injury. Brain Res 2004;1019:68–76.

Suzuki R, Rahman W, Rygh LJ, Webber M, Hunt SP, Dickenson AH. Spinal-supraspinal serotonergic circuits regulating neuropathic pain and its treatment with gabapentin. Pain 2005;117:292–303.

Todd AJ. Anatomy of primary afferents and projection neurones in the rat spinal dorsal horn with particular emphasis on substance P and the neurokinin 1 receptor. Exp Physiol 2002;87:245–249.

Todd AJ, McGill MM, Shehab SA. Neurokinin 1 receptor expression by neurons in laminae I, III and IV of the rat spinal dorsal horn that project to the brainstem. Eur J Neurosci 2000;12:689–700.

Urban MO, Gebhart GF. Supraspinal contributions to hyperalgesia. Proc Natl Acad Sci USA 1999;96:7687–7692.

Yu XM, Hua M, Mense S. The effects of intracerebroventricular injection of naloxone, phentolamine and methysergide on the transmission of nociceptive signals in rat dorsal horn neurons with convergent cutaneous-deep input. Neuroscience 1991;44:715–723.

Zeitz KP, Guy N, Malmberg AB, Dirajlal S, Martin WJ, Sun L, Bonhaus DW, Stucky CL, Julius D, Basbaum AI. The 5-HT$_3$ subtype of serotonin receptor contributes to nociceptive processing via a novel subset of myelinated and unmyelinated nociceptors. J Neurosci 2002;22:1010–1019.

Correspondence to: Wahida Rahman, PhD, Department of Pharmacology, University College London, Gower Street, London WC1E 6BT, United Kingdom. Tel: 44-207-679-3737; fax: 44-207-679-0181; email: w.rahman@ucl.ac.uk.

Peripheral Aspects of Cytokines in Musculoskeletal Pain

Sigvard Kopp and Per Alstergren

Department of Clinical Oral Physiology, Institute of Odontology,
Karolinska Institute, Huddinge, Sweden

Cytokines are extracellular peptides that mediate potent stimulatory or inhibitory biological effects on most cell types. Cytokines play an important role in the pathology of rheumatoid arthritis (RA) by taking part in the mediation of acute and chronic pain and in the ensuing destruction of connective tissue. Originally identified as being important in inflammatory processes and immune responses, cytokines are now recognized to be involved in most physiological processes. Their essential role in homeostasis involves activating inflammatory and nociceptive mechanisms and modulating the repair and remodeling of damaged tissue. In inflammatory conditions, a dramatic increase in cytokine production can be seen, and at the same time the balance between the production and control of cytokines is disturbed (Jouvenne et al., 1998; Fig.1). Indeed, it appears that the balance of pro- and anti-inflammatory cytokines is at least as important as absolute levels of individual cytokines (Kopp and Sommer, 2007). The available knowledge about musculoskeletal pain and cytokines is in general very limited, except for the cytokines interleukin-1β (IL-1β) and tumor necrosis factor-α (TNF-α).

Fundamentals of Musculoskeletal Pain
edited by Thomas Graven-Nielsen, Lars Arendt-Nielsen, and Siegfried Mense
IASP Press, Seattle, © 2008

119

Local joint and muscle pain is frequently associated with the activation of joint and muscle nociceptors by a variety of inflammatory mediators such as cytokines, neuropeptides, and arachidonic acid derivatives (Kopp and Sommer, 2007). Evidence shows that inflammation in the synovial tissues, such as those of the temporomandibular joint (TMJ), and probably in the surrounding musculature plays an important role in determining whether a painful condition will develop; it also determines the prognosis of different treatment strategies.

Model of Cytokine Modulation of Joint Pain

Balanced Cytokine Release

When balanced cytokine release occurs in healthy tissue or during remissions of inflammatory disease, the deleterious effects of proinflammatory cytokines are endogenously controlled by the effects of anti-inflammatory factors. Examples of the latter are anti-inflammatory cytokines (e.g., IL-10), receptor antagonists (e.g., IL-1ra), soluble receptors (e.g., TNFsRII, IL-1sRII) and decoy receptors (IL-1RII). Balanced release at a low level enables tissue repair and remodeling, while at a high level it can reduce an ongoing inflammatory process (Fig. 1A).

Unbalanced Cytokine Release

Unbalanced cytokine release means that the amount of proinflammatory cytokines released exceeds the ability of the endogenous control factors to counteract the proinflammatory effects, which results in increased inflammatory activity (Fig. 1B). The cytokines TNF-α, IL-1β, and IL-6 not only have direct proinflammatory effects but also exert indirect effects by stimulating the release of inflammatory mediators including other cytokines, prostanoids, bradykinin, and serotonin.

Peripheral nociceptive neurons are sensitized or activated directly by TNF-α, IL-1β, and IL-6 via binding to their respective receptors. Cell-surface bound receptors on nociceptive afferents have been identified for

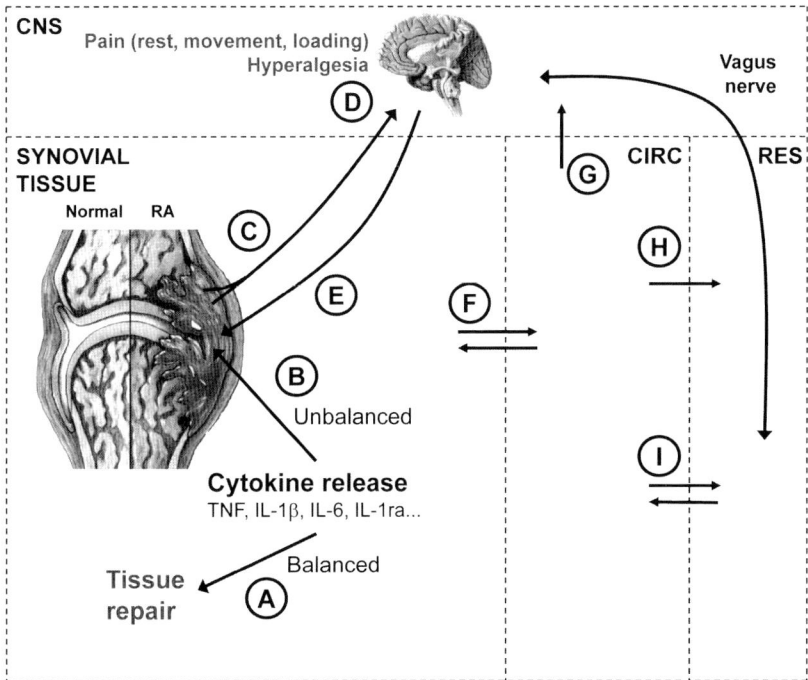

Fig. 1. A model for cytokine modulation of joint pain. (A) Balanced cytokine release, where the deleterious effects of the proinflammatory cytokines are endogenously controlled by the effects of the anti-inflammatory factors. (B) Unbalanced cytokine release, where the effects of the released proinflammatory cytokines exceed those of the endogenous control factors to counteract the proinflammatory effects, resulting in increased inflammatory activity. (C) Peripheral nociceptive neurons are sensitized or activated; repeated activity in peripheral nociceptive neurons may trigger neurogenic inflammation via the axon reflex. (D) The increase of nociceptive signaling to the central nervous system (CNS) due to the effects of the proinflammatory cytokines amplifies pain sensations from the joint region and causes hyperalgesia over the joint. (E) Extensive nociceptive input to the CNS may increase sympathetic activity, which in turn causes release of norepinephrine and neuropeptide Y from sympathetic nerve efferents in the synovial tissue that further amplify the nociceptive signaling of the nerve endings. (F) During inflammation, cytokines from the joint tissues enter the blood circulation (CIRC), via lymphatic drainage, endothelial leakage, or capillary diffusion. The increased plasma levels may in turn influence distant synovial and other tissues. (G) Circulating tumor necrosis factor-α (TNF-α), interleukin-1 (IL-1), and IL-6 have direct effects on the CNS via receptors in periventricular regions that cause fever and generalized hyperalgesia. (H) Cytokines in the circulation may also influence the CNS via activation of receptors on the vagus nerve in the reticuloendothelial system (RES), including the liver and spleen. Afferent signaling in the vagus elicits fever and generalized hyperalgesia. (I) Activity in the cholinergic anti-inflammatory pathway (the vagus nerve and RES) may downregulate cytokine release from major producers such as the liver and spleen and also redirect leucocyte trafficking away from the periphery, thereby reducing peripheral inflammatory activity.

TNF and IL-1β. Peripheral nociceptive neurons have no cell surface IL-6 receptors, but instead they express the cell surface gp130 protein, which links the soluble part of the IL-6 receptor to the cell surface. IL-6 thus binds to the soluble form of its receptor, and this complex then binds to the gp130 protein, which in turn causes a cellular response.

Increased or repeated activity in peripheral nociceptive neurons may trigger neurogenic inflammation via the axon reflex, causing release of neuropeptides such as substance P and calcitonin-gene related peptide. These mediators may then amplify nociceptor sensitization as well as other aspects of the inflammatory process (Fig. 1C). The increase in nociceptive signal influx into the central nervous system (CNS) due to the effects of the proinflammatory cytokines amplifies pain sensations from the joint region and causes hyperalgesia over the joint. TNF and IL-1β have been related to resting pain and pain on movement of the joint (Fig. 1D).

Extensive nociceptive input to the CNS may increase sympathetic activity, which in turn may cause release of norepinephrine and neuropeptide Y from sympathetic nerve efferents in the synovial tissue. These mediators may in turn modulate nociceptive nerve endings and impair blood circulation (Fig. 1E). During inflammation, cytokines from the joint tissues enter the blood circulation via lymphatic drainage, endothelial leakage, or capillary diffusion, which results in elevated plasma levels of these cytokines. Elevated plasma levels may in turn influence distant synovial and other tissues (Fig. 1F). Circulating TNF-α, IL-1β, and IL-6 have direct effects on the CNS via receptors in periventricular regions, leading to fever and generalized hyperalgesia (Fig. 1G).

Cytokines in the circulation may also influence the CNS by activating receptors on the vagus nerve in the reticuloendothelial system, including the liver and spleen. Afferent signaling in the vagus may elicit fever and generalized hyperalgesia (Fig. 1H). Activity in the cholinergic anti-inflammatory pathway (the vagus nerve and reticuloendothelial system) may downregulate cytokine release from major systemic producers as the liver and spleen and redirect leukocyte trafficking away from the periphery to the spleen and lymphatic nodes, thereby reducing peripheral inflammatory activity (Fig. 1I). For an excellent review of the cholinergic anti-inflammatory pathway, see Tracey (2007).

Specific Cytokines

Interleukin-1

The molecule and its mechanisms of action. IL-1 (molecular weight 15 kDa) is mainly derived from macrophages and plays a key role in amplifying and perpetuating peripheral inflammation. Two subtypes of IL-1 have been identified: IL-1α and IL-1β. Most of the IL-1α remains inside the cell or on the surface of the cell membrane, where it functions more as an autocrine messenger rather than as an extracellular mediator, whereas most IL-1β is transported out of the cell, where it acts locally or enters the blood circulation (Dinarello, 1994). Both subtypes are involved in inflammatory reactions, but only IL-1β has been found in synovial fluid from patients with RA (Ruschen et al., 1989). The IL-1 family also includes an IL-1 receptor antagonist (IL-1ra). IL-1ra competes with IL-1α and IL-1β for receptor binding and is produced in much higher concentrations than IL-1β. However, IL-1ra does not elicit a biological response when coupled to an IL-1 receptor and is therefore anti-inflammatory (Dinarello, 1996). The inflammatory process causes increased local IL-1ra production, but the amount produced is probably insufficient to inhibit the effects of IL-1β in active inflammation.

Antigen presentation to T cells in joint tissues by dendritic cells or macrophages activates the T cells to produce cytokines including IL-1, resulting in an inflammatory reaction and pain. After recognizing the antigen, the presenting macrophage also secretes IL-1 (Verbruggen et al., 1991). IL-1 then induces several inflammatory events. It activates lymphocytes and stimulates the release of cytokines, prostaglandins, and collagenase from connective tissue cells. It also has systemic effects by stimulating the production and release of C-reactive protein, eliciting fever, causing malaise and somnolence, and leading to sickness-related behaviors such as decreased social interaction and sexual activity, weakness, and depression (Barbe and Barr, 2006).

There are two IL-1 receptors: IL-1RI with low/high affinity for IL-1β/IL-1ra, respectively, and IL-1RII with high/low affinity for

IL-1β/IL-1ra. IL-1RII causes no signal transduction when stimulated and is therefore considered a "decoy receptor." Soluble IL-1RI (IL-1sRI) and IL-1RII (IL-1sRII) are present in the extracellular matrix and blood both in healthy individuals and in patients with inflammatory disorders. Levels of IL-1sRII are elevated in the blood plasma and synovial fluid of patients with inflammatory joint disease (Arend et al., 1994). Upregulation of these soluble receptors is assumed to have an anti-inflammatory effect (Dinarello, 1996). Together, the IL-1 receptor antagonist, the endogenous soluble IL-1 receptors, and the inactive form of the receptors modulate the effects of IL-1.

Interleukin-1β is capable of decreasing nociceptive thresholds in peripheral tissues by a direct excitatory, sensitizing action on nociceptive fibers (Fukuoka et al., 1994). When given systemically to rats, IL-1β is a potent hyperalgesic agent, partly by peripheral action (Ferreira et al., 1988). Jeanjean et al. (1995) showed that intraplantar injections of IL-1β in rats were able to sensitize nociceptors by a long-term increase of neuronal synthesis and axonal transport of substance P as well as its release from the axons. In chronic peripheral neurogenic inflammation, this effect could increase sensitivity to nociceptive stimuli. IL-1β may also cause a general decrease of nociceptive thresholds by a central action, either directly or via actions on the hepatic vagus nerve (Watkins et al., 1994).

Clinical aspects. IL-1β is undetectable in the TMJ synovial fluid from healthy individuals, but levels are significant in patients with polyarthritis (Alstergren et al., 1999a). IL-1β was detected in the synovial fluid of 34% of patients with TMJ arthritis in a study by Alstergren et al. (1998); these levels were within the range for synovial fluid levels found in other joints of patients with RA in a previous study (Holt et al., 1992). The IL-1β in the synovial fluid of the TMJ in patients with inflammatory disorder seems to originate locally because the correlation between plasma and synovial fluid levels is poor and the level is much higher in the synovial fluid than in the plasma. In patients with RA, the synovial fluid level of IL-1β in the knees also showed a poor correlation with plasma levels; it correlated better with local disease activity as measured by the Ritchie score (indicating joint tenderness) and joint circumference (indicating swelling) than with systemic disease activity (Rooney et al., 1990).

In patients with arthritis of the TMJ, there was a strong positive correlation between the right and left sides regarding synovial fluid IL-1β, which indicates that inflammatory conditions of the TMJ involving IL-1β often are bilateral (Alstergren et al., 1998). The same situation was reported in the study mentioned above by Rooney et al. (1990), who found almost identical levels of IL-1β in the synovial fluid from the right and left knee joint in RA patients with clinical signs (pain and swelling) of symmetrical joint involvement but different levels in patients with asymmetrical involvement. There are no published results indicating a difference in IL-1β levels between patients with specific inflammatory conditions such as RA, psoriatic arthritis, or ankylosing spondylitis compared to unspecific systemic inflammatory joint conditions. However, patients with local TMJ monoarthritis had no detectable IL-1β in the synovial fluid, whereas IL-1β was found in 34% of TMJ synovial fluid samples from patients with chronic systemic inflammatory joint conditions (Alstergren et al., 1999b).

Levels of IL-1β in the synovial fluid from the arthritic TMJ showed significant positive correlations to resting pain and tenderness to digital palpation and a negative correlation to pressure-pain tolerance level (Alstergren et al., 1998; Fig. 2). It therefore seems that IL-1β is one of the determinants of pain and sensitization of the TMJ. Patients with high IL-1ra and low IL-1β concentrations in the synovial fluid show a more rapid resolution of arthritis, and the balance between synovial fluid IL-1β and IL-1ra concentrations thus seems to determine the progression of the inflammatory process. Indeed, high levels of IL-1ra in TMJ synovial fluid are associated with little or no pain with mandibular movement (Alstergren et al., 2003).

Detectable plasma levels of IL-1β were found in 79% of 14 patients with rheumatoid factor positive RA and in 33% of 9 patients with rheumatoid factor negative RA, as compared with 22% of healthy individuals (Alstergren et al., 1999b). The plasma level of IL-1β has been associated with general inflammatory joint disease activity, as indicated by Ritchie score (tenderness), pain, and erythrocyte sedimentation rate in patients with RA (Eastgate et al., 1988). The study by Alstergren et al. (1999a) did not support a relationship between circulating IL-1β and TMJ pain.

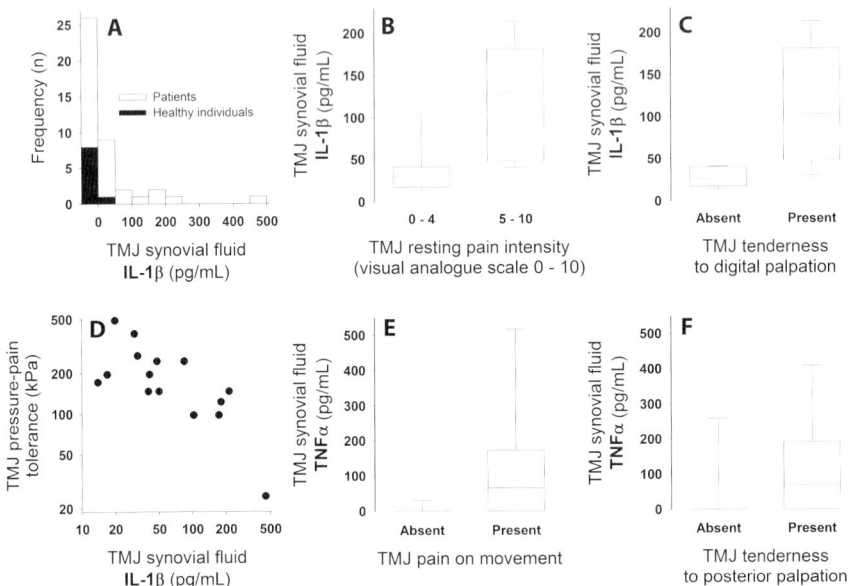

Fig. 2. Panel showing temporomandibular joint (TMJ) synovial fluid levels of interleukin-1β (IL-1β) and tumor necrosis factor-α (TNF-α) in relation to TMJ pain and hyperalgesia. (A) Distribution of IL-1β-levels in 41 synovial fluid samples from 29 patients with TMJ arthritis and 9 samples from 7 healthy individuals (Alstergren et al., 1998). (B) Relation between TMJ synovial fluid levels of IL-1β and TMJ resting pain intensity ($r_s = 0.62$, $n = 13$, $P = 0.020$; Alstergren et al., 1998). (C) Relation between TMJ synovial fluid levels of IL-1β and presence or absence of TMJ tenderness to digital palpation ($r_s = 0.80$, $n = 15$, $P < 0.000$; Alstergren et al., 1998). (D) Relation between TMJ synovial fluid levels of IL-1β and TMJ pressure-pain tolerance pressure ($r = -0.60$, $n = 15$, $P = 0.016$; Alstergren et al., 1998). (E) Higher TMJ synovial fluid levels of TNF-α in patients with TMJ pain on mandibular movement compared to those without such pain ($P = 0.010$, $n = 24$; Nordahl et al., 2000). (F) Higher TMJ synovial fluid levels of TNF-α in patients with tenderness to posterior palpation of the joint compared to those without such tenderness ($P = 0.040$, $n = 24$; Nordahl et al., 2000).

Tumor Necrosis Factor Alpha

The molecule and its mechanisms of action. TNF-α is a pleiotropic cytokine (17 kDa) that is produced by a number of cell types including activated macrophages and monocytes. It has biological activities similar to those of IL-1β. However, many other cells can produce TNF-α upon adequate stimulation. TNF-α is not considered to be produced by normal cells but rather by cells stimulated by neoplastic or infectious disease (Feldmann et al., 1992). Synthesis of TNF-α is triggered by immune complexes, complement components, IL-1, and TNF-α itself. The main physiological role of TNF-α is activation of the first-line reaction to microbial, viral, and mechanical stress. TNF-α rapidly induces synthesis of other mediators such as IL-1, IL-6, and prostaglandins. In RA, TNF-α is often present at the site of inflammation (synovial membrane lining cells, endothelial cells, and cells in the junction between cartilage and pannus), and it also seems to be responsible for the systemic inflammation in this disease (Bayaert and Fiers, 1998). Animal research indicates that TNF-α induces mechanical hyperalgesia with rapid onset (within 30 minutes) when administered subcutaneously. The hyperalgesia appears to result from sensitization of cutaneous C fibers, which may persist for 30 days or more; it is associated with signs of inflammation and increased levels of inflammatory mediators such as prostaglandins (Sommer and Kress, 2004; Cunha et al., 2005). In addition, local TNF-α administration evokes spontaneous activity in afferent C and Aδ nerve fibers that results in low-grade nociceptive input, contributing to central sensitization (Sorkin et al., 1997; Junger and Sorkin, 2000; Özakatay et al., 2006). However, injection of TNF-α into the muscle tissue of rats did not excite group IV muscle afferents but had desensitizing effects (Hoheisel et al., 2005). In addition, intramuscular levels of TNF-α did not increase in a rat model of muscle inflammation (Loram et al., 2007).

TNF-α appears to be one of the mediators involved in several animal models of arthritis (Cunha et al., 2005). Subcutaneous administration of the TNF-α inhibitor etanercept decreased mechanical hyperalgesia when administered prior to induction of arthritis by injection of complete Freund's adjuvant into the rat knee joint (Inglis et al., 2005). In contrast to its effects on cutaneous and articular tissues, TNF-α injected into the rat gastrocnemius muscle induced prolonged mechanical sensitization that was associated with increased tissue levels of prostaglandin E_2, calcitonin-gene related peptide, and nerve growth factor, although there was no significant muscle inflammation or recruitment of inflammatory cells (Schäfers et al., 2003).

Two TNF-α receptors have been identified: the 55-kDa TNFRII receptor and the 75-kDa TNFRII receptor. These receptors have been found on most cells, including nerve cells. They activate different intracellular signaling pathways, although no significant functional difference between the two receptor types has been found. The binding of TNF-α to its cell surface receptors activates several complex signaling pathways that include the activation of transcription factors (such as nuclear factor κB), mitogen-activated protein kinases, and proteases, which eventually cause changes in protein expression and activity (Pickering et al., 2005).

Clinical aspects. TNF-α has been detected in the synovium and synovial fluid of patients with RA (Chu et al., 1991) and in patients with other inflammatory diseases such as psoriatic arthritis, pelvospondylitis, osteoarthritis (degenerative joint disease), and reactive arthritis (Partsch et al., 1997). TNF-α has also been found in the synovial fluid of patients with internal derangement of the TMJ (Sandler et al., 1998), as well as in patients with unspecified TMJ disorders (Takahashi et al., 1998). In our clinic, TNF-α was detectable in 33% of the TMJ synovial fluid samples taken from patients with chronic connective tissue diseases involving joints, including RA, psoriatic arthropathy, pelvospondylitis, chronic unspecific arthritis, osteoarthritis, and Sjögren's syndrome (Nordahl et al., 2000). The data from our clinic agree with the results of Di Giovine et al. (1988), who also found detectable levels of TNF-α in 30% of knee synovial fluid samples from 93 individuals with chronic connective tissue diseases. In a study of patients with a diagnosis of internal derangement of the TMJ without systemic disease, TNF-α was detected in 8% of 62 synovial fluid samples (Sandler et al., 1998). Levels of TNF-α in the synovial fluid significantly exceeded those in the plasma. The concentration of circulating TNF-α in the blood is usually low (25th–75th percentile: 8–12 pg/mL). Therefore, in most pathological states, measurements of systemic cytokine levels do not adequately reflect local pathology. As in the example of TMJ disease, local cytokine levels are higher and are probably of more diagnostic value than circulating blood levels.

Studies of TNF-α in relation to nociception have shown that experimental hyperalgesia can be caused by local or systemic administration of the cytokine (Watkins et al., 1995). TNF-α may have an indirect effect in receptor sensitization by increasing the production and release of other pain mediators such as IL-1β, serotonin, and prostaglandins, which cause pain and hyperalgesia (Watkins et al., 1995). IL-1β results in upregulation of the neurotrophic nerve growth factor that mediates inflammatory hyperalgesia (Woolf et al., 1997). TNF-α also induced ectopic activity in nociceptive primary afferent fibers in rats when applied directly on the sciatic nerve trunk (Sorkin et al., 1997).

The role of cytokines in muscle pain is largely unknown. In a study of delayed-onset muscle soreness in healthy males, administration of etanercept, a TNF-α blocker, did not affect muscle soreness, but muscle strength improved more rapidly (Rice et al., 2007), suggesting that muscle soreness is not modulated by TNF-α. However, proinflammatory cytokines such as TNF-α have been associated with muscle pathology in conditions such as inflammatory myopathies (Lundberg, 2000) and fibromyalgia (Wallace et al., 2001). TNF-α and IL-1β levels were elevated in microdialysates from the trapezius muscle in patients with idiopathic cervical pain associated with myofascial trigger points compared to healthy controls (Shah et al., 2005). Elevated levels of TNF-α, IL-1β, and IL-6 in plasma have been associated with more pronounced upper-body symptoms in patients with musculoskeletal disorders from overuse (Carp et al., 2007). An additional systemic response may be evoked by cytokines released into the blood from the injured muscle tissue, where circulating cytokines such as TNF-α, IL-1β, and IL-6 may stimulate a global response of widespread tissue sensitization (Barbe and Barr, 2006).

Synovial fluid TNF-α levels are significantly higher in individuals with TMJ pain, including pain upon mandibular movement, than in those without such pain (Nordahl et al., 2000; Fig. 2). In addition, synovial fluid TNF-α levels were associated with tenderness to palpation of the posterior aspect of the TMJ, which corresponds to sensitization of afferent nerves in the synovial tissues and other tissues surrounding the TMJ. TNF-α, or agents induced by this mediator, are thus contributors to pain of the arthritic TMJ. Elevated levels of TNF-α induced by glutamate release from neural cells or macrophages may cause a prolonged period of muscle or joint mechanical sensitization, according to findings that glutamate can induce release of TNF-α from synoviocytes in vitro (McNearney et al., 2004; Takeuchi et al., 2006). A recent study of RA in patients with TMJ involvement found that concentrations of glutamate and

TNF-α were positively correlated in the TMJ synovial fluid but not in the plasma (P. Alstergren, A.-K. Hajati, B. Sessle, and S. Kopp, unpublished data). These findings suggest that glutamate released in muscle and joint tissues may excite nociceptors and induce mechanical sensitization by local elevation of tissue levels of TNF-α.

As can be expected, TNF-α levels in synovial fluid and plasma appear to be predictive for the treatment response to intra-articular administration of glucocorticoid into the TMJ. A high pretreatment level of TNF-α in the TMJ synovial fluid was a positive predictor for TMJ pain relief after intra-articular administration of glucocorticoid (Fredriksson et al., 2006). Pain relief was associated with reduced TNF levels after treatment. It is thus likely that TNF-α is involved in the modulation of TMJ pain. There was no correlation between synovial fluid and plasma levels of TNF-α, but higher levels in the synovial fluid than in the plasma indicate local production of the mediator in the TMJ synovial tissues.

Interleukin-4

Interleukin-4 (IL-4) is anti-inflammatory and is mainly produced by T lymphocytes, mast cells, and basophils. IL-4 reduces pain in various models (Hao et al., 2006).

Interleukin-6

Interleukin-6 (IL-6) is proinflammatory and causes pain as well as degradation of cartilage and bone (Watkins et al., 1994). Its production in monocytes and macrophages is strongly induced by TNF-α and IL-1β. IL-6 induces circulating levels of IL-1ra and the soluble receptor TNFs-RI. IL-6 is the major cytokine to initiate the acute phase response in the liver and the production of acute phase proteins such as C-reactive protein. IL-6 has been found more often in the synovial fluid from patients with TMJ pain than in healthy controls; the levels of IL-6 correlated with pain intensity (Shinoda and Takaku, 2000). In an arthroscopic study of TMJ internal derangement, IL-6 showed the closest correlation with the level of synovitis, and it correlated with the degree of vascularity of the synovial membrane (Sandler et al., 1998). IL-6 is significantly elevated in RA. Plasma levels of IL-6 were reduced after systemic administration of infliximab in parallel with a reduction of C-reactive protein and global joint pain intensity (Kopp et al., 2005).

Interleukin-10, Interleukin-13, and Transforming Growth Factor Beta

These cytokines have anti-inflammatory properties. Interleukin-10 (IL-10) is a suppressor of monocyte and macrophage function and therefore inhibits production of TNF, IL-1, and IL-6 (Fang et al., 1999). A deficiency in the production of the anti-inflammatory mediators IL-10, and transforming growth factor β (TGF-β) was found in patients with TMJ pain (Fang et al., 1999; Tominaga et al., 2004). The related cytokine interleukin-13 (IL-13) reduces pain in various models (Hao et al., 2006). IL-10 pretreatment reduces hyperalgesic responses to intraplantar injections of carrageenan, IL-1β, IL-6, and TNF-α (Poole et al., 1995) and to nerve injury (Wagner et al., 1998). Plasma levels of IL-10 were raised after systemic infliximab treatment in parallel with reduction of TMJ pain in patients with RA (Kopp et al., 2005).

Anticytokine Therapy

Of the many cytokines present in the synovial fluid from patients with RA, IL-1β and TNF are considered to have particular importance in the inflammatory disease process, and blocking the effects of these potent cytokines has met with success as a therapeutic approach (Elliot et al., 1993).

Blocking Interleukin-1β

Treatment with systemic IL-1ra elicited a dose-dependent reduction in the number of swollen joints and new bone erosions, levels of C-reactive protein, and erythrocyte sedimentation rate in RA patients (Bresnihan et al., 1998). In addition, the new nonsteroidal anti-inflammatory drug diacerein inhibits IL-1 production but has no effect on prostaglandin synthesis. Diacerein is as effective as piroxicam in reducing pain and improving function in osteoarthritis (Nicolas et al., 1998).

In an animal model of chronic arthritis, administration of IL-1sRII showed a marked and dose-related inhibition of joint swelling and reduction of plasma prostaglandin E_2 and synovial fluid IL-1β. In addition, an inhibitory effect on joint damage was observed histologically (Dawson et al., 1999).

Blocking Tumor Necrosis Factor

Blocking TNF-α in RA with anti-TNF antibodies or soluble receptors, i.e., infliximab or etanercept, is now commonly used to treat RA patients (Bankhurst, 1999). Intravenous infusion with the chimeric mouse/human monoclonal antibody against TNF-α, infliximab, reduces disease activity including arthritic pain and joint destruction in RA patients (Lipsky et al., 2000).

Blocking of the effects of TNF-α, systemically or locally, may be a rational therapy to alleviate severe TMJ inflammation and pain, both in generalized and localized types of arthritis (Choy et al., 2005). Systemic treatment with a combination of infliximab and methotrexate reduced TMJ pain in RA and increased anti-inflammatory cytokines in synovial fluid and blood plasma (Kopp et al., 2005). TMJ pain intensity at rest and on movement as well as tenderness to digital palpation of the TMJ (hyperalgesia/allodynia) decreased in parallel with global joint pain intensity, while TMJ pressure pain thresholds remained normal. Both erythrocyte sedimentation rate and C-reactive protein decreased, which indicates that the local improvement occurred together with reduced systemic inflammatory activity. Both local and global decrease of pain intensity probably resulted from the elimination of biologically active TNF-α (Charles et al., 1999). However, the reduction of TMJ pain was associated with raised synovial fluid levels of TNFsRII and IL-1sRII as well as raised plasma levels of IL-1ra and IL-10. This increase in anti-inflammatory cytokine and soluble receptor levels indicates that endogenous cytokine control mechanisms also influence the response to infliximab treatment.

The effect of systemic treatment with a combination of infliximab and methotrexate therefore seems to depend partly on an increase of anti-inflammatory cytokines and receptors in synovial fluid and blood plasma.

In about one-third of patients, systemic administration of infliximab and methotrexate has no effect or only minor effects on TMJ pain intensity (Kopp et al., 2006). The effect of infliximab on TMJ pain was predicted by pretreatment plasma levels of IL-1β, IL-1ra, and IL-10 and by pretreatment levels of TMJ synovial fluid IL-1sRII. High pretreatment levels of these cytokines and receptors as well as the presence of rheumatoid factor were associated with no or minor reduction of TMJ pain after treatment. This negative effect of IL-1β was independent of TNF-α because infliximab specifically inhibits TNF-α (van den Berg, 2001), and because the plasma level of IL-1β was unchanged during follow-up of treatment. In agreement with the results from the TMJ study, a high pretreatment level of IL-1β in the synovial fluid of the knee was a negative predictor for reduction of the number of tender and swollen joints after systemic treatment with a combination of infliximab and methotrexate (S. Kopp, P. Alstergren, S. Ernestam, S. Nordahl, and J. Bratt, unpublished data). Furthermore, a low pretreatment level of IL-1sRII in the knee synovial fluid was associated with a reduction in global pain intensity, and a low pretreatment level of IL-10 was associated with a reduced number of tender and swollen joints.

Local Treatment with Infliximab

A few case reports have been published about single intra-articular administration of infliximab into the knee joint in cases of persistent inflammation due to RA. Intra-articular administration of infliximab seems to be effective and safe in patients with persistent monoarthritis due to RA (Nikas et al., 2004) and ankylosing spondylitis (Schatteman et al., 2006), but opinions differ about the long-term outcome of the treatment and whether the effect is superior to intra-articular glucocorticosteroids (Bokarewa and Tarkowski, 2003).

There is one case report presenting the clinical and radiographic course of TMJ involvement in a patient with severe TMJ symptoms from psoriatic arthritis resistant to both systemic infliximab and intra-articular glucocorticoid. The patient received multiple bilateral intra-articular infliximab injections during 36 weeks. TMJ symptoms (pain and movement capacity) improved after the first injection and even more after the second injection. A considerable improvement remained after 36 weeks of follow-up (Alstergren et al., 2008).

Summary

TNF-α and IL-1-β are (at present) the most important cytokines known to be involved in the development and maintenance of musculoskeletal inflammation and pain. However, a balance between these proinflammatory cytokines and anti-inflammatory cytokines is essential for health and disease. In the future, more treatment modalities for chronic and severe musculoskeletal pain of inflammatory nature can be expected to be based on the use of cytokine agonists or antagonists.

References

Alstergren P, Ernberg M, Kopp S, Lundeberg T, Theodorsson E. TMJ pain in relation to circulating neuropeptide Y, serotonin and interleukin-1β in rheumatoid arthritis. J Orofac Pain 1999a;13:49–55.

Alstergren P, Ernberg M, Kvarnström M, Kopp S. Interleukin-1β in synovial fluid from the arthritic temporomandibular joint and its relation to pain, mobility and anterior open bite. J Oral Maxillofac Surg 1998;56:1059–1065.

Alstergren P, Kopp S, Theodorsson E. Synovial fluid sampling from the temporomandibular joint: sample quality criteria and levels of interleukin-1β and serotonin. Acta Odontol Scand 1999b;57:16–22.

Alstergren P, Larsson P, Kopp S. Successful treatment with multiple intraarticular injections of infliximab in a patient with psoriatic arthritis. Scand J Rheumatol 2008; 37:155–157.

Arend WP, Malyak M, Smith MF Jr, Whisenand TD, Slack JL, Sims JE, Giri JG, Dower SK. Binding of IL-1α, IL-1β and IL-1 receptor antagonist by soluble IL-1 receptors and levels of soluble IL-1 receptors in synovial fluids. J Immunol 1994;153:4766–4774.

Bankhurst AD. Etanercept and methotrexate combination therapy. Clin Exp Rheumatol 1999;17: S69–72.

Barbe MF, Barr AE. Inflammation and the pathophysiology of work-related musculoskeletal disorders. Brain Behav Immun 2006;20:423–429.

Beyaert R, Fiers W. Tumor necrosis factor and lymphotoxin. In: Mire-Sluis AR, Thorpe R, editors. Cytokines. London: Academic Press; 1998. p 335–360.

Bokarewa M, Tarkowski A. Local infusion of infliximab for the treatment of acute joint inflammation. Ann Rheum Dis 2003;62:783–784.

Bresnihan B, Alvaro-Gracia JM, Cobby M, et al. Treatment of rheumatoid arthritis with recombinant human interleukin-1 receptor antagonist. Arthritis Rheum 1998;41:2196–2204.

Carp SJ, Barbe MF, Winter KA, Amin M, Barr AE. Inflammatory biomarkers increase with severity of upper-extremity overuse disorders. Clin Sci (Lond) 2007;112:305–314.

Charles P, Elliott MJ, Davis D, Potter A, et al. Regulation of cytokines, cytokine inhibitors, and acute-phase proteins following anti-TNF-alpha therapy in rheumatoid arthritis. J Immunol 1999;163:1521–1528.

Choy EH, Smith C, Dore CJ, Scott DL. A meta-analysis of the efficacy and toxicity of combining disease-modifying anti-rheumatic drugs in rheumatoid arthritis based on patient withdrawal. Rheumatology (Oxford) 2005;44:1414–1421.

Chu CQ, Field M, Feldmann M, Maini RN. Localization of tumor necrosis factor alpha in synovial tissues and at the cartilage-pannus junction in patients with rheumatoid arthritis. Arthritis Rheum 1991;34:1125–1132.

Cunha TM, Verri WA Jr, Silva JS, Poole S, Cunha FQ, Ferreira SH. A cascade of cytokines mediates mechanical inflammatory hypernociception in mice. Proc Natl Acad Sci USA 2005;102:1755–1760.

Dawson J, Engelhardt P, Kastelic T, Cheneval D, MacKenzie A, Ramage P. Effects of soluble interleukin-1 type II receptor on rabbit antigen-induced arthritis: clinical, biochemical and histological assessment. Rheumatology (Oxford) 1999;38:401–406.

Di Giovine FS, Nuki G, Duff GW. Tumour necrosis factor in synovial exudates. Ann Rheum Dis 1988;47:768–772.

Dinarello CA. Interleukin-1. Dig Dis Sci 1988;33:25S–35S.

Dinarello CA. The biological properties of interleukin-1. Eur Cytokine Netw 1994;5:517–531.

Dinarello CA. Biologic basis for interleukin-1 in disease. Blood 1996;87:2095–2147.

Eastgate JA, Symons JA, Wood NC, Grinlinton FM, di Giovine FS, Duff GW. Correlation of plasma interleukin 1 levels with disease activity in rheumatoid arthritis. Lancet 1988;ii:706–709.

Elliot M, Maini RN, Feldmann M, et al. Treatment of rheumatoid arthritis with chimeric monoclonal antibodies to tumor necrosis factor α. Arthritis Rheum 1993;36:1681–1690.

Fang PK, Ma XC, Ma DL, Fu KY. Determination of interleukin-1 receptor antagonist, interleukin-10, and transforming growth factor-beta1 in synovial fluid aspirates of patients with temporomandibular disorders. J Oral Maxillofac Surg 1999;57:922–929.

Feldmann M, Brennan FM, Field M, Maini RN. Pathogenesis of rheumatoid arthritis: cellular and cytokine interactions. In: Smolen JS, Kalden JR, Maini RN, editors. Rheumatoid arthritis. Berlin: Springer-Verlag; 1992. p 41–54.

Ferreira SH, Lorenzetti BB, Bristow AF, Poole S. Interleukin-1 beta as a potent hyperalgesic agent antagonized by a tripeptide analogue. Nature 1988;334:698–700.

Fredriksson L, Alstergren P, Kopp S. Tumor necrosis factor alpha in temporomandibular joint synovial fluid predicts treatment effects on pain by intra-articular glucocorticoid treatment. Mediators Inflamm 2006;6:1–7.

Fukuoka H, Kawatani M, Hisamitsu T, Takeshige C. Cutaneous hyperalgesia induced by peripheral injection of interleukin-1β in the rat. Brain Res 1994;657:133–140.

Hao S, Mata M, Glorioso JC, Fink DJ. HSV-mediated expression of interleukin-4 in dorsal root ganglion neurons reduces neuropathic pain. Mol Pain 2006;2:6.

Hoheisel U, Unger T, Mense S. Excitatory and modulatory effects of inflammatory cytokines and neurotrophins on mechanosensitive group IV muscle afferents in the rat. Pain 2005;114:168–176.

Holt I, Cooper RG, Denton J, Meager A, Hopkins SJ. Cytokine inter-relationships and their association with disease activity in arthritis. Br J Rheumatol 1992;31:725–733.

Inglis JJ, Nissim A, Lees DM, Hunt SP, Chernajovsky Y, Kidd BL. The differential contribution of tumour necrosis factor to thermal and mechanical hyperalgesia during chronic inflammation. Arthritis Res Ther 2005;7:R807–816.

Jeanjean AP, Moussaoui SM, Maloteaux JM, Laduron PM. Interleukin-1 beta induces long-term increase of axonally transported opiate receptors and substance P. Neurosci 1995;68:151–157.

Jouvenne P, Vannier E, Dinarello CA, Miossec P. Elevated levels of soluble interleukin-1 receptor type II and interleukin-1 receptor antagonist in patients with chronic arthritis: correlations with markers of inflammation and joint destruction. Arthritis Rheum 1998;41:1083–1089.

Junger H, Sorkin LS. Nociceptive and inflammatory effects of subcutaneous TNF-alpha. Pain 2000;85:145–151.

Kopp S, Alstergren P, Ernestam S, Nordahl S, Bratt J. Interleukin-1beta influenced the effect of inflix-
    imab on temporomandibular joint pain in rheumatoid arthritis. Scand J Rheumatol 2006;35:182–
    188.
Kopp S, Alstergren P, Ernestam S, Nordahl S, Morin P, Bratt J. Reduction of temporomandibular
    joint pain after treatment with a combination of methotrexate and infliximab is associated with
    changes in synovial fluid and plasma cytokines in rheumatoid arthritis. Cells Tissues Organs
    2005;180:22–30.
Kopp S, Sommer C. Inflammatory mediators in temporomandibular joint pain. In: Türp JC, Sommer
    C, Hugger A, editors. The puzzle of orofacial pain: integrating research into clinical manage-
    ment. Pain and Headache, Vol. 15. Basel: Karger; 2007. p. 28–43.
Lipsky PE, van der Heijde DM, St Clair EW, et al. Anti-tumor necrosis factor trial in rheumatoid
    arthritis with concomitant therapy study group. infliximab and methotrexate in the treatment of
    rheumatoid arthritis. anti-tumor necrosis factor trial in rheumatoid arthritis with concomitant
    therapy study group. N Engl J Med 2000;343:1594–1602.
Loram LC, Fuller A, Fick LG, Cartmell T, Poole S, Mitchell D. Cytokine profiles during carrageenan-
    induced inflammatory hyperalgesia in rat muscle and hind paw. J Pain 2007;8:127–136.
Lundberg IE. The role of cytokines, chemokines, and adhesion molecules in the pathogenesis of id-
    iopathic inflammatory myopathies. Curr Rheumatol Rep 2000;2:216–224.
McNearney T, Baethge BA, Cao S, Alam R, Lisse JR, Westlund KN. Excitatory amino acids, TNF-
    alpha, and chemokine levels in synovial fluids of patients with active arthropathies. Clin Exp Im-
    munol 2004;137:621–627.
Nicolas P, Tod M, Padoin C, Petitjean O. Clinical pharmacokinetics of diacerein. Clin Pharmacokinet
    1998;35:347–359.
Nikas SN, Temekonidis TI, Zikou AK, Argyropoulou MI, Efremidis S, Drosos AA. Treatment of re-
    sistant rheumatoid arthritis by intra-articular infliximab injections: a pilot study. Ann Rheum
    Dis 2004;63:102–103.
Nordahl S, Alstergren P, Kopp S. Tumor necrosis factor α in synovial fluid and plasma from patients
    with chronic connective tissue disease and its relation to temporomandibular joint pain. J Oral
    Maxillofac Surg 2000;58:525–530.
Özaktay AC, Kallakuri S, Takebayashi T, Cavanaugh JM, Asik I, DeLeo JA, Weinstein JN. Effects of
    interleukin-1 beta, interleukin-6, and tumor necrosis factor on sensitivity of dorsal root ganglion
    and peripheral receptive fields in rats. Eur Spine J 2006;15:1529–1537.
Partsch G, Steiner G, Leeb BF, Dunky A, Broll H, Smolen JS. Highly increased levels of tumor ne-
    crosis factor-alpha and other proinflammatory cytokines in psoriatic arthritis synovial fluid. J
    Rheumatol 1997;24:518–523.
Pickering M, Cumiskey D, O'Connor JJ. Actions of TNF-alpha on glutamatergic synaptic transmis-
    sion in the central nervous system. Exp Physiol 2005;90:663–670.
Poole S, Cunha FQ, Selkirk S, Lorenzetti BB, Ferreira SH. Cytokine-mediated inflammatory hyperal-
    gesia limited by interleukin-10. Br J Pharmacol 1995;115:684–688.
Rice TL, Chantler I, Loram LC. Neutralization of muscle tumour necrosis factor alpha does not at-
    tenuate exercise-induced muscle pain but does improve muscle strength in healthy male volun-
    teers. Br J Sports Med 2007;Aug 23.
Rooney M, Symons JA, Duff GW. Interleukin 1 beta in synovial fluid is related to local disease activ-
    ity in rheumatoid arthritis. Rheumatol Int 1990;10:217–219.
Ruschen S, Lemm G, Warnatz H. Spontaneous and LPS-stimulated production of intracellular IL-1
    beta by synovial macrophages in rheumatoid arthritis is inhibited by IFN-gamma. Clin Exp Im-
    munol 1989;76:246–251.
Sandler NA, Buckley MJ, Cillo JE, Braun TW. Correlation of inflammatory cytokines with ar-
    throscopic findings in patients with temporomandibular joint internal derangements. J Oral
    Maxillofac Surg 1998;56:534–543.
Schäfers M, Sorkin LS, Sommer C. Intramuscular injection of tumor necrosis factor-alpha induces
    muscle hyperalgesia in rats. Pain 2003;104:579–588.
Schatteman L, Gyselbrecht L, De Clercq L, Mielants H. Treatment of refractory inflammatory
    monoarthritis in ankylosing spondylitis by intraarticular injection of infliximab. J Rheumatol
    2006;33:82–85.

Shah JP, Phillips TM, Danoff JV, Gerber LH. An in vivo microanalytical technique for measuring the local biochemical milieu of human skeletal muscle. J Appl Physiol 2005;99:1977–1984.

Shinoda C, Takaku S. Interleukin-1 beta, interleukin-6, and tissue inhibitor of metalloproteinase-1 in the synovial fluid of the temporomandibular joint with respect to cartilage destruction. Oral Dis 2000;6:383–390.

Sommer C, Kress M. Recent findings on how proinflammatory cytokines cause pain: peripheral mechanisms in inflammatory and neuropathic hyperalgesia. Neurosci Lett 2004;361:184–187.

Sorkin LS, Xiao WH, Wagner R, Myers RR. Tumour necrosis factor-alpha induces ectopic activity in nociceptive primary afferent fibers. Neuroscience 1997;81:255–262.

Takahashi T, Kondoh T, Fukuda M, Yamazaki Y, Toyosaki T, Suzuki R. Proinflammatory cytokines detectable in synovial fluids from patients with temporomandibular disorders. Oral Surg Oral Med Oral Pathol Oral Radiol Endod 1998;85:135–141.

Takeuchi H, Jin S, Wang J, Zhang G, Kawanokuchi J, Kuno R, Sonobe Y, Mizuno T, Suzumura A. Tumor necrosis factor-alpha induces neurotoxicity via glutamate release from hemichannels of activated microglia in an autocrine manner. J Biol Chem 2006;281:21362–21368.

Tominaga K, Habu M, Sukedai M, Hirota Y, Takahashi T, Fukuda J. IL-1 beta, IL-1 receptor antagonist and soluble type II IL-1 receptor in synovial fluid of patients with temporomandibular disorders. Arch Oral Biol 2004;49:493–499.

Tracey KJ. Physiology and immunology of the cholinergic antiinflammatory pathway. J Clin Invest 2007;117:289–296.

van den Berg WB. Anti-cytokine therapy in chronic destructive arthritis. Arthritis Res 2001;3:18–26.

Verbruggen G, Veys EM, Malfait AM, De Clerq L, Van den Bosch F, de Vlam K. Influence of human recombinant interleukin 1beta on human articular cartilage. Mitotic activity and proteoglycan metabolism. Clin Exp Rheumatol 1991;9:481–488.

Wagner R, Janjigian M, Myers RR. Anti-inflammatory interleukin-10 therapy in CCI neuropathy decreases thermal hyperalgesia, macrophage recruitment, and endoneurial TNF-alpha expression. Pain 1998;74:35–42.

Wallace DJ, Linker-Israeli M, Hallegua D, Silverman S, Silver D, Weisman MH. Cytokines play an aetiopathogenic role in fibromyalgia: a hypothesis and pilot study. Rheumatology (Oxford) 2001;40:743–749.

Watkins LR, Goehler LE, Relton J, Brewer MT, Maier SF. Mechanisms of tumor necrosis factor-alpha (TNF-alpha) hyperalgesia. Brain Res 1995;692:244–250.

Watkins LR, Wiertelak EP, Goehler LE, Smith KP, Martin D, Maier SF. Characterization of cytokine-induced hyperalgesia. Brain Res 1994;654:15–26.

Woolf CJ, Allchorne A, Safieh-Garabedian B, Poole S. Cytokines, nerve growth factor and inflammatory hyperalgesia: the contribution of tumor necrosis factor alpha. Br J Pharmacol 1997;121:417–424.

Correspondence to: Professor Sigvard Kopp, DDS, PhD, Department of Clinical Oral Physiology, Institute of Odontology, Karolinska Institutet, 14104 Huddinge, Sweden. Email: sigvard.kopp@ki.se.

Serotonergic Receptor Involvement in Muscle Pain and Hyperalgesia

Malin Ernberg

*Department of Clinical Oral Physiology, Institute of Odontology,
Karolinska Institutet, Huddinge, Sweden*

This chapter describes the current knowledge of the role of serotonin (5-HT) in muscle pain and hyperalgesia, focusing on 5-HT receptor involvement in human pain mediation and modulation.

Serotonin

Serotonin, or 5-hydroxytryptamine (5-HT), is a member of the monoamine family. This small molecule (molecular weight 176.2 Da) exerts a range of biological effects in the human body and modulates physiological processes in both the central and peripheral nervous systems. It is synthesized both peripherally and in the central nervous system (CNS) from the essential amino acid tryptophan, which is derived from the diet (Hindle, 1994). Peripherally, 5-HT (90%) is found in the enterochromaffin cells of the small intestines, in enteric neurons, and in mast cells and platelets. There is also a small unbound portion (less than 5%) in the blood. In the CNS, 5 HT is found in serotonergic neurons, including those in the nucleus raphe magnus (NRM).

Peripherally, 5-HT is released from its neural stores and platelets following tissue trauma or inflammation. Tissue trauma may cause
a direct release of 5-HT due to disruption of blood vessels and neurons,
but it may also lead to an indirect release of 5-HT due to production of
pro-inflammatory vasodilative substances such as arachidonic acid, prostaglandins, and cytokines (Giordano and Schultea, 2004; Coutaux et al.,
2005). The released 5-HT then exerts its biological effects by acting on
several receptors that are distributed throughout the human body. The
effects of 5-HT are terminated by reuptake that is mediated through 5-
HT binding to a specific 5-HT transporter (SERT) and through metabolism. SERT has been identified on platelets, on presynaptic nerve terminals, and on endothelial cells (Brenner et al., 2007). SERT has also been
found on the endothelial cells that make up the blood-brain barrier , suggesting that it plays a role in the inactivation of 5-HT from brain paren-
chyma into endothelial cells, and also that it mediates the uptake of 5-HT
from the circulating blood (Wakayama et al., 2002). This finding refutes
the previous belief that 5-HT cannot pass through the blood-brain barrier.

Serotonin and Pain Transduction

The involvement of 5-HT in pain processing is well known. Peripherally, it seems to act as a pronociceptive substance (Giordano and Schultea, 2004), both by direct activation of peripheral afferents and also by
the release of other mediators, such as substance P (SP) and glutamate
(Saria et al., 1990). 5-HT also sensitizes peripheral mechanoreceptive afferent fibers to other chemicals by enhancing the efficiency of tetrodotoxin (TTX)-resistant sodium channels and by lowering the threshold
of the vanilloid receptor (TRPV1), which results in primary hyperalgesia
(Coutaux et al., 2005).

It has long been acknowledged that centrally, 5-HT has analgesic actions as part of the descending endogenous pain-inhibitory system.
Large quantities of 5-HT are found in the NRM, and stimulation of this
area releases 5-HT, activating inhibitory interneurons and thus inhibiting
pain transduction (Sommer, 2006). However, recent research suggests

that 5-HT has both anti- and pronociceptive effects in the endogenous pain-inhibitory system, depending on which receptor it activates (Suzuki et al., 2004). It is now believed that tonic activation of central 5-HT neurons that mediate facilitatory responses may contribute to central sensitization in chronic pain conditions (Porreca et al., 2002).

Effects of 5-HT on Muscle Pain and Hyperalgesia

Several studies have investigated the effect of peripheral administration of 5-HT on muscle pain and allodynia. Injection of 5-HT (0.1–10 mM) into the rat masseter muscle dose-dependently increased afferent discharge, but did not affect mechanical pain threshold (Sung et al., 2008). In humans, one study found that 5-HT (10 µM) injected into the temporalis muscle did not affect pain or pressure pain threshold (PPT), whereas a combination of 5-HT (5 µM) and bradykinin induced pain and reduced PPT (Jensen et al., 1990). Another study reported that injection of 5-HT (4–40 µM) into the tibialis anterior muscle induced mild pain, but did not affect PPT (Babenko et al., 1999a). However, a combination of 5-HT (20 nM) and bradykinin induced even more pain and also reduced PPT (Babenko et al., 1999b). Injection of 5-HT (1 mM) into the masseter muscle induced pain and reduced PPT (Ernberg et al., 2000a). The discrepancy in the results can probably be attributed to the different concentrations of 5-HT used in the studies, but it may also be caused by anatomical or physiological differences between the muscles. Gender differences offer a third explanation, given that such differences have been reported for intramuscular injection of glutamate into the masseter muscle (Svensson et al., 2003). In the two former studies, all subjects were men (Jensen et al., 1990; Babenko et al., 1999a,b), whereas only women participated in the latter study (Ernberg et al., 2000a).

Patients with fibromyalgia are reported to show decreased cerebrospinal fluid (CSF) levels of 5-hydroxyindoleacetic acid (5-HIAA) (Russell et al., 1992b; Legangneux et al., 2001) and reduced serum levels of 5-HT (Russell et al., 1992a). Reduced serum levels of 5-HT, which may mirror levels in the CNS (Bianchi et al., 2002), were positively correlated to hyperalgesia in fibromyalgia and localized craniofacial myalgia (Ernberg et al., 1999). In patients with fibromyalgia, researchers have found a negative correlation between plasma tryptophan and the level of pain (Moldofsky and Warsh, 1978), as well as a reduced level of plasma tryptophan and a decreased transport ratio of tryptophan across the blood-brain barrier (Yunus et al., 1992). Together, these results suggest that descending pain inhibition may be disturbed due to reduced central 5-HT in chronic muscle pain states, perhaps as a consequence of an interaction between 5-HT and SP (Yunus et al., 1992). This suggestion is supported by findings of elevated levels of SP in the CSF of patients with fibromyalgia (Vaerøy et al., 1988; Russell et al., 1994). A possible explanation for the reduced 5-HT in the CNS is enhanced reuptake of 5-HT, given that platelet [^{3}H]-imipramine binding was reported to be increased in fibromyalgia patients (Russell et al., 1992a). However, another study could not confirm this finding (Legangneux et al., 2001).

The Serotonin Receptor Family

The first classification of 5-HT receptors was described in the 1950s. At that time two receptors were identified, the D receptor and the M receptor. The classification was later revised when studies using radioligand binding identified 5-HT$_1$ and 5-HT$_2$ receptors. It then became apparent that these receptors were not identical to the D and M receptors (Hindle, 1994).

Currently, seven 5-HT receptor classes have been identified (5-HT$_{1-7}$). Within these classes, several receptor subclasses have been identified (5-HT$_{1A-B, D-F}$, 5-HT$_{2A-C}$, 5-HT$_{3A-B,}$ and 5-HT$_{5A-B}$) (Boess and Martin, 1994). The 5-HT$_{2C}$ receptor was primarily classified as 5-HT$_{1C}$, but due to its sequence and functional similarity with the 5-HT$_2$ receptors it has been reclassified. The majority of 5-HT receptors are linked to a G protein and affect neuronal activity through a second messenger, but the 5-HT$_3$ receptor is a ligand-gated ion channel.

Serotonin Receptors Involved in Pain Transduction and Modulation

Identification of 5-HT$_{1-4}$ and 5-HT$_7$ receptors peripherally on sensory afferent nerves and in dorsal root ganglia points to a possible role of these receptors in pain transduction (Sommer, 2006). Most of these receptors are pronociceptive in the periphery. For example, the nociceptive response to intraplantar injections of 5-HT in rats increased with higher concentrations of 5-HT and was blocked by 5-HT$_1$, 5-HT$_2$, and 5-HT$_3$ receptor antagonists (Sufka et al., 1992). The hypothetical influence of 5-HT on muscle pain mediation and modulation is shown in Fig. 1.

Pharmacological tests in animal experiments indicate that the 5-HT$_{1A}$ receptor mediates peripheral hyperalgesia to chemical (inflammatory) and thermal stimuli (Sufka et al., 1992; Taiwo and Levine, 1992). However, 5-HT$_{1B/D}$ receptors are reported to reduce neurogenic inflammation and thus may reduce pain (Sommer, 2006).

The 5-HT$_{2A}$ receptor seems to be involved in peripheral thermal and chemical hyperalgesia. Intraplantar injection of 5-HT and the 5-HT$_2$ agonist α-methyl-5-HT in rats induced behavioral signs of pain that were attenuated by the 5-HT$_{2A}$ antagonists ketanserin, ritanserin, and spiperone (Abbott et al., 1996). Similarly, intradermal injection of 5-HT and α-methyl-5-HT into the rat hindpaw increased thermal hyperalgesia, which was attenuated by ketanserin (Tokunaga et al., 1998). Both primary thermal hyperalgesia and secondary mechanical allodynia were attenuated by the 5-HT$_{2A}$ antagonist sarpogrelate (Sasaki et al., 2006). In 5-HT$_{2A}$ mutant mice, a dramatic increase of the late-phase formalin-induced nociceptive response was reported compared to wild-type mice (Kayser et al., 2007). Intravenous administration of ketanserin in patients with complex regional pain syndrome reduced pain during exercise, but did not relieve pain at rest (Moesker, 2000). The author found a positive effect on pain at rest and upon movement as well as an increase in skin temperature after long-term treatment.

Several animal reports indicate that peripheral 5-HT$_3$ receptors mediate inflammatory pain. An early study reported that 5-HT$_3$ antagonists

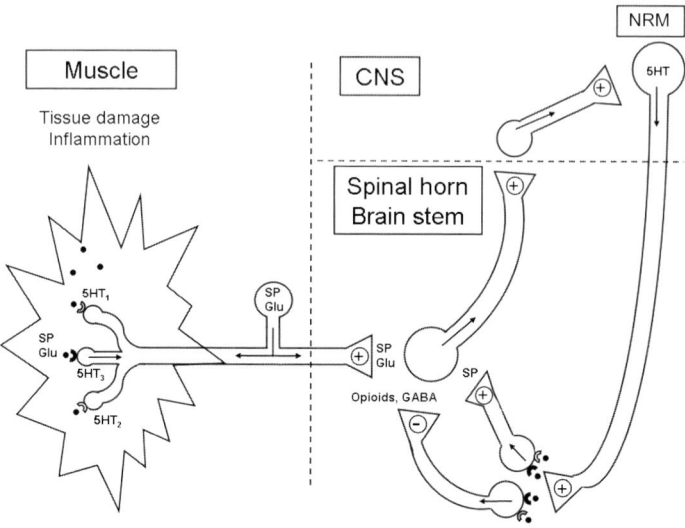

Fig. 1. Hypothetical influence of serotonin (5-HT) on muscle pain mediation and modulation. The figure is simplified, and central 5-HT receptor mechanisms are not shown. Tissue trauma or inflammation releases 5-HT from platelets and damaged neurons. Serotonin may also be released secondary to release of neuropeptides, causing vasodilation and plasma extravasation, which in turn leads to the production of interleukins and causes platelet degradation. The liberated 5-HT activates receptors on peripheral afferents (5-HT$_3$, and possibly 5-HT$_1$ and 5-HT$_2$). Activation of these receptors depolarizes the afferent fiber and leads to the release of glutamate (GLU) and substance P (SP) from the central terminals of the afferent fiber onto second-order neurons in the spinal cord dorsal horn or trigeminal sensory nucleus to propagate the pain signal to the central nervous system (CNS). Under certain circumstances, SP and GLU may also be transported antidromically and released from the peripheral nerve terminal. Centrally, serotonergic descending pathways from the nucleus raphe magnus (NRM) are activated to release 5-HT, which activates 5-HT receptors located on interneurons containing endogenous opioids (enkephalins and dynorphins) or gamma-aminobutyric acid (GABA), thus inhibiting nociception. Serotonin from the endogenous system may also activate excitatory interneurons to enhance nociception.

reduced behavioral effects in acute inflammation induced by complete Freund's adjuvant (CFA), but was even more effective in reducing behavioral effects to chronic inflammation induced by formalin (Giordano and Rogers, 1989). In 5-HT$_3$ knockout mice, no difference was found compared to wild-type mice in acute thermal, inflammatory, or mechanical nociception or in mechanical allodynia as a result of CFA administration or partial nerve ligation. However, there was a difference in the response to chronic inflammation (late-phase formalin test), which was attenuated by the 5-HT_3 antagonist ondansetron (Zeitz et al., 2002). In contrast, another study reported that nociceptive responses to intraplantar injection of 5-HT were reduced by ondansetron (Sufka et al., 1992). 5-HT_3 antagonists also reduce inflammatory pain by diminishing 5-HT-induced release of SP (Giordano and Schultea, 2004). In humans, 5-HT applied to a blister caused pain that was attenuated by a 5-HT_3 antagonist (Richardson et al., 1985), and topical administration of ondansetron reduced inflammatory pain induced by intradermal capsaicin (Giordano et al., 1998).

Peripheral 5-HT_4 receptors seem to reduce visceral nociception, given that the 5-HT_4 agonist tegaserod reduces the response to colonic distension (Greenwood-Van Meerveld et al., 2004). The role peripheral 5-HT_7 receptors play in pain mediation is unclear, but one study suggests that they may be involved in migraine headache (Terron, 2002). Another study reported that a 5-HT_7 antagonist reduced 5-HT-induced knee joint nociception (Meuser et al., 2002).

As mentioned previously, 5-HT at spinal and central levels may be both anti- and pronociceptive (Fig. 1). Stimulation of 5-HT_{1A} receptors in the spinal cord seems to inhibit nociceptive transduction (Hains et al., 2003). These receptors are also reported to be involved in opioid-mediated analgesia (Liu et al., 2002). In contrast, 5-HT_{2A} receptors at the spinal level are reported to increase nociception, an effect that may be related to release of SP from presynaptic terminals (Honda et al., 2006).

Spinal 5-HT_3 receptors are reported to be antinociceptive and to reduce hyperexcitability after spinal cord hemisection (Hains et al., 2003), but they are also reported to enhance nociception (Zeitz et al., 2002), depending on whether excitatory or inhibitory interneurons are activated (Fig. 1).

5-HT Receptors and Muscle Pain

Of the few studies that have tested the effect of 5-HT antagonists on muscle pain, the vast majority have used a 5-HT_3 antagonist (Table I). However, one study in humans reported no effect of intramuscular injection

Table I

Studies that have investigated the effect of 5-HT antagonists for muscle pain and hyperalgesia

Receptor	Subj.	N	Study Type	Antagonist	Dose	Route	Reference
Mechanical Allodynia							
5-HT$_3$	HI	20	R, C, DB, CO	Granisetron	2 mg/day, 3 days	oral	Christidis et al. 2005
5-HT$_3$	HI	24	R, C, DB	Granisetron	1 mg, single dose	i.m.	Christidis et al. 2007
Experimental Pain and Hyperalgesia							
5-HT-Induced							
5-HT$_{1A/B}$	HI	24	R, C, DB	Propranolol#	0.2 mg, single dose	i.m.	Ernberg et al. 2000b
5-HT$_3$	HI	24	R, C, DB	Granisetron	0.2 mg, single dose		Ernberg et al. 2000b
Hypertonic Saline-Induced							
5-HT$_3$	HI	30	R, C, DB	Granisetron	0.5 mg, single dose		Christidis et al., unpubl.
Clinical Pain and Hyperalgesia							
5-HT$_3$	FM	18	R, C, DB	Granisetron	1 mg, single dose	i.m.	Ernberg et al. 2003
5-HT$_3$	FM	10	open	Tropisetron	5 mg/day, 4 weeks	oral	Papadopoulos et al. 2000
5-HT$_3$	FM	30	open	Tropisetron	5 mg/day, 4 weeks	oral	Haus et al. 2000
5-HT$_3$	FM	21	R, C, DB, CO	Ondansetron	16 mg/day, 5 days	oral	Hrycaj et al 1996
5-HT$_3$	FM	418	R, C, DB	Tropisetron	5, 10, or 15 mg/day, 10 days	oral	Färber et al. 2001
5-HT$_3$	FM	21	R, C, DB	Tropisetron	2 mg, 5 days	i.v.	Späth et al. 2004
5-HT$_3$	LM	18	R, C, DB	Granisetron	1 mg, single dose	i.m.	Christidis et al. 2007
5-HT$_3$	LM	12	open	Tropisetron	5 mg x 1–2, TrP	i.m.	Stratz and Müller 2004
5-HT$_3$	LM	20	open	Tropisetron	5 mg, multiple doses, TrP	i.m.	Ettlin 2005
5-HT$_3$	LM	33	R, C, DB	Tropisetron	5 mg, single dose, TrP	i.m.	Müller and Stratz 2005

Abbreviations C = controlled, CO = crossover, DB = double blind, FM = fibromyalgia, HI = healthy individuals, i.m = intramuscular, i.v. = intravenous, LM = localized myalgia, R = randomized, TrP = trigger point.
A nonselective antagonist that is also an adrenergic receptor antagonist.

of the nonselective $5\text{-HT}_{1A/B}$ antagonist propranolol into the masseter muscle on 5-HT-induced pain or allodynia in healthy subjects (Ernberg et al., 2000b).

A recent study investigated the presence of 5-HT_3 receptors in trigeminal ganglion cells from masticatory afferent fibers and their role in muscle nociception and hyperalgesia (Sung et al., 2008). The authors found that 52% of the cell bodies expressed 5-HT_3 receptors. Further, afferent discharge induced by intramuscular injection of 5-HT and the 5-HT_3 agonist 2-methyl-5-HT into the masseter muscle was reduced by tropisetron.

The 5-HT_3 receptor may further be involved in determining the mechanical pain threshold of muscles, given that oral granisetron increased PPT over healthy muscles (Christidis et al., 2005). However, the effect of granisetron differed among muscles, with a significant increase of PPT in the trapezius and anterior tibialis muscles, but not in the masseter or anterior temporalis muscles. On the other hand, intramuscular injection of granisetron into the masseter muscle of healthy subjects increased PPT significantly more than did normal saline (Christidis et al., 2007). The difference between these two studies with respect to the masseter muscle may be attributed to a difference in dose. Recently, we investigated the effect of granisetron on muscle pain induced by hypertonic saline in a randomized and double-blind study in 30 healthy subjects (Christidis et al., unpublished data). Subjects received simultaneous injection (0.2 mL) with hypertonic saline (5.8%) into the masseter muscles after pretreatment (2 minutes prior to injection) with granisetron on one side and isotonic saline on the other. We found that pretreatment with granisetron significantly reduced pain and increased PPT compared with isotonic saline.

Several studies have investigated the role of 5-HT_3 antagonists in clinical muscle pain (Table I). Some of these studies were randomized controlled trials (RCTs). In a treatment trial in fibromyalgia patients, oral tropisetron reduced pain score, tender point count, fatigue, and sleep disturbances in 50% of the patients (Papadopoulos et al., 2000). In another study in fibromyalgia patients, oral tropisetron reduced pain intensity on a visual analogue scale (VAS) and pain score (sum of pain on a 0–5-

point scale for 24 body regions) in 72% of the patients (Haus et al., 2000). Ondansetron also significantly reduced VAS pain intensity, pain score, tender point score, PPT, and functional symptoms (e.g., sleep disturbances and anxiety) in fibromyalgia (Hrycaj et al., 1996). Half of the patients were responders. Serum 5-HT increased significantly for the whole group, but this increase was due to an increase in the nonresponders.

Finally, in a large-scale multicenter study comprising fibromyalgia patients, 5 mg oral tropisetron significantly decreased VAS pain intensity and pain score as well as tender point count (although with only a minor decrease of 7.4%) and ancillary symptoms in 39.2% of the patients. Tropisetron at 10 mg had less effect, while 15 mg had no effect (Färber et al., 2001). Blood levels of dopamine, norepinephrine, epinephrine, and serotonin did not differ between the patients and age- and sex-matched healthy controls, but patients with reduced serum serotonin level or elevated dopamine levels tended to show a higher response rate (Höcherl et al., 2000). Adverse events (mostly constipation) were frequent, but were mostly mild to moderate. The authors concluded that short-term treatment of fibromyalgia with tropisetron 5 mg was efficacious and well-tolerated. Further, patients who responded to tropisetron were followed up to 12 months. Although pain intensity increased within 1 month after treatment, it was still reduced 12 months after treatment compared to before treatment (Färber et al., 2000).

Intravenous tropisetron has also been shown to be effective for fibromyalgia in a few studies. A placebo-controlled study reported that VAS pain scores decreased significantly more after tropisetron than after placebo (Späth et al., 2004). The same research group investigated the effect of intravenous tropisetron on serum SP levels in fibromyalgia patients (Stratz et al., 2004). Patients who considered that they were "clearly better" or "better" (responders) showed higher serum SP levels before treatment than those who considered themselves to be "unchanged" or "worse" (nonresponders), although not significantly. The SP level was decreased directly after the first injection and was still lower before the last injection compared to baseline in the responders, but it did not change significantly after the last injection. The nonresponders had no significant changes in serum SP levels. The authors concluded that more extensive studies are needed to verify these results. To date, no such study has been published.

Several studies have used local administration of 5-HT$_3$ antagonists to treat muscle pain conditions. One study did not show any effect of intramuscular administration of granisetron on masseter muscle pain and hyperalgesia (assessed as PPT) in patients with fibromyalgia (Ernberg et al., 2003). In contrast, there was an increase in pain after both granisetron and placebo, with a greater increase with placebo. However, the patients who showed an increase of PPT after granisetron had a lower increase in pain with granisetron compared to saline. In patients with low back myofascial pain, on the other hand, one study reported that one or two intramuscular trigger-point injections of tropisetron significantly decreased VAS pain ratings (by 35.7%). No side effects were reported, with the exception of short-term burning pain at the injection site (Stratz and Müller, 2005).

Trigger-point injections with tropisetron have also been used in patients with whiplash-associated pain in the head and neck region (Ettlin, 2004). An average of 15 trigger-points were injected with tropisetron (0.5–1 mL) at each session. Treatment was repeated an average 1 week after pain renewal. Each trigger point received a maximum of five injections, and a total of 73 sessions were performed. In 84% of the sessions, more than 50% pain reduction was achieved. The duration of pain relief was more than 2 weeks in 52% of the sessions and more than 2 months in 10%. However, there was great intra- and interindividual variation in treatment effect.

Finally, in another study, tropisetron was compared with prilocaine for treatment of myofascial pain in the neck shoulder region (Müller and Stratz, 2005). Pain was assessed on a VAS before and 3 hours after treatment and then daily for 7 days. If symptoms improved, the patient was followed weekly for 3 months. VAS pain decreased significantly after tropisetron, while it decreased nonsignificantly after prilocaine. The response rate (reduction of pain by at least 30% 3 hours after injections) was 53% in the group that received tropisetron and 50% in the prilocaine group. Seven days after treatment, the pain had decreased even further in the patients who responded to tropisetron.

Future Perspectives and Conclusion

Increasing evidence shows that 5-HT has an impact on muscle pain and hyperalgesia. Several 5-HT receptors might be involved at spinal and higher central levels, and drugs that target central 5-HT receptors are thus of interest. Among these are the selective serotonin reuptake inhibitors (SSRIs), which are reported to exert their effects by blocking the 5-HT transporter SERT, thus increasing the amount of 5-HT in the synaptic cleft. However, recent studies suggest that SSRIs also bind directly to 5-HT$_{2A/C}$ receptors and perhaps also 5-HT$_7$ receptors, thereby blocking the pain signal, and that this effect may be more potent than the effect on SERT (Dempsey et al., 2005; Honda et al., 2006). On the other hand, the SSRIs seem to be less effective in reducing chronic pain than amitriptyline, which inhibits the reuptake of both 5-HT and norepinephrine.

Given that animal experiments indicate that peripheral 5-HT$_2$ and 5-HT$_1$ receptors mediate pain, drugs that target these receptors (and perhaps also 5-HT$_4$ and 5-HT$_7$ receptors) might be interesting for treatment of clinical muscle pain. However, this approach has not been investigated. On the other hand, 5-HT$_2$ and 5-HT$_1$ receptors seem to be involved mainly in (superficial) chemical and thermal hyperalgesia, which indicates that such drugs may not be effective for muscle pain. Experimental and clinical studies are needed before a clinical role for these receptors in peripheral pain mediation can be excluded.

Among the 5-HT receptors, the 5-HT$_3$ receptor seems to be specifically important for pain mediation in the periphery. Antagonists to this receptor may therefore be promising new analgesics for treatment of muscle pain. A few 5-HT$_3$ antagonists are used clinically to treat chemotherapy- and radiotherapy-induced emesis, including ondansetron, tropisetron, granisetron, and alosetron (Hindle, 1994). These drugs freely penetrate the blood-brain barrier, and by blocking central 5-HT$_3$ receptors in the area postrema, hippocampus, and limbic regions of the brain, they efficiently reduce emesis and anxiety. These drugs are now also used for nausea and vomiting induced by general anesthesia. Although they all block the 5-HT$_3$ receptor, they have a somewhat different pharmacological profile and affinity to the receptor. Granisetron is reported to have an effect that is equivalent to or better than that of ondansetron and tropisetron and is specific to the 5-HT$_3$ receptor, whereas ondansetron and tropisetron also show affinity for the 5-HT$_4$ receptor (Gyermek, 1996). Although the side effects are mostly mild, constipation occurs frequently. These drugs may be of specific value for local treatment of chronic myalgia. However, large-scale RCTs are needed before any firm conclusions can be drawn regarding their efficacy.

In conclusion, the 5-HT$_1$, 5-HT$_2$, and especially the 5-HT$_3$ receptor may be involved in muscle pain and hyperalgesia, and drugs that target these receptors might offer an additional treatment approach.

References

Abbott FV, Hong Y, Blier P. Activation of 5-HT2A receptors potentiates pain produced by inflammatory mediators. Neuropharmacology 1996;35:99–110.

Babenko V, Graven-Nielsen T, Svensson P, Drewes AM, Jensen TS, Arendt-Nielsen L. Experimental human muscle pain induced by intramuscular injections of bradykinin, serotonin, and substance P. Eur J Pain 1999a;3:93–102.

Babenko V, Graven-Nielsen T, Svensson P, Drewes AM, Jensen TS, Arendt-Nielsen L. Experimental human muscle pain and muscular hyperalgesia induced by combinations of serotonin and bradykinin. Pain 1999b;82:1–8.

Bianchi M, Moser C, Lazzarini C, Vecchiato E, Crespi F. Forced swimming test and fluoxetine treatment: In vivo evidence that peripheral 5-HT in rat platelet-rich plasma mirrors cerebral extracellular 5-HT levels, whilst 5-HT in isolated platelets mirrors neuronal 5-HT changes. Exp Brain Res 2002;143:191–197.

Boess FG, Martin IL. Molecular biology of 5-HT receptors. Neuropharmacology 1994;33:275–317.

Brenner B, Harney JT, Ahmed BA, Jeffus BC, Unal R, Mehta JL, Kilic F. Plasma serotonin levels and the platelet serotonin transporter. J Neurochem 2007;102:206–215.

Christidis N, Kopp S, Ernberg M. The effect on mechanical pain threshold over human muscles by oral administration of granisetron and diclofenac-sodium. Pain 2005;113:265–270.

Christidis N, Nilsson A, Kopp S, Ernberg M. Intramuscular injection of granisetron into the masseter muscle increases the pressure pain threshold in healthy subjects and patients with localized myalgia. Clin J Pain 2007;23:467–472.

Coutaux A, Adam F, Willer JC, Le Bars D. Hyperalgesia and allodynia: peripheral mechanisms. Joint Bone Spine 2005;72:359–371.

Dempsey CM, Mackenzie SM, Gargus A, Blanco G, Sze JY. Serotonin (5HT), fluoxetine, imipramine and dopamine target distinct 5HT receptor signaling to modulate *Caenorhabditis elegans* egg-laying behavior. Genetics 2005;169:1425–1436.

Ernberg M, Hedenberg-Magnusson B, Alstergren P, Lundeberg T, Kopp S. Pain, allodynia, and serum serotonin level in orofacial pain of muscular origin. J Orofac Pain 1999;13:56–62.

Ernberg M, Lundeberg T, Kopp S. Pain and allodynia/hyperalgesia induced by intramuscular injection of serotonin in patients with fibromyalgia and healthy individuals. Pain 2000a;85:31–39.

Ernberg M, Lundeberg T, Kopp S. Effect of propranolol and granisetron on experimentally induced pain and allodynia/hyperalgesia by intramuscular injection of serotonin into the human masseter muscle. Pain 2000b;84:339–346.

Ernberg M, Lundeberg T, Kopp S. Effects on muscle pain by intramuscular injection of granisetron in patients with fibromyalgia. Pain 2003;101:275–282.

Ettlin T. Trigger point injection treatment with the 5-HT3 receptor antagonist tropisetron in patients with late whiplash-associated disorder. First results of a multiple case study. Scand J Rheumatol Suppl 2004;119:49–50.

Färber L, Stratz T, Bruckle W, et al. German Fibromyalgia Study Group. Efficacy and tolerability of tropisetron in primary fibromyalgia—a highly selective and competitive 5-HT3 receptor antagonist. Scand J Rheumatol Suppl 2000;113:49–54.

Färber L, Stratz TH, Bruckle W, et al. German Fibromyalgia Study Group. Short-term treatment of primary fibromyalgia with the 5-HT3-receptor antagonist tropisetron. results of a randomized, double-blind, placebo-controlled multicenter trial in 418 patients. Int J Clin Pharmacol Res 2001;21:1–13.

Giordano J, Daleo C, Sacks SM. Topical ondansetron attenuates nociceptive and inflammatory effects of intradermal capsaicin in humans. Eur J Pharmacol 1998;354:R13–R14.

Giordano J, Rogers LV. Peripherally administered serotonin 5-HT3 receptor antagonists reduce inflammatory pain in rats. Eur J Pharmacol 1989;170:83–86.

Giordano J, Schultea T. Serotonin 5-HT3 receptor mediation of pain and anti-nociception: Implications for clinical therapeutics. Pain Physician 2004;7:141–147.

Greenwood-Van Meerveld B, Venkova K, Hicks G, Dennis E, Crowell MD. Activation of peripheral 5-HT4 receptors attenuates colonic sensitivity to intraluminal distension. Neurogastroenterol Motil 2006;18:76– 86.

Gyermek L. Pharmacology of serotonin as related to anesthesia. J Clin Anesth 1996;8:402–425.

Höcherl K, Färber L, Ladenburger S, Vosshage D, Stratz T, Müller W, Grobecker H. Effect of tropisetron on circulating catecholamines and other putative biochemical markers in serum of patients with fibromyalgia. Scand J Rheumatol Suppl 2000;113:46–48.

Hains BC, Willis WD, Hulsebosch CE. Serotonin receptors 5-HT1A and 5-HT3 reduce hyperexcitability of dorsal horn neurons after chronic spinal cord hemisection injury in rat. Exp Brain Res 2003;149:174–186.

Haus U, Varga B, Stratz T, Späth M, Müller W. Oral treatment of fibromyalgia with tropisetron given over 28 days: Influence on functional and vegetative symptoms, psychometric parameters and pain. Scand J Rheumatol Suppl 2000;113:55–58.

Hindle AT. Recent developments in the physiology and pharmacology of 5-hydroxytryptamine. Br J Anaesth 1994;73:395–407.

Honda M, Uchida K, Tanabe M, Ono H. Fluvoxamine, a selective serotonin reuptake inhibitor, exerts its antiallodynic effects on neuropathic pain in mice via 5-HT2A/2C receptors. Neuropharmacology 2006;51:866–872.

Hrycaj P, Stratz T, Mennet P, Müller W. Pathogenetic aspects of responsiveness to ondansetron (5-hydroxytryptamine type 3 receptor antagonist) in patients with primary fibromyalgia syndrome: a preliminary study. J Rheumatol 1996;23:1418–1423.

Jensen K, Tuxen C, Pedersen-Bjergaard U, Jansen I, Edvinsson L, Olesen J. Pain and tenderness in human temporal muscle induced by bradykinin and 5-hydroxytryptamine. Peptides 1990;11:1127–1132.

Kayser V, Elfassi IE, Aubel B, Melfort M, Julius D, Gingrich JA, Hamon M, Bourgoin S. Mechanical, thermal and formalin-induced nociception is differentially altered in 5-HT(1A)-/-, 5-HT(1B)-/-, 5-HT(2A)-/-, 5-HT(3A)-/- and 5-HTT-/- knock-out male mice. Pain 2007;130:235–248.

Legangneux E, Mora JJ, Spreux-Varoquaux O, Thorin I, Herrou M, Alvado G, Gomeni C. Cerebrospinal fluid biogenic amine metabolites, plasma-rich platelet serotonin and [3H]imipramine reuptake in the primary fibromyalgia syndrome. Rheumatology (Oxford) 2001;40:290–296.

Liu ZY, Zhuang DB, Lunderberg T, Yu LC. Involvement of 5-hydroxytryptamine (1A) receptors in the descending anti-nociceptive pathway from periaqueductal gray to the spinal dorsal horn in intact rats, rats with nerve injury and rats with inflammation. Neuroscience 2002;112:399–407.

Meuser T, Pietruck C, Gabriel A, Xie GX, Lim KJ, Pierce Palmer P. 5-HT7 receptors are involved in mediating 5-HT-induced activation of rat primary afferent neurons. Life Sci 2002;71:2279–2289.

Moesker A. Treatment of CRPS patients with ketanserin. Thesis. Rotterdam: Erasmus University; 2000. p 37–51.

Moldofsky H, Warsh JJ. Plasma tryptophan and musculoskeletal pain in non-articular rheumatism ("fibrositis syndrome"). Pain 1978;5:65–71.

Müller W, Stratz T. The use of the 5-HT3 receptor antagonist tropisetron in trigger point therapy: a pilot study. J Musculoskel Pain 2005;13:43–48.

Papadopoulos IA, Georgiou PE, Katsimbri PP, Drosos AA. Treatment of fibromyalgia with tropise-tron, a 5HT3 serotonin antagonist: a pilot study. Clin Rheumatol 2000;19:6–8.

Porreca F, Ossipov MH, Gebhart GF. Chronic pain and medullary descending facilitation. Trends Neurosci 2002;25:319–325.

Richardson BP, Engel G, Donatsch P, Stadler PA. Identification of serotonin M-receptor subtypes and their specific blockade by a new class of drugs. Nature 1985;316:126–131.

Russell IJ, Michalek JE, Vipraio GA, Fletcher EM, Javors MA, Bowden CA. Platelet 3h-imipramine uptake receptor density and serum serotonin levels in patients with fibromyalgia/fibrositis syn-drome. J Rheumatol 1992a;19:104–109.

Russell IJ, Orr MD, Littman B, Vipraio GA, Alboukrek D, Michalek JE, Lopez Y, MacKillip F. Elevat-ed cerebrospinal fluid levels of substance P in patients with the fibromyalgia syndrome. Arthritis Rheum 1994;37:1593–1601.

Russell IJ, Vaeroy H, Javors M, Nyberg F. Cerebrospinal fluid biogenic amine metabolites in fibromy-algia/fibrositis syndrome and rheumatoid arthritis. Arthritis Rheum 1992b;35:550–556.

Saria A, Javorsky F, Humpel C, Gamse R. 5-HT3 receptor antagonists inhibit sensory neuropeptide release from the rat spinal cord. Neuroreport 1990;1:104–106.

Sasaki M, Obata H, Kawahara K, Saito S, Goto F. Peripheral 5-HT2A receptor antagonism attenu-ates primary thermal hyperalgesia and secondary mechanical allodynia after thermal injury in rats. Pain 2006;122:130–136.

Sommer C. Is serotonin hyperalgesic or analgesic? Curr Pain Headache Rep 2006;10:101–106.

Späth M, Stratz T, Neeck G, Kotter I, Hammel B, Amberger CC, Haus U, Färber L, Pongratz D, Mül-ler W. Efficacy and tolerability of IV tropisetron in the treatment of fibromyalgia. Scand J Rheu-matol 2004;33:267–270.

Stratz T, Fiebich B, Haus U, Müller W. Influence of tropisetron on the serum substance P levels in fibromyalgia patients. Scand J Rheumatol Suppl 2004;119:41–43.

Stratz T, Müller W. Treatment of chronic low back pain with tropisetron. Scand J Rheumatol Suppl 2004;119:76–78.

Sufka KJ, Schomburg FM, Giordano J. Receptor mediation of 5-HT-induced inflammation and noci-ception in rats. Pharmacol Biochem Behav 1992;41:53–56.

Sung D, Dong X, Ernberg M, Kumar U, Cairns BE. Serotonin (5-HT) excites rat masticatory muscle afferent fibers through activation of peripheral 5-HT$_3$ receptors. Pain 2008;134:41–50.

Suzuki R, Rygh LJ, Dickenson AH. Bad news from the brain: Descending 5-HT pathways that con-trol spinal pain processing. Trends Pharmacol Sci 2004;25:613–617.

Svensson P, Cairns BE, Wang K, Hu JW, Graven-Nielsen T, Arendt-Nielsen L, Sessle BJ. Glutamate-evoked pain and mechanical allodynia in the human masseter muscle. Pain 2003;101:221–227.

Taiwo YO, Levine JD. Serotonin is a directly-acting hyperalgesic agent in the rat. Neuroscience 1992;48:485–490.

Terron JA. Is the 5-HT$_7$ receptor involved in the pathogenesis and prophylactic treatment of mi-graine? Eur J Pharmacol 2002;439:1–11.

Tokunaga A, Saika M, Senba E. 5-HT2A receptor subtype is involved in the thermal hyperalgesic mechanism of serotonin in the periphery. Pain 1998;76:349–355.

Vaerøy H, Helle R, Førre Ø, Kåss E, Terenius L. Elevated CSF levels of substance P and high inci-dence of Raynaud phenomenon in patients with fibromyalgia: new features for diagnosis. Pain 1988;32:21–26.

Wakayama K, Ohtsuki S, Takanaga H, Hosoya K, Terasaki T. Localization of norepinephrine and se-rotonin transporter in mouse brain capillary endothelial cells. Neurosci Res 2002;44:173–180.

Yunus MB, Dailey JW, Aldag JC, Masi AT, Jobe PC. Plasma tryptophan and other amino acids in primary fibromyalgia: A controlled study. J Rheumatol 1992;19:90–94.

Zeitz KP, Guy N, Malmberg AB, Dirajlal S, Martin WJ, Sun L, Bonhaus DW, Stucky CL, Julius D, Basbaum AI. The 5-HT3 subtype of serotonin receptor contributes to nociceptive processing via a novel subset of myelinated and unmyelinated nociceptors. J Neurosci 2002;22:1010–1019.

Correspondence to: Malin Ernberg, DDS, PhD, Department of Clinical Oral Physiology, Institute of Odontology, Karolinska Institute, 14104 Huddinge, Swe-den. Tel: +468 524 882 36; fax +468 601 08 80; email: malin.ernberg@ki.se.

Human Models and Clinical Manifestations of Musculoskeletal Pain and Pain-Motor Interactions

Thomas Graven-Nielsen and Lars Arendt-Nielsen

Center for Sensory-Motor Interaction (SMI), Laboratory for Musculoskeletal Pain and Motor Control, Aalborg University, Denmark

Pain from deep tissues is generally accepted to constitute a special diagnostic and therapeutic challenge. Insight into the peripheral and central neurobiological mechanisms of such pain is necessary to improve diagnosis and management strategies. Human experimental pain models applied to healthy volunteers are a potential strategy by which to investigate aspects of the neurobiological mechanisms involved in muscle pain. Experimental muscle pain research involves two separate topics: (1) standardized activation of the nociceptive system and (2) quantitative assessment of the evoked sensory and motor responses. One important advantage of experimental muscle pain studies is that the cause-and-effect relationship is known. In this situation, healthy volunteers transiently become patients with well-defined muscle pain to allow assessment of sensory manifestations and sensory-motor interactions.

Sensory manifestations of muscle pain are reported as a diffuse aching pain in the muscle, pain referred to distant somatic structures, and sensitivity modifications in the painful areas. The sensation of acute muscle pain is the result of activation of group III and group IV muscle receptors (nociceptors) responding to strong (noxious) mechanical or chemical stimulation. Nociceptors can be sensitized by the release of substances from glial cells, neurons, and muscular tissues. Eventually, peripheral sensitization may lead to hyperalgesia and central sensitization of dorsal horn neurons, manifested as prolonged neuronal discharges, increased responses to defined noxious stimuli, nociceptive responses to non-noxious stimuli, and expansion of the receptive field (see Chapters 1 and 5 by Mense and Hoheisel). In humans, limited information is available on the peripheral neuronal correlate of muscle nociceptor activation. Few microneurographic studies have been published, the main reasons being difficulties in recording from muscle nociceptors. Therefore, other quantitative techniques are needed. Quantitative sensory testing may help to assess muscle pain, muscle hyperalgesia, temporal summation, referred pain, and pain-motor interactions.

Experimental Muscle Pain Modalities

Several procedures can induce muscle pain (Graven-Nielsen, 2006), and they can be divided into endogenous and exogenous techniques. Endogenous techniques are methods that induce muscle pain by natural stimuli, for example by ischemia or by exercise. Exogenous techniques are external interventions, such as electrical stimulation of muscle afferents or injection of pain-producing substances. In general, the endogenous experimental techniques induce widespread deep pain in muscles and other somatic structures, and they may be used in studies that require non-tissue-specific deep pain assessment. Experimental muscle pain modalities include ischemia, exercise, and electrical, mechanical and chemical techniques, which will be introduced in this section along with muscle pain assessment methods. The relevance and applicability of the various models are outlined in Table I.

Table I
Applicability of some experimental models for induction and assessment
of sensory characteristics and pain-motor interaction in muscle pain

Modality		Localized Muscle Pain	Referred Pain	Hyperalgesia	Temporal Summation	Pain-Motor Interaction
Ischemic contractions		Tonic	(Yes)	-	-	-
Exercise	Concentric	Tonic	-	Assessment*	-	-
	Eccentric	(Tonic)	-	Induction*	-	Yes
Electrical		Tonic	Yes	Assessment	Yes	-
Mechanical	Pressure	Phasic and tonic	Yes	Assessment	Yes	-
	Cuff	Phasic and tonic	-	Assessment	-	-
Chemical	Hypertonic saline	Tonic	Yes	(Induction)	(Yes)	Yes
	Glutamate	Tonic	Yes	Induction	-	Yes
	Capsaicin	Tonic	Yes	Induction	-	Yes
	Acidic saline	Tonic	Yes	(Induction)	-	Yes
	Nerve growth factor	-	-	Induction	-	Yes

* Indicates that the model can be used to induce or assess muscle hyperalgesia.

Assessment of Muscle Pain

Verbal assessments of muscle pain intensity and other subjective characteristics of muscle pain are necessary in all clinical and experimental muscle pain studies. Pain intensity is usually scored in a continuous mode on an electronic visual electronic scale (VAS) to characterize the time profile of experimental muscle pain. Pain drawings, verbal descriptor scales, the McGill Pain Questionnaire, and similar scales and questionnaires may be very helpful for the assessment of perceived pain location and quality (Gracely, 2006).

Ischemia

Repeated contractions of limb muscles under ischemia created by application of a tourniquet produce a deep pain sensation of moderate to high pain intensity in the entire occluded limb (including skin, periosteum, and muscles) (Lewis, 1932). The level of force, the number of contractions, and the duration of ischemia are important determinants of pain. The mechanisms of deep pain after ischemic contractions are not fully understood. Lewis (1932) suggested that the pain induced by ischemic contractions might be due to a physical or chemical mechanism termed "factor P." "Factor P" is formed under ischemic contractions and remains unchanged or intensifies with each contraction (Lewis, 1932). Accumulation of various substances (potassium, adenosine, and lactate) may excite muscle nociceptors or sensitize them to respond to muscle contractions that are normally nonpainful.

Lactate increases during ischemia combined with exercise (Saltin et al., 1981), but it probably is not involved in ischemic pain because patients with McArdle disease, who do not produce lactate, experience muscle pain during fatiguing contractions (McArdle, 1951). Furthermore, animal studies have shown that lactate is a poor activator of muscle receptors (Kniffki et al., 1978). Potassium concentration is increased during muscle exercise, and so potassium has been suggested to be the main substance involved in pain following ischemic contractions (Harpuder and Stein, 1943). However, muscle interstitial potassium concentration is significantly lower during ischemic exercise compared with a similar nonischemic exercise, unlike pain intensity, which is higher during ischemic contractions compared with control contractions (Green et al., 2000). Similarly, the role of tissue acidosis is unclear. During high-intensity exercise, muscle pH drops below 6.6, and the time for recovery of muscle pH to baseline levels is much longer (Allsop et al., 1990) than the immediate decrease of pain when the tourniquet is released after ischemic contractions (Graven-Nielsen et al., 2003). Progressively increasing work rate escalates the concentration of skeletal muscle interstitial adenosine, and a further increase is found during exercise combined with ischemia (Costa et al., 1999). Nonetheless, experimentally elevated adenosine levels did not induce muscle pain (Graven-Nielsen et al., 2003).

The qualities of pain after ischemic contractions are similar to those of hypertonic saline (HS)-induced muscle pain, but study participants were significantly more likely to rate the former as "stabbing," "burning," "heavy," and "exhausting" (Graven-Nielsen et al., 2003). The "stabbing" and "burning" pain qualities indicate that ischemic pain is not exclusively muscle pain because these descriptors are frequently used for more superficial pain conditions (Graven-Nielsen et al., 1997a). Intravenous administrations of drugs such as propofol are known to induce pain with a burning quality (Eriksson et al., 1997), which suggests that the ischemic pain might originate from the vascular system in addition to the pain mediated by muscle nociceptors. However, to qualify such a suggestion, the algesic substances must diffuse from the muscle to other tissues (e.g., the skin or vascular systems), because short-term ischemia without contractions does not induce pain. Alternatively, ischemic pain might be mediated by a subset of nociceptors that are not excited by i.m. HS.

Exercise

Muscle pain induced by concentric exercise results from impaired blood flow during concentric muscle work (shortening contractions) and is normally short-lasting. Therefore, it may resemble ischemic muscle pain. As an example, moderate quadriceps muscle pain was induced in volunteers who performed a cycle ergometry task involving cycling at different power outputs (O'Connor and Cook, 2001). Eccentric muscle work (lengthening contractions) may cause delayed onset of muscle soreness, with peak soreness after 24 to 48 hours. Delayed-onset muscle soreness (DOMS) has been widely used to explore pathophysiological components of the musculoskeletal system and gender-related issues (see Chapter 16 by Dannecker). A model of deep tissue hyperalgesia based on DOMS in the wrist extensors has characteristics similar to tennis elbow pain (Slater et al., 2005). The mechanism underlying DOMS is not clear (see Chapter 4 by Mizumura and Taguchi), but it is probably related to ultrastructural damage resulting in the release of algesic substances. An inflammatory reaction may result, given that nonsteroidal anti-inflammatory drugs (NSAIDs) appear to have an effect on this type of muscle soreness.

Electrical Stimulation

In human studies, intramuscular (i.m.) electrical stimulation can be used to assess the sensitivity of muscles, to study basic aspects of deep pain, and to investigate the electrophysiological properties of muscle afferent fibers by microneurography. Intramuscular electrical stimulation is a tissue-specific (although non-receptor-specific) and reliable method, but it is confounded by concurrently activated muscle twitches. Moreover, electrical stimulation is a nonphysiological technique that bypasses receptor transduction and depolarizes the afferent fibers directly. As thick myelinated (non-nociceptive) afferent fibers are activated at lower stimulus intensities than unmyelinated fibers, electrical stimuli are not specifically nociceptive. At pain threshold levels, electrically induced muscle pain is probably mediated by group III afferent fibers. In a series of studies, electrically induced muscle pain was reduced by more than 70% during a differential block where myelinated afferent fibers were progressively blocked and thin nonmyelinated afferent fibers were not affected (Laursen et al., 1999b). The effect of simultaneous excitation of myelinated and unmyelinated afferent fibers is not clear.

Laursen and colleagues (1999a) used the phasic nature of electrical stimulation to explore mechanisms of referred pain. Electrical stimulation also offers a unique possibility to compare both muscle and cutaneous tissues using the same stimulus modality. For example, a systemically administered anesthetic drug (remifentanil) caused a higher increase in the pain threshold to i.m. electrical stimulation compared with the relative increase in pain threshold induced by cutaneous stimulation (Curatolo et al., 2000).

Mechanical Stimulation

Mechanical painful stimulation can be achieved with pressure algometers (Fig. 1A). The most widely used technique is manual pressure algometry (Jensen et al., 1986). Methodological concerns include short-term and long-term reproducibility on pain thresholds, as well as the influence of pressure rates, duration, muscle contraction levels, and interexaminer variability or examiner expectancy; these concerns have all been addressed carefully (for references see Graven-Nielsen 2006). In

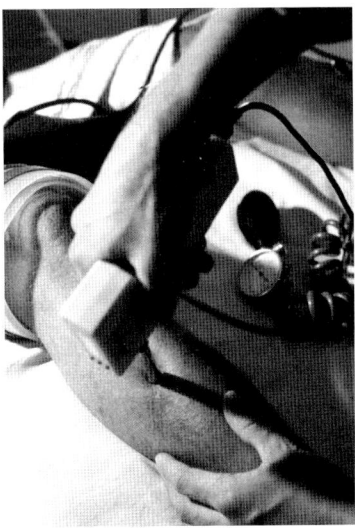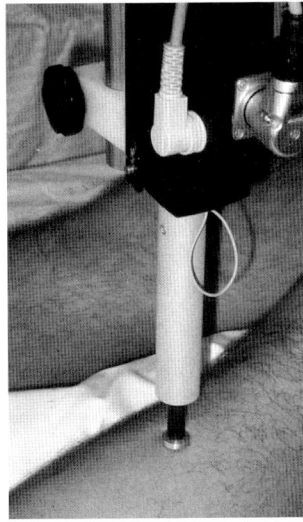

Fig. 1. Assessment of deep tissue sensitivity by manual (A) and automated (B) pressure algometry. Application of pressure and control of increment rate are manually controlled when using the handheld algometer. In contrast, these parameters are computer-controlled in the automated version, which increases the reproducibility of assessments. Reprinted with permission from Arendt-Nielsen and Graven-Nielsen (2005).

line, equipment can be used to ensure standardized finger pressure during muscle palpation (Bendtsen et al., 1997). An alternative to pressure algometry, with the inherent variability related to manual pressure application, is computer-controlled pressure algometry (Fig. 1B), where the rate and peak pressure can be predefined and automatically controlled (Graven-Nielsen et al., 2004). This method allows estimation of the stimulus-response function between pressure and pain intensities. In most human studies, investigators have tacitly assumed that stimulation with local pressure excites receptors in deep somatic tissues such as muscles, fascia, and aponeuroses. However, pressure stimulation obviously also excites cutaneous receptors. A study carefully applying cutaneous anesthesia clearly demonstrated that the mechanically elicited pain sensation originated mainly from deep tissue and only to a minor degree from the skin (Graven-Nielsen et al., 2004). Interestingly, when the thick afferent fibers from the muscle was blocked and simultaneously anesthetize the skin, subjects still have a nonpainful sensation of pressure (Graven-Nielsen et al., 2004). This finding illustrates that the large proportion of group III and IV afferent fibers with low mechanical thresholds (see Chapter 1 by Mense and Hoheisel) might mediate this pressure sensation from muscle.

Pressure algometry assesses a relatively small volume of tissue. A larger volume can be assessed by a computer-controlled cuff-algometry technique. Pain intensity related to inflation of a tourniquet applied around an extremity is used to establish stimulus-response curves, which allow the investigator to assess somatosensory sensitivity. After i.m. injections of lidocaine, the stimulus-response curve between tourniquet pressure and pain intensity was right-shifted, indicating that this technique can be used to assess the sensitivity of muscles (Polianskis et al., 2002).

Chemical Stimulation

Exogenous and endogenous algesic substances have been used to induce experimental muscle pain in humans (Graven-Nielsen, 2006). The hypertonic saline model has been used extensively to characterize the sensory and motor effects involved in muscle pain, as the quality of the induced pain is comparable to acute clinical muscle pain and shows localized and referred pain characteristics (Kellgren, 1938). The work of Kellgren (1938) and Lewis (1938) in the late 1930s introduced the method of inducing muscle pain by HS. Most of the earlier studies used manual bolus injections of HS. Later, the model was improved by computer-controlled infusions of HS, which provide greater standardization and allow the induction of tonic muscle pain by continuous infusion (Fig. 2). Saline-induced muscle pain intensity is dependent on volume, concentration, and infusion rate. The quality of saline-induced muscle pain is typically described as "aching," "cramping," "boring," "drilling," "taut," "tight," "spreading," and "radiating." Injections of hypotonic saline may have similar nociceptive capabilities, but this method has not been extensively used (Jarvik and Wolff, 1962), probably due to the relatively short duration of pain with this model compared to the HS model. The HS-induced pain model has been used extensively, and no side effects have been reported (Graven-Nielsen, 2006). Recent animal studies have shown no muscle

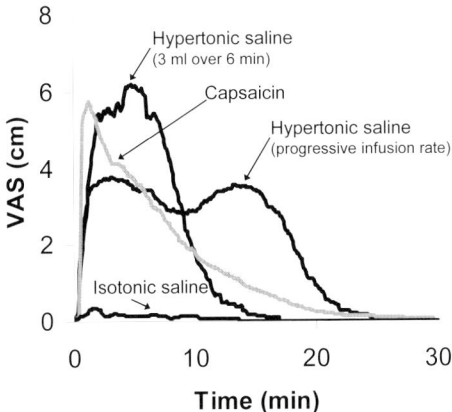

Fig. 2. Muscle pain intensity profiles (averaged across 11–15 subjects) after bolus injections of capsaicin (0.5 mL, 330 μM), hypertonic saline (3 mL, 1 M, 6 min) and continuous infusion of hypertonic saline with progressive infusion rate (7.1 mL, 1 M, 15 min). The low-level pain intensity of continuous infusion of isotonic saline (7.1 mL, 0.15 M, 15 min) is also illustrated. Pain intensity was assessed on a 10-cm electronic visual analogue scale (VAS) where 0 cm indicated "no pain" and 10 cm "most intense pain." The profile of pain is characteristically different between different substances and infusion paradigms. Reprinted from Graven-Nielsen (2006), with permission from Taylor & Francis.

toxicity with this method (Svendsen et al., 2005), and therefore it is appropriate for human experimentation.

Animal studies have shown a robust excitation of group III and IV afferent fibers by HS (Cairns et al., 2003; Hoheisel et al., 2005) in contrast to the thick, fast afferent fibers (Cairns et al., 2003). Iggo (1961) reported that in addition to group III and IV fibers, other afferent fibers (such as those related to muscle spindles) were excited by HS, but no specific details were given. Afferent fibers excited by HS showed an inverse relationship between nerve conduction velocity and saline-evoked cumulative afferent discharges (Cairns et al., 2003). Within group IV afferent fibers, HS excites both low- and high-threshold mechanosensitive units, indicating the nonspecific characteristics of this model (Cairns et al., 2003; Hoheisel et al., 2005). The nonspecificity of HS is well known in other animal models of muscle nociception. Capsaicin (Hoheisel et al., 2004) and bradykinin (Mense and Meyer, 1985) excite thin muscle afferent fibers with both low and high mechanical thresholds. The receptor type involved in saline-induced muscle pain is still not apparent, but the stretch-inactivated ion channel is a potential candidate. The stretch-inactivated channel (a subtype of the transient receptor potential vanilloid receptor 1, TRPV1) is expressed in small-diameter sensory neurons and elicits an inward current in response to cell shrinkage following exposure to hypertonic solutions (Schumacher et al., 2000). Alternatively, it may be the penetration of high sodium concentrations into the nerve fiber that excites the fiber.

Capsaicin (a TRPV1 agonist) has been widely used to induce cutaneous pain by topical application or intradermal injection, and more recently it has been used to induce muscle pain (Marchettini et al., 1996) (Fig. 2). Human microneurographic recordings show immediate excitation of group III and IV afferent fibers with medium to high mechanical thresholds (Marchettini et al., 1996). In animals, group III and IV afferent activity after i.m. injections of capsaicin was reduced by capsazepine, an antagonist to TRPV1 (Takeda et al., 2005), indicating that the TRPV1 receptor is present on muscle nociceptors. The specificity is unclear, however, because both low- and high-threshold mechanosensitive group IV units are excited by capsaicin (Hoheisel et al., 2004).

Peripheral glutamate receptors are potential receptors for mediation of muscle pain (see Chapter 2 by Cairns; Chapter 3 by Ro). An NMDA-receptor antagonist when co-injected with glutamate attenuates glutamate-induced muscle pain in humans or decreases the afferent activity recorded in animals (Cairns et al., 2003). This finding indicates that activation of peripheral NMDA receptors may contribute to glutamate-evoked muscle pain. However, glutamate is not nociceptor specific because the cumulative afferent discharge evoked by glutamate did not correlate with the mechanical threshold for these afferent fibers (Cairns et al., 2003).

Acidic buffers have also been used to induce muscle pain in humans. Constant infusion of isotonic phosphate-buffered saline induces a steady level of pain intensity (Steen et al., 2001), in contrast to infusion of HS, where the infusion rate needs to be increased to maintain steady pain (Graven-Nielsen et al., 1998a). Whether this difference is due to the acidity is not clear because bolus injections of levo-ascorbic acid (pH 6.3) create a pain profile (Rossi and Decchi, 1997) that is similar to that following bolus injections of HS, with a fast increase and a slow decline in pain intensity. Acidity seems to excite afferent fibers with both low and high mechanosensitivity (Hoheisel et al., 2004), so the stimulus is not nociceptive specific. Acid-induced muscle pain is probably mediated by acid-sensing ion channels (ASICs). The ASIC3 channel has been found especially important for evoking hyperexcitability in dorsal horn neurons (central sensitization) after repeated i.m. injections of acid saline in animals (see Chapter 6 by Walder and Sluka).

The endogenous nature of bradykinin and serotonin and the effective excitation or sensitization of animal afferent fibers with these substances form the background for using them in experimental models (Babenko et al., 1999; Chapters 1 and 2). In humans, these substances should be given in high doses with respect to physiological levels or in combination to induce a reliable pain intensity (Babenko et al., 1999). Serotonin-induced muscle pain has been carefully described elsewhere (see Chapter 10 by Ernberg). Other substances that are known to be inflammatory mediators or that are released after tissue injury (i.e., adenosine triphosphate) will induce muscle pain when injected into muscle (Mørk et al., 2003).

Referred Pain

Referred pain has been described for more than a century, but there is still no strict definition. Originally, Head (1893) used "referred tenderness and pain" to describe pain perceived remote from the site of origin or pain locus. This definition does not allow a distinction between spread of pain and actual referred pain. An operational definition of referred pain is pain occurring outside and remote from the local pain area. Accordingly, referred hyperalgesia is defined as increased sensitivity occurring in association with the referred pain area and outside the local muscle pain area.

Assessment of Referred Pain

Assessment of referred pain includes a detailed description of the location, pain intensity, and changes in somatosensory sensitivity. Adequate assessment requires evaluation of the muscle pain (local pain) and of the somatic structures related to the referred pain area; ongoing pain intensity and sensitivity must be described for both areas.

Experimental Referred Pain

Referred pain can be induced by chemical, electrical, and mechanical stimulation. The tibialis anterior, brachioradialis, and infraspinatus muscles typically refer pain to distinct areas not included in the local pain area (Fig. 3), whereas saline-induced biceps brachii muscle pain only occurs locally. Referred pain is probably due to a combination of central processing and peripheral input because it is possible to induce referred pain in limbs with complete sensory loss resulting from an anesthetic block. However, the involvement of peripheral input from the referred pain area is not clear because anesthetizing this area shows inhibitory or no effects on the intensity of referred pain. As illustrated in Fig. 4, central sensitization may be involved in the mechanisms of referred pain (Graven-Nielsen, 2006). Each muscle afferent fiber is assumed to have a complex network of extensive collateral synaptic connections onto multiple

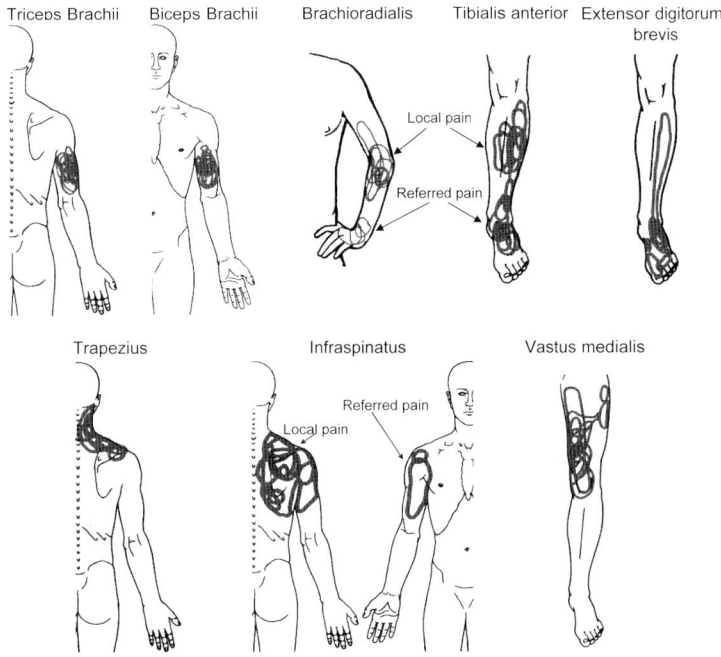

Fig. 3. Distribution of experimentally induced local and referred pain. Hypertonic saline (0.5 to 1 mL, 1M) was injected into the triceps brachii, biceps brachii, brachioradialis, tibialis anterior, extensor digitorum brevis, trapezius, infraspinatus, and vastus medialis muscles. The subjects ($n = 9$–15) outlined the area of pain. Saline-induced pain in the tibialis anterior, brachioradialis and infraspinatus muscles showed distinct referred pain areas (not included in the local pain area), whereas the other muscles show more localized pain around the injection site.

dorsal horn neurons (Mense and Simons, 2001). Under normal conditions, the afferent fibers have fully functional synaptic connections with dorsal horn neurons, as well as latent synaptic connections to other neurons within the same region of the spinal cord. Following ongoing strong noxious input, latent synaptic connections become operational, thereby allowing for the convergence of input from more than one source.

The area of referred pain is correlated with the intensity of muscle pain, and the appearance of referred pain is delayed by 20 to 40 seconds compared with local muscle pain (Graven-Nielsen, 2006), indicating the involvement of a time-dependent process, perhaps the unmasking of new synaptic connections, in the neural mediation of referred pain. The

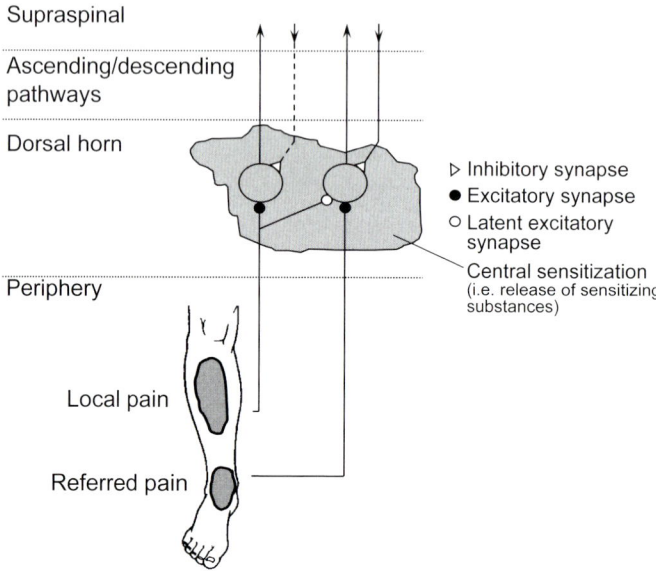

Fig. 4. A neurophysiological model for referred muscle pain based on two pools of dorsal horn neurons with receptive fields in the local muscle pain area and in the area of referred pain (Graven-Nielsen 2006). The neuronal diagram is schematic and illustrates functional properties and not direct connections (e.g., interneurons are probably involved). Local muscle pain will excite the pathway normally mediating pain from this structure. At the same time a sensitizing process (gray area) is initiated that will open latent synaptic connections to the neurons normally mediating pain from the referred area. The perception of referred pain is caused either by direct excitation of these neurons due to collaterals from the muscle afferent fibers or by facilitation of afferent input from the referred area. The neurons involved in mediating referred pain are suggested to be affected by descending inhibition, in contrast to the neurons mediating local pain, with a relatively smaller degree of descending inhibition (indicated by a dashed line). Parts of this model are derived from an animal-based model on referred pain (Mense 1994). Reprinted from Graven-Nielsen (2006), with permission from Taylor & Francis.

frequency of referred pain from prolonged mechanical stimulation on the anterior tibial muscle is significantly higher than for brief stimulation (Fig. 5), again indicating the time dependency of referred pain (Gibson et al., 2006). Moreover, saline-induced referred pain occurred less frequently in healthy subjects treated with ketamine compared with those receiving a placebo treatment (Schulte et al., 2003), indicating the involvement of central sensitization.

Clinical Presentations of Referred Pain

Substantial clinical knowledge exists on the patterns of referred muscle pain from various skeletal muscles after the activation of trigger points (Simons et al., 1999); these descriptions generally fit the experimental referred pain pattern shown in Fig. 3. Typically, the referral of muscle pain is described as a sensation from deep structures, in contrast to visceral referred pain, which is both superficially and deeply located. The pattern and size of referral seem to be different in chronic musculoskeletal pain conditions. For example, patients with fibromyalgia syndrome experience stronger pain and larger referred areas after exogenous muscle pain (induced by HS) compared with matched controls (Sörensen et al., 1998). Interestingly, these manifestations occurred in lower limb muscles, where patients typically do not experience ongoing pain. Normally, pain from the tibialis anterior is projected distally to the ankle and only rarely proximally. However, the fibromyalgia patients showed substantial proximal spread of the areas of experimentally induced referred pain. Enlarged

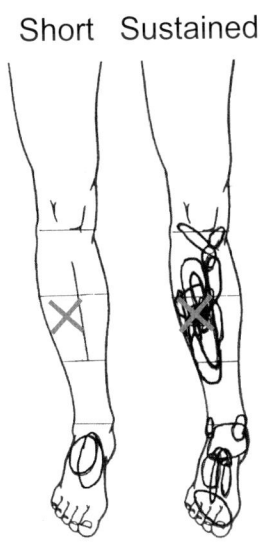

Short Sustained

Fig. 5. Subjects (*n* = 18) outlined the referred pain area evoked by short pressure stimulation versus stimulation sustained for 2 minutes on the tibialis anterior muscle. The frequency of referred pain from the sustained mechanical stimulation is higher than for the brief stimulation. Based on data from Gibson et al. (2006).

referred pain areas in pain patients suggest that the efficacy of central processing is increased (central sensitization). Moreover, the expansion of areas of referred pain in fibromyalgia patients was partly inhibited by an NMDA-receptor antagonist (ketamine), which was thus shown to inhibit central sensitization (Graven-Nielsen et al., 2000). Extended areas of referred pain from the tibialis anterior muscle, indicating central sensitization, have also been shown in patients suffering from other chronic musculoskeletal pain conditions (Arendt-Nielsen and Graven-Nielsen, 2003).

Muscle Hyperalgesia

Deep tissue hyperalgesia characterizes "an increased response to a stimulus which is normally painful," as opposed to allodynia, which describes "pain due to a stimulus which does not normally provoke pain." According to these definitions, a decreased pain threshold should be defined as allodynia. Nonetheless, the nomenclature used in numerous psychophysical studies is hyperalgesia in the case of decreased pain thresholds and also often in the case of pain due to a nonpainful stimulus, such as in secondary hyperalgesia, where pain can be evoked by weak mechanical stimulation.

Assessment of Muscle Hyperalgesia

Psychophysical determinations can be divided into response-dependent and stimulus-dependent methods (Gracely, 2006). Response-dependent methods are constructed by a series of fixed stimulus intensities with a score for each stimulus. The score can be determined using a visual analogue scale (VAS), a verbal descriptor scale, magnitude estimation, or cross-modality matching. The stimulus-dependent methods are based on adjustment of the stimulus intensity until a predefined response, typically a threshold (e.g., detection, pain, or tolerance), is reached.

Stimulus-response functions are more informative than a threshold determination because suprathreshold response characteristics can be derived from the data. For example, stimulus-response functions clearly differentiate between low- and high-intensity stimuli. Nevertheless, the stimulus-response function can often be established with stimulus intensities around the pain threshold, and therefore both assessment methods are needed. Assessments of sensory aspects involve evaluations both of the muscle pain (local pain) and of the somatic structures related to the referred pain area. As mentioned above in the section on assessment of referred pain, ongoing pain intensity and sensitivity must be described for both areas.

Experimental Models of Muscle Hyperalgesia

In humans, decreased pressure pain thresholds have been reported after i.m. injections of capsaicin (Witting et al., 2000) and after injections of bradykinin together with serotonin (Babenko et al., 1999). Intra-arterial injections of serotonin, bradykinin, and prostaglandin have been found effective in sensitizing animal nociceptors (Mense and Simons, 2001); the relevance of this finding is further discussed in Chapter 22 (Arendt-Nielsen and Graven-Nielsen). The sensitization lasts for less than an hour. In human studies, i.m. injections of glutamate produce local hyperalgesia to pressure stimuli outlasting the muscle pain (Svensson et al., 2003b). Capsaicin-induced muscular hyperalgesia in healthy subjects, assessed by cuff algometry, produces a characteristic leftward shift in the stimulus-response curve (the pressure pain curve) (Polianskis et al., 2002).

Some studies report deep-tissue hyperalgesia at the injection site during saline-induced muscle pain, but not all of them used comparisons with injection of isotonic saline (Graven-Nielsen, 2006). Hyperalgesia to pressure was found immediately after injection of 0.9% or 9% saline into the tibialis anterior muscle (Graven-Nielsen et al., 1998b), but another study noted hyperalgesia at the injection site after injection of 1.8% and not after 0.9% saline (Jensen and Norup, 1992). During saline-induced muscle pain, findings of hyperalgesia to pressure at a short distance from the injection site are patchy. Only one quantitative study has reported greater hyperalgesia after HS than after infusion of a nonpainful control substance (Graven-Nielsen et al., 2003). Other quantitative studies controlling for the effect of isotonic saline find either unchanged sensitivity or hypoalgesia. Interestingly, in many studies reporting decreased or unchanged sensitivity, the maximal pain intensity scores were moderate, whereas another study demonstrating increased sensitivity to pressure stimulations reported on average high pain intensity scores (Graven-Nielsen, 2006). The relation between pain intensity and sensitivity changes is illustrated by the correlation between individual maximal pain intensity and the decrease in pressure pain threshold (Graven-Nielsen et al., 2003).

The DOMS model, described above, is an endogenous model of deep-tissue hyperalgesia. A detailed evaluation of pressure pain sensitivity along the musculoskeletal unit (from the proximal to the distal tendon) did not find general hyperalgesia, but rather an increased sensitivity to pressure at various sites that differed among subjects (Andersen et al., 2006) (Fig. 6). These sites of reversible muscle hyperalgesia might involve mechanisms similar to those underlying the initial development of trigger points seen in myofascial pain patients (Simons et al., 1999), and further studies should explore this possibility in detail. Interestingly, assessment of pain after injections of HS into deep and superficial structures in both control and DOMS muscles found hyperalgesia in the superficial structures with DOMS (Gibson and Graven-Nielsen, unpublished observations). In DOMS, peripheral sensitization is probably the main mechanism responsible for hyperalgesia to pressure. However, the hyperalgesic component in DOMS has been suggested to be mediated in part by the thick myelinated afferent fibers and not exclusively by the thin unmyelinated nociceptive afferent fibers (Barlas et al., 2000). A comparable model of delayed-onset hyperalgesia consists of i.m. injection of nerve growth factor (Svensson et al., 2003a). This model is interesting because no pain occurs immediately after the injection, but hyperalgesic reactions develop after a few hours and last for weeks. Recent data indicate that the hyperalgesic area expands over time and reaches its maximum one day after the administration of nerve growth factor.

Referred hyperalgesia of deep tissue has been reported both in quantitative studies (Madeleine et al., 1998; Graven-Nielsen et al., 2002a) and in case reports, although it is also described as inconsistent in other case reports. When testing deep tissue sensitivity by pressure stimulation, it is critical to consider the influence of cutaneous sensitivity.

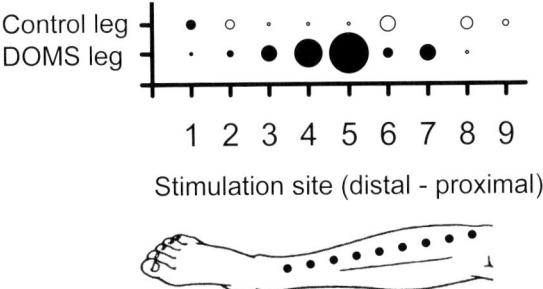

Fig. 6. Sites of hyperalgesia to pressure stimulation after induction of delayed-onset muscle soreness (DOMS) induced by eccentric exercise in one subject. Each circle represents the change of pressure pain thresholds for the DOMS leg and the control leg. The width of the circles represents the amount of either hyperalgesia (filled circles) or hypoalgesia (open circles) compared to pre-exercise recordings taken 2 days previously. Interestingly, one site with extensive hyperalgesia is located close to a site with no or very little change in deep tissue sensitivity. Based on data from Andersen et al. (2006). Reprinted with permission from Graven-Nielsen et al. (2006).

Anesthetic skin above the referred pain area does not change the referred deep-tissue hyperalgesia to palpation (Kellgren, 1938). Decreased sensitivity to pressure stimulation in the referred pain area is a typical finding, but this effect is most likely generalized rather than restricted to the referred pain areas. In fact, contralateral or extrasegmental sites show similar decreased sensitivity, probably due to a general descending inhibitory mechanism.

Kellgren (1938) concluded that hyperalgesia could often be found in areas with referred pain except when pain was felt deeply in the joints, and this proposal is consistent with studies on referred pain to the ankle area (Graven-Nielsen, 2006). The accessibility of joint receptors to stimulation by pressure may provide a physiological explanation for this observation. However, hyperalgesia to pressure distal to the referred pain at the ankle has been reported (Graven-Nielsen et al., 2002a). The referred hyperalgesic area is innervated by the deep peroneal nerve, which also innervates the tibialis anterior muscle. The deep peroneal nerve also innervates the referred pain area but is probably not accessible by pressure stimulation, in contrast to the distal area tested. These findings suggest involvement of summation between muscle afferent fibers and the somatosensory afferent fibers from the hyperalgesic area.

Clinical Deep-Tissue Hyperalgesia

Mechanical stimuli have been used extensively to assess the sensitization of musculoskeletal tissues in humans, such as tender points, fibromyalgia, work-related myalgia, myofascial pain, strain injuries, myositis, arthritis/arthroses, and other inflammatory conditions of the muscles, tendons, and joints. Pressure algometry is adequate to quantify and follow the development of given diseases, but it has also proven instrumental for documenting the outcome of treatments such as local or systemic administration of NSAIDs. Stimulus-response functions relating pressure intensity to pain intensity showed a parallel shift toward the left together with an increased slope for myofascial pain patients (Svensson et al., 1995). When the muscle was anesthetized, the curve shifted toward the right, with a reduced slope.

Tender points are anatomically determined soft-tissue body sites where, among other criteria, the patients must be sensitive to 4 kg pressure at 11 out of 18 points to conform with the American College of Rheumatology criteria for fibromyalgia (Wolfe et al., 1990). Trigger points are localized hardening of muscle tissue that is hypersensitive and located in a tense band of muscle fibers (Simons et al., 1999). In contrast to tender points, pressure stimulation on trigger points is typically characterized by referral of pain. Pressure algometry has been widely used to assess trigger and tender point sensitivity in musculoskeletal pain patients. In patients with tension-type headache and fibromyalgia, there was a qualitative difference in the stimulus-response functions (pressure versus pain intensity scores) when pressure was assessed with a palpometer (Bendtsen et al., 1997). The widespread hyperalgesia in fibromyalgia has also been demonstrated with the cuff algometry method, for example in a study that found pain and pain tolerance thresholds assessed on the lower leg to be significantly decreased compared with control subjects (Jespersen et al., 2007).

Electrical pain thresholds were recorded from myofascial trigger points in the trapezius in myofascial pain patients, from tender points (also in the trapezius) in fibromyalgia patients, from control points in patients, and from control subjects (Vecchiet et al., 1994). Reduced pain thresholds were found for trigger points as well as for tender points with cutaneous, subcutaneous, and muscle stimulation, indicating that the hyperalgesia was not specific to deep tissue. In myofascial pain patients, hyperalgesia was not detected outside the trigger point area, in contrast to fibromyalgia patients, who showed a more generalized hyperalgesia.

Few clinical studies have focused on referred hyperalgesia. Leffler et al. (2002b) assessed somatosensory function in referred pain in patients with long-term trapezius myalgia. Hyperalgesia to pressure and hypoalgesia to light mechanical stimulation were found in the referred pain area, suggesting a modality-specific or tissue-specific change of somatosensory function, similar to previous experimental findings. However, in patients with lateral epicondylalgia, only hypoalgesia to light mechanical stimulation was found in the referred pain area (Leffler et al., 2000). A factor that might influence the somatosensory changes is the duration of habitual pain. Increased sensitivity to pressure in a nonpainful area was found in patients who had rheumatoid arthritis for more than 5 years, but not in patients who had experienced pain for less than 1 year (Leffler et al., 2002a). This finding fits well with the concept of central sensitization, because a certain period of nociceptive input is needed to induce central sensitization. Interestingly, widespread pain in musculoskeletal pain disorders is frequently initiated by localized deep pain, indicating the development of central sensitization over time.

Another manifestation of central sensitization may be the number of palpable trigger points. A significantly higher number of such points were found in the lower limb muscles in patients suffering from knee osteoarthritis compared to controls (Bajaj et al., 2001). Central sensitization may facilitate low-intensity input and result in the experience of pain when a latent trigger point is activated. This may also be one of the reasons why a localized painful condition can spread and become generalized.

A dysfunction of the descending inhibitory control systems might have effects similar to those of central sensitization (see Chapter 8 by Rahman and Dickinson). In healthy subjects, generalized hypoalgesia to pressure is found during strong experimentally induced pain. In contrast, fibromyalgia patients do not show such modulation, indicating a dysfunction of descending inhibitory control (Kosek and Hansson, 1997). The mechanism of descending inhibition is not different in short- and long-term rheumatoid arthritis patients compared to controls (Leffler et al., 2002a). Before surgery (e.g., hip replacement), osteoarthritis patients lacked the generalized hypoalgesic effect to pressure during strong experimental pain, in contrast to the normalized descending inhibition after hip surgery (Kosek and Ordeberg, 2000). This finding might indicate that the descending system is maximally involved in the condition with continuous pain (before surgery), and after surgery the dynamics of the system are reestablished, allowing it to effectively modulate sensitivity to pressure. Thus, a dysfunction of the descending inhibitory control system might be involved in chronic musculoskeletal pain conditions, although it has not been a systematic finding in different groups of patients.

Temporal Summation

A facilitated pain response to sequential stimuli of equal strength is defined as temporal summation. To elicit temporal summation, a stimulus is repeated at constant intervals, e.g., five times at a frequency of 1 Hz, at constant intensity. The neurophysiological correlate from animal studies is discussed in Chapter 22 (Arendt-Nielsen and Graven-Nielsen).

Assessment of Temporal Summation

Temporal summation is typically determined by stimulus-dependent methods in which the intensity of all stimuli is adjusted until the subject feels pain at the last stimulus and not at previous stimuli. Alternatively, a fixed stimulus intensity (i.e., the intensity sufficient to induce pain at a single stimulus) is used, and the subject scores the sensation on a VAS.

Experimental Manifestations of Temporal Summation

Temporal summation of muscle pain has been assessed by intramuscular electrical stimulation, by focused ultrasound, by mechanical stimulation, and by sequential injections of algesic substances. Repeated tapping on a muscle with a pressure probe was the assessment method used in a recent study (Fig. 7). The study found temporal summation to be more potent for deep tissue stimulation compared with skin stimulation (Nie et al., 2005). This finding illustrates the importance of testing the temporal summation from deep tissue, which might specifically be affected by central sensitization in musculoskeletal pain conditions. Temporal summation to pressure stimulation was facilitated in DOMS (Nie et al. 2006), indicating that central changes occur in this condition.

Temporal Summation in Clinical Studies

In fibromyalgia patients, intramuscular electrical stimulation was used to assess the efficacy of temporal summation of painful muscle stimuli; temporal summation was more pronounced in the patients compared with control subjects (Sörensen et al., 1998). Moreover, temporal summation after i.m. stimulation was attenuated by the NMDA-receptor antagonist ketamine (Graven-Nielsen et al., 2000). The increased efficacy of temporal summation in fibromyalgia patients has been reproduced with repeated pressure stimulation (Staud et al., 2003). Moreover, the threshold for the withdrawal reflex during repeated stimulation was significantly lower in fibromyalgia and whiplash patients compared with healthy controls, indicating spinal cord hyperexcitability in these patients (Banic et al., 2004). Facilitated temporal summation might explain the pain after minimal ongoing nociceptive input arising from minimally damaged tissues. This possibility is an attractive explanation for cases in which there is pain, but no clear evidence of tissue damage.

Pain-Motor Interaction

It is well known from activities of daily life that muscle pain interacts with movement. This section illustrates how muscle pain affects muscle control in different ways depending on the specific motor task. The functional effects of muscle pain can be assessed by electromyographic (EMG), kinematic, and force recordings.

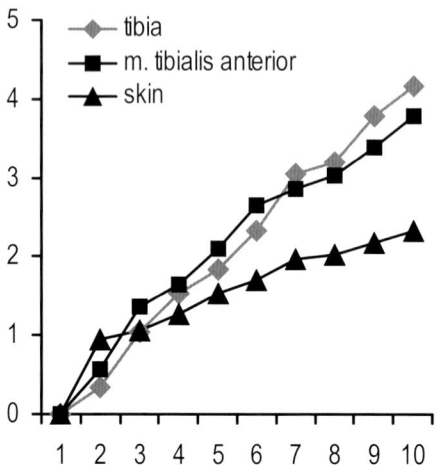

Fig. 7. Mean visual analogue scale (VAS) scores after pressure stimuli applied to the tibialis anterior muscle, the tibia, and the skin (web) with a 1-second interstimulus interval at an intensity equal to the pressure-pain threshold for one stimulation. The subject scored the pain intensity on a VAS after each stimulus. VAS scores are normalized to the first stimulus (by subtraction). Temporal summation was clearly seen by the increase in VAS scores during sequential stimulation and was most pronounced for deep tissue. Based on data from Nie el al. (2005).

Resting Muscle Activity and Muscle Pain

Resting muscle activity after saline-induced muscle pain was found to be increased compared with baseline recordings, but not compared with a sham pain condition in which subjects recalled a painful condition without receiving any painful stimulation (Stohler et al., 1996). This finding indicates that hyperactivity does not result from muscle pain per se. In another study, a transient increase in resting EMG activity during infusion of HS was recorded, in contrast to no change with a control infusion of isotonic saline (Svensson et al., 1998). Importantly, ongoing muscle pain did not produce a sustained increase in EMG activity. Moreover, experimental muscle pain does not cause any changes in resting EMG activity between repeated, maximal voluntary contractions (Graven-Nielsen et al., 1997b). In musculoskeletal pain patients both increased and unchanged resting EMG activities have been reported.

Static Muscle Activity and Muscle Pain

The maximal voluntary contraction (MVC) during saline-induced muscle pain is significantly lower than in the control condition (Graven-Nielsen et al., 2002b). The attenuation of MVC force during experimental muscle pain was not associated with changes in the contractile properties of muscle fibers, but was attributed to a purely central effect, i.e., a modulation of motor control.

During a static contraction (i.e., 80% of the MVC before pain), experimental muscle pain significantly reduced endurance time (Ciubotariu et al., 2004). The different findings between submaximal and maximal contractions may be explained by changes in the descending neural drive to motor neurons. Descending neural drive cannot be voluntarily increased during MVC, and therefore, an inhibitory mechanism controlling the motor neurons might explain the decreases in MVC. When submaximal contractions are performed, the voluntary neural drive may be increased and thus may compensate for potential inhibitory mechanisms. Experimental muscle pain delays the recovery phase after fatiguing contractions (Ciubotariu et al., 2007); obviously, the combination of fatigue and pain is a detrimental condition. Decreased surface EMG activity is detected for contraction levels above 25% of MVC (Falla et al., 2007a), but at low contraction levels, attenuations are also detectable by slow firing of single motor unit activity (Farina et al., 2004). An interesting observation is that muscle pain during static contractions not only decreases the activity of the painful muscle, but also attenuates the activity of synergistic muscles (Ciubotariu et al., 2004; Falla et al., 2007a). The modulating effect of muscle pain on motor control is highlighted by a correlation between pain intensity and motor unit firing inhibition (Farina et al., 2004). To produce the necessary force, generalized inhibition requires changes in muscle coordination and eventual overload of otherwise nonpainful muscles. The spatial distribution of muscle activity can be assessed by surface matrix EMG electrodes and based on this method one study found that trapezius muscle activity was completely reorganized and decreased by experimental muscle pain (Madeleine et al., 2006).

A clinical demonstration of the observed decrease in muscle strength during voluntary isometric contractions of a painful muscle has also been made in musculoskeletal pain patients. In fibromyalgia patients, the reduction in strength may be due to deficient central activation of motor units, based on a study that found no difference in the strength of the adductor pollicis muscle between patients and a control group after supramaximal stimulation of the ulnar nerve (Bäckman et al., 1988). In accordance with experimental findings, endurance time was decreased in musculoskeletal pain patients performing a submaximal contraction compared with age- and sex-matched control subjects (Bengtsson et al., 1994). If submaximal contractions during muscle pain are obtained by increased voluntary neural drive, the decreased endurance time may alternatively be due to more pronounced central fatigue. In clinical studies, various physiological factors within the muscle (e.g., the microcirculation) could influence endurance time, but these factors are not likely to affect healthy volunteers exposed to acute muscle pain.

Dynamic Muscle Activity and Muscle Pain

To better understand the effect of muscle pain on motor performance, the activity of lumbar muscles in volunteers walking on a treadmill was evaluated during HS-induced experimental low back muscle pain. Lumbar muscle activity was increased in one phase where EMG activity is normally silent, and was unaffected in the phases with strong EMG activity (Arendt-Nielsen et al., 1996). During dynamic contractions, muscle pain typically causes decreased EMG in the agonistic phase and increased EMG in the antagonistic phase of muscle activity in painful muscles. Decreased activity in both the agonistic and antagonistic muscles during muscle pain has been found without significant impairment of movement amplitude or acceleration (Ervilha et al., 2004). In particular, the initial (100 ms) agonistic EMG burst activity was decreased, illustrating that motor strategy was affected by muscle pain. This finding might be highly important in occupational settings, where such a change may elicit compensatory action from other muscles to carry out the required movement and could contribute to the development of musculoskeletal pain problems. Increased trapezius activity during contractions has been found during biceps muscle pain that might illustrate a compensatory action (Ervilha et al., 2004). Reorganization of trapezius muscle activity during repetitive shoulder flexion took the form of increased activity in the lower trapezius to compensate for decreased activity of the upper trapezius, where pain was induced (Falla et al., 2007b).

Muscle pain can have a strong biomechanical impact on the other skeletal structures. A recent study assessed the functional significance of muscle pain on knee joint control when walking by conducting three-dimensional gait analyses in subjects exposed to experimental pain induced in the vastus medialis muscle. Muscle pain modulated the function of the quadriceps muscle, resulting in impaired knee joint control and joint instability during walking (Henriksen et al., 2007). These changes are similar to those observed in patients with osteoarthritic knee pain. The loss of joint control may leave the knee joint prone to injury, may participate in the chronicity of musculoskeletal problems, and may have clinically important implications for rehabilitation and training of patients with knee pain of musculoskeletal origin.

Lumbar muscle EMG activity during a flexion-extension exercise was higher in low back pain patients in full extension than in control subjects, where EMG activity was normally silent (Ahern et al., 1988). This finding indicates that the modulation of muscle activity by pain is dependent on the specific muscle function (agonist versus antagonist phases). Findings were similar in several previous clinical studies (Lund et al., 1993). Reduced movement amplitudes have been reported in many experimental and clinical musculoskeletal pain conditions such as low back pain (Arendt-Nielsen et al., 1996). The increased EMG activity of the muscle (in the antagonistic phase) opposite to the painful muscle and the decreased EMG activity of the painful muscle (in the agonistic phase) are probably a functional adaptation of muscle coordination to limit movement. This adaptation may protect the painful muscle by reducing its activity and contraction force.

Pain-Motor Interaction Models

Muscle hyperactivity initiated by a vicious cycle due to ischemia was one of the first theories put forward to explain the cause of muscle pain (Travell et al., 1942). Another theory proposed muscle hyperactivity due to facilitation of the muscle-spindle system by muscle pain (Johansson and Sojka, 1991). However, the evidence for human muscle hyperactivity is not convincing. Lund et al. (1993) suggested the pain-adaptation model to explain the interrelationship among activity in nociceptive afferents, a central pattern generator, motor function, and coordination of muscles. This pain-adaptation model predicts increased muscle activity in the antagonistic phases and decreased muscle activity in the agonistic phases during muscle pain. Such coordination may decrease movement amplitude and velocity. Challenging and novel explanatory models linking muscle pain and motor function are further discussed by Ro et al. (Chapter 23), Madeleine (Chapter 25), Falla (Chapter 26), Svensson (Chapter 27), Hodges (Chapter 28), and Farina (Chapter 29).

Conclusion

Peripheral and central sensitization may explain a significant part of the manifestations of myofascial pain (e.g., hyperalgesia and referred pain) in chronic musculoskeletal disorders. Quantitative induction and assessment techniques are available for muscle pain, muscle hyperalgesia, referred pain, and temporal summation.

The interaction between muscle pain and motor control depends on the specific motor task. Muscle pain causes no increase in EMG activity at rest and reduces maximal voluntary contraction and endurance time during submaximal contractions. Moreover, muscle pain causes a change in coordination during dynamic exercises. Functional adaptation to muscle pain may also involve increased muscle activity, reflecting changed muscle coordination and motor strategy.

Sensory and motor control assessment procedures can provide complementary clinical information that may help to revise and optimize treatment regimes. Moreover, these experimental techniques are needed to translate basic findings into clinical manifestations and mechanisms.

References

Ahern DK, Follick MJ, Council JR, Laser-Wolston N, Litchman H. Comparison of lumbar paravertebral EMG patterns in chronic low back pain patients and non-patient controls. Pain 1988;34:153–160.

Allsop P, Cheetham M, Brooks S, Hall GM, Williams C. Continuous intramuscular pH measurement during the recovery from brief, maximal exercise in man. Eur J Appl Physiol Occup Physiol 1990;59:465–470.

Andersen H, Arendt-Nielsen L, Danneskiold-Samsoe B, Graven-Nielsen T. Pressure pain sensitivity and hardness along human normal and sensitized muscle. Somatosens Mot Res 2006;23:97–109.

Arendt-Nielsen L, Graven-Nielsen T. Central sensitization in fibromyalgia and other musculoskeletal disorders. Curr Pain Headache Rep 2003;7:355–361.

Arendt-Nielsen L, Graven-Nielsen T. Assessing muscle pain mechanisms in humans. In: Justins DM, editor. Pain 2005—an updated review: refresher course syllabus. Seattle: IASP Press; 2005. p 355–365.

Arendt-Nielsen L, Graven-Nielsen T, Svarrer H, Svensson P. The influence of low back pain on muscle activity and coordination during gait: a clinical and experimental study. Pain 1996;64:231–240.

Babenko V, Graven-Nielsen T, Svensson P, Drewes AM, Jensen TS, Arendt-Nielsen L. Experimental human muscle pain and muscular hyperalgesia induced by combinations of serotonin and bradykinin. Pain 1999;82:1–8.

Bäckman E, Bengtsson A, Bengtsson M, Lennmarken C, Henriksson KG. Skeletal muscle function in primary fibromyalgia. Effect of regional sympathetic blockade with guanethidine. Acta Neurol Scand 1988;77:187–191.

Bajaj P, Graven-Nielsen T, Arendt-Nielsen L. Trigger points in patients with lower limb osteoarthritis. J Musculoskel Pain 2001;9:17–33.

Banic B, Petersen-Felix S, Andersen OK, Radanov BP, Villiger PM, Arendt-Nielsen L, Curatolo M. Evidence for spinal cord hypersensitivity in chronic pain after whiplash injury and in fibromyalgia. Pain 2004;107:7–15.

Barlas P, Walsh DM, Baxter GD, Allen JM. Delayed onset muscle soreness: effect of an ischaemic block upon mechanical allodynia in humans. Pain 2000;87:221–225.

Bendtsen L, Nørregaard J, Jensen R, Olesen J. Evidence of qualitatively altered nociception in patients with fibromyalgia. Arthritis Rheum 1997;40:98–102.

Bengtsson A, Bäckman E, Lindblom B, Skogh T. Long term follow-up of fibromyalgia patients: Clinical symptoms, muscular function, laboratory test—an eight year comparison study. J Musculoskel Pain 1994;2:67–80.

Cairns BE, Svensson P, Wang K, Hupfeld S, Graven-Nielsen T, Sessle BJ, Berde CB, Arendt-Nielsen L. Activation of peripheral NMDA receptors contributes to human pain and rat afferent discharges evoked by injection of glutamate into the masseter muscle. J Neurophysiol 2003;90:2098–2105.

Ciubotariu A, Arendt-Nielsen L, Graven-Nielsen T. The influence of muscle pain and fatigue on the activity of synergistic muscles of the leg. Eur J Appl Physiol 2004;91:604–614.

Ciubotariu A, Arendt-Nielsen L, Graven-Nielsen T. Localized muscle pain causes prolonged recovery after fatiguing isometric contractions. Exp Brain Res 2007;181;147–158.

Costa F, Sulur P, Angel M, Cavalcante J, Haile V, Christman B, Biaggioni I. Intravascular source of adenosine during forearm ischemia in humans: implications for reactive hyperemia. Hypertension 1999;33:1453–1457.

Curatolo M, Petersen-Felix S, Gerber A, Arendt-Nielsen L. Remifentanil inhibits muscular more than cutaneous pain in humans. Br J Anaesth 2000;85:529–532.

Eriksson M, Englesson S, Niklasson F, Hartvig P. Effect of lignocaine and pH on propofol-induced pain. Br J Anaesth 1997;78:502–506.

Ervilha UF, Arendt-Nielsen L, Duarte M, Graven-Nielsen T. Effect of load level and muscle pain intensity on the motor control of elbow-flexion movements. Eur J Appl Physiol 2004;92:168–175.

Falla D, Farina D, Dahl MK, Graven-Nielsen T. Muscle pain induces task-dependent changes in cervical agonist/antagonist activity. J Appl Physiol 2007a;102:601–609.

Falla D, Farina D, Graven-Nielsen T. Experimental muscle pain results in reorganization of coordination among trapezius muscle subdivisions during repetitive shoulder flexion. Exp Brain Res 2007b;178:385–393.

Farina D, Arendt-Nielsen L, Merletti R, Graven-Nielsen T. Effect of experimental muscle pain on motor unit firing rate and conduction velocity. J Neurophysiol 2004;91:1250–1259.

Gibson W, Arendt-Nielsen L, Graven-Nielsen T. Referred pain and hyperalgesia in human tendon and muscle belly tissue. Pain 2006;120:113–123.

Gracely RH. Studies of pain in human subjects. In: McMahon SB, Koltzenburg M, editors. Textbook of pain. Edinburgh: Churchill Livingstone; 2006. p 267–289.

Graven-Nielsen T. Fundamentals of muscle pain, referred pain, and deep tissue hyperalgesia. Scand J Rheumatol 2006;35(Suppl 122):1–43.

Graven-Nielsen T, Arendt-Nielsen L, Svensson P, Jensen TS. Experimental muscle pain: a quantitative study of local and referred pain in humans following injection of hypertonic saline. J Musculoskel Pain 1997a;5:49–69.

Graven-Nielsen T, Svensson P, Arendt-Nielsen L. Effects of experimental muscle pain on muscle activity and co-ordination during static and dynamic motor function. Electroencephalogr Clin Neurophysiol 1997b;105:156–164.

Graven-Nielsen T, Babenko V, Svensson P, Arendt-Nielsen L. Experimentally induced muscle pain induces hypoalgesia in heterotopic deep tissues, but not in homotopic deep tissues. Brain Res 1998a;787:203–210.

Graven-Nielsen T, Fenger-Grøn LS, Svensson P, Steengaard-Pedersen K, Arendt-Nielsen L, Jensen TS. Quantification of deep and superficial sensibility in saline-induced muscle pain—a psychophysical study. Somatosens Mot Res 1998b;15:46–53.

Graven-Nielsen T, Kendall SA, Henriksson KG, Bengtsson M, Sörensen J, Johnson A, Gerdle B, Arendt-Nielsen L. Ketamine reduces muscle pain, temporal summation, and referred pain in fibromyalgia patients. Pain 2000;85:483–491.

Graven-Nielsen T, Gibson SJ, Laursen RJ, Svensson P, Arendt-Nielsen L. Opioid-insensitive hypoalgesia to mechanical stimuli at sites ipsilateral and contralateral to experimental muscle pain in human volunteers. Exp Brain Res 2002a;146:213–222.

Graven-Nielsen T, Lund H, Arendt-Nielsen L, Danneskiold-Samsøe B, Bliddal H. Inhibition of maximal voluntary contraction force by experimental muscle pain: a centrally mediated mechanism. Muscle Nerve 2002b;26:708–712.

Graven-Nielsen T, Jansson Y, Segerdahl M, Kristensen JD, Mense S, Arendt-Nielsen L. Experimental pain by ischaemic contractions compared with pain by intramuscular infusions of adenosine and hypertonic saline. Eur J Pain 2003;7:93–102.

Graven-Nielsen T, Mense S, Arendt-Nielsen L. Painful and non-painful pressure sensations from human skeletal muscle. Exp Brain Res 2004;159:273–283.

Graven-Nielsen T, Curatolo M, Mense S. Central sensitization, referred pain, and deep tissue hyperalgesia in musculoskeletal pain. In: Flor H, Kalso E, Dostrovsky JO (Eds). Proceedings of the 11th World Congress on Pain. Seattle: IASP Press; 2006. p 217–230.

Green S, Langberg H, Skovgaard D, Bülow J, Kjær M. Interstitial and arterial-venous [K$^+$] in human calf muscle during dynamic exercise: effect of ischaemia and relation to muscle pain. J Physiol (Lond) 2000;529:849–861.

Harpuder K, Stein ID. Studies on the nature of pain arising from an ischemic limb. Am Heart J 1943;25:429–448.

Head H. On disturbances of sensation with especial reference to the pain of visceral disease. Brain 1893;16:1–133.

Henriksen M, Alkjaer T, Lund H, Simonsen EB, Graven-Nielsen T, Danneskiold-Samsoe B, Bliddal H. Experimental quadriceps muscle pain impairs knee joint control during walking. J Appl Physiol 2007;103:132–139.

Hoheisel U, Reinöhl J, Unger T, Mense S. Acidic pH and capsaicin activate mechanosensitive group IV muscle receptors in the rat. Pain 2004;110:149–157.

Hoheisel U, Unger T, Mense S. Excitatory and modulatory effects of inflammatory cytokines and neurotrophins on mechanosensitive group IV muscle afferents in the rat. Pain 2005;114:168–176.

Iggo A. Non-myelinated afferent fibres from mammalian skeletal muscle. J Physiol 1961;155:52P–53P.

Jarvik ME, Wolff BB. Differences between deep pain responses to hypertonic and hypotonic saline solutions. J Appl Physiol 1962;17:841–843.

Jensen K, Andersen HØ, Olesen J, Lindblom U. Pressure-pain threshold in human temporal region. Evaluation of a new pressure algometer. Pain 1986;25:313–323.

Jensen K, Norup M. Experimental pain in human temporal muscle induced by hypertonic saline, potassium and acidity. Cephalalgia 1992;12:101–106.

Jespersen A, Dreyer L, Kendall S, Graven-Nielsen T, Arendt-Nielsen L, Bliddal H, Danneskiold-Samsoe B. Computerized cuff pressure algometry: A new method to assess deep-tissue hypersensitivity in fibromyalgia. Pain 2007;131:57–62.

Johansson H, Sojka P. Pathophysiological mechanisms involved in genesis and spread of muscular tension in occupational muscle pain and in chronic musculoskeletal pain syndromes: a hypothesis. Med Hypotheses 1991;35:196–203.

Kellgren JH. Observations on referred pain arising from muscle. Clin Sci 1938;3:175–190.

Kniffki K-D, Mense S, Schmidt RF. Responses of group IV afferent units from skeletal muscle to stretch, contraction and chemical stimulation. Exp Brain Res 1978;31:511–522.

Kosek E, Hansson P. Modulatory influence on somatosensory perception from vibration and heterotopic noxious conditioning stimulation (HNCS) in fibromyalgia patients and healthy subjects. Pain 1997;70:41–51.

Kosek E, Ordeberg G. Abnormalities of somatosensory perception in patients with painful osteoarthritis normalize following successful treatment. Eur J Pain 2000;4:229–238.

Laursen RJ, Graven-Nielsen T, Jensen TS, Arendt-Nielsen L. The effect of compression and regional anaesthetic block on referred pain intensity in humans. Pain 1999a;80:257–263.

Laursen RJ, Graven-Nielsen T, Jensen TS, Arendt-Nielsen L. The effect of differential and complete nerve block on experimental muscle pain in humans. Muscle Nerve 1999b;22:1564–1570.

Leffler A-S, Kosek E, Hansson P. The influence of pain intensity on somatosensory perception in patients suffering from subacute/chronic lateral epicondylalgia. Eur J Pain 2000;4:57–71.

Leffler A-S, Kosek E, Lerndal T, Nordmark B, Hansson P. Somatosensory perception and function of diffuse noxious inhibitory controls (DNIC) in patients suffering from rheumatoid arthritis. Eur J Pain 2002a;6:161–176.

Leffler AS, Hansson P, Kosek E. Somatosensory perception in a remote pain-free area and function of diffuse noxious inhibitory controls (DNIC) in patients suffering from long-term trapezius myalgia. Eur J Pain 2002b;6:149–159.

Lewis T. Pain in muscular ischemia. Arch Int Med 1932;49:713–727.

Lewis T. Suggestions relating to the study of somatic pain. Br Med J 1938;1:321–325.

Lund JP, Stohler CS, Widmer CG. The relationship between pain and muscle activity in fibromyalgia and similar conditions. In: Værøy H, Merskey H, editors. Progress in fibromyalgia and myofascial pain. Amsterdam: Elsevier; 1993. p 311–327.

Madeleine P, Lundager B, Voigt M, Arendt-Nielsen L. Sensory manifestations in experimental and work-related chronic neck-shoulder pain. Eur J Pain 1998;2:251–260.

Madeleine P, Leclerc F, Arendt-Nielsen L, Ravier P, Farina D. Experimental muscle pain changes the spatial distribution of upper trapezius muscle activity during sustained contraction. Clin Neurophysiol 2006;117:2436–2445.

Marchettini P, Simone DA, Caputi G, Ochoa JL. Pain from excitation of identified muscle nociceptors in humans. Brain Res 1996;740:109–116.

McArdle B. Myopathy due to a defect in muscle glycogen breakdown. Clin Sci 1951;10:13–33.

Mense S. Referral of muscle pain: new aspects. Am Pain Soc J 1994;3:1–9.

Mense S, Meyer H. Different types of slowly conducting afferent units in cat skeletal muscle and tendon. J Physiol (Lond) 1985;363:403–417.

Mense S, Simons DG. Muscle pain: understanding its nature, diagnosis, and treatment. Philadelphia: Lippincott Williams & Wilkins; 2001.

Mørk H, Ashina M, Bendtsen L, Olesen J, Jensen R. Experimental muscle pain and tenderness following infusion of endogenous substances in humans. Eur J Pain 2003;7:145–153.

Nie H, Arendt-Nielsen L, Andersen H, Graven-Nielsen T. Temporal summation of pain evoked by mechanical stimulation in deep and superficial tissue. J Pain 2005;6:348–355.

Nie H, Arendt-Nielsen L, Madeleine P, Graven-Nielsen T. Enhanced temporal summation of pressure pain in the trapezius muscle after delayed onset muscle soreness. Exp Brain Res 2006;170:182–190.

O'Connor PJ, Cook DB. Moderate-intensity muscle pain can be produced and sustained during cycle ergometry. Med Sci Sports Exerc 2001;33:1046–1051.

Polianskis R, Graven-Nielsen T, Arendt-Nielsen L. Pressure-pain function in desensitized and hypersensitized muscle and skin assessed by cuff algometry. J Pain 2002;3:28–37.

Rossi A, Decchi B. Changes in Ib heteronymous inhibition to soleus motoneurones during cutaneous and muscle nociceptive stimulation in humans. Brain Res 1997;774:55–61.

Saltin B, Sjøgaard G, Gaffney FA, Rowell LB. Potassium, lactate, and water fluxes in human quadriceps muscle during static contractions. Circ Res 1981;48(Suppl I):I18–I24.

Schulte H, Graven-Nielsen T, Sollevi A, Jansson Y, Arendt-Nielsen L, Segerdahl M. Pharmacological modulation of experimental phasic and tonic muscle pain by morphine, alfentanil and ketamine in healthy volunteers. Acta Anaesthesiol Scand 2003;47:1020–1030.

Schumacher MA, Jong BE, Frey SL, Sudanagunta SP, Capra NF, Levine JD. The stretch-inactivated channel, a vanilloid receptor variant, is expressed in small-diameter sensory neurons in the rat. Neurosci Lett 2000;287:215–218.

Simons DG, Travell JG, Simons L. Myofascial pain and dysfunction: the trigger point manual. Philadelphia: Lippincott Williams & Wilkins; 1999.

Slater H, Arendt-Nielsen L, Wright A, Graven-Nielsen T. Sensory and motor effects of experimental muscle pain in patients with lateral epicondylalgia and controls with delayed onset muscle soreness. Pain 2005;114:118–130.

Staud R, Cannon RC, Mauderli AP, Robinson ME, Price DD, Vierck Jr CJ. Temporal summation of pain from mechanical stimulation of muscle tissue in normal controls and subjects with fibromyalgia syndrome. Pain 2003;102:87–95.

Steen KH, Wegner H, Meller ST. Analgesic profile of peroral and topical ketoprofen upon low pH-induced muscle pain. Pain 2001;93:23–33.

Stohler CS, Zhang X, Lund JP. The effect of experimental jaw muscle pain on postural muscle activity. Pain 66:215–221.

Svendsen O, Edwards CN, Lauritzen B, Rasmussen AD. Intramuscular injection of hypertonic saline: in vitro and in vivo muscle tissue toxicity and spinal neurone c-fos expression. Basic Clin Pharmacol Toxicol 2005;97:52–57.

Svensson P, Arendt-Nielsen L, Nielsen H, Larsen JK. Effect of chronic and experimental jaw muscle pain on pain-pressure thresholds and stimulus-response curves. J Orofac Pain 1995;9:347–356.

Svensson P, Graven-Nielsen T, Matre D, Arendt-Nielsen L. Experimental muscle pain does not cause long-lasting increases in resting electromyographic activity. Muscle Nerve 1998;21:1382–1389.

Svensson P, Cairns BE, Wang K, Arendt-Nielsen L. Injection of nerve growth factor into human masseter muscle evokes long-lasting mechanical allodynia and hyperalgesia. Pain 2003a;104:241–247.

Svensson P, Cairns BE, Wang K, Hu JW, Graven-Nielsen T, Arendt-Nielsen L, Sessle BJ. Glutamate-evoked pain and mechanical allodynia in the human masseter muscle. Pain 2003b;101:221–227.

Sörensen J, Graven-Nielsen T, Henriksson KG, Bengtsson M, Arendt-Nielsen L. Hyperexcitability in fibromyalgia. J Rheumatol 1998;25:152–155.

Takeda M, Tanimoto T, Ito M, Nasu M, Matsumoto S. Role of capsaicin-sensitive primary afferent inputs from the masseter muscle in the C1 spinal neurons responding to tooth-pulp stimulation in rats. Exp Brain Res 2005;160:107–117.

Travell JG, Rinzler S, Herman M. Pain and disability of the shoulder and arm. JAMA 1942;120:417–422.

Vecchiet L, Giamberardino MA, de Bigontina P, Dragani L. Comparative sensory evaluation of pa-
    rietal tissues in painful and nonpainful areas in fibromyalgia and myofascial pain syndrome. In:
    Gebhart GF, Hammond DL, Jensen TA, editors. Proceedings of the 7th World Congress on Pain.
    Seattle: IASP Press; 1994. p 177–185.
Witting N, Svensson P, Gottrup H, Arendt-Nielsen L, Jensen TS. Intramuscular and intradermal in-
    jection of capsaicin: a comparison of local and referred pain. Pain 2000;84:407–412.
Wolfe F, Smythe HA, Yunus MB, Bennett RM, Bombardier C, Goldenberg DL, Tugwell P, Camp-
    bell SM, Abeles M, Clark P. The American College of Rheumatology 1990 Criteria for the Clas-
    sification of Fibromyalgia. Report of the Multicenter Criteria Committee. Arthritis Rheum
    1990;33:160–172.

Correspondence to: Thomas Graven-Nielsen, PhD, Dr Med Sci, Center for Sensory-Motor Interaction (SMI), Laboratory for Experimental Pain Research, Aalborg University, Fredrik Bajers Vej 7D-3, DK-9220 Aalborg E, Denmark. Tel:
+4596359832; fax: +4598154008; email: tgn@hst.aau.dk.

Central Representation of Muscle Pain and Hyperalgesia

Peter Svensson[a,b,c] and Randi Abrahamsen[a]

aDepartment of Clinical Oral Physiology, School of Dentistry, University of Aarhus, Aarhus, Denmark;
bDepartment of Oral and Maxillofacial Surgery, Aarhus University Hospital, Aarhus, Denmark;
cOrofacial Pain Laboratory, Center for Sensory-Motor Interaction,
Aalborg University, Aalborg, Denmark

There is good evidence to suggest that many chronic musculoskeletal pain conditions, including myofascial temporomandibular disorders (TMD), involve a significant dysfunction of the central nociceptive pathways (Sarlani and Greenspan, 2005). Nevertheless, most pain imaging studies have studied the cerebral processing of either cutaneous or visceral types of pain, with a relative paucity of data on muscle pain. This is surprising because from a clinical point of view, muscle pain represents a much greater diagnostic and therapeutic problem than, for example, cutaneous pain. Studies on the cerebral processing of muscle pain indicate close similarity between the "pain matrix" for muscle pain and cutaneous pain (Table I); however, there are several important questions to address with respect to the cerebral processing of muscle pain. This chapter will mainly focus on positron emission tomography (PET) and functional magnetic resonance imaging (fMRI) studies and restrict the discussion to three topics: (1) studies on experimental muscle pain in comparison with cutaneous pain, (2) studies on processing of experimental muscle hyperalgesia, and (3) studies on the influence of modulatory effects on experimental muscle

Table I
Meta-analysis of brain activation areas derived from positron emission
tomography (PET) and functional magnetic resonance imaging (fMRI) studies

	ACC	S1	S2	IC	Th	PFC
PET (*n* = 32 studies)	94%	69%	68%	88%	84%	39%
fMRI (*n* = 36 studies)	81%	76%	81%	100%	81%	70%

Source: Table modified from Apkarian et al. (2005) and reproduced with
permission from Elsevier.
Note: ACC = anterior cingulate cortex, S1 = primary somatosensory cortex,
S2 = secondary somatosensory cortex, IC = insular cortex, Th = thalamus,
PFC = prefrontal cortex. A Fisher´s exact test did not indicate significant
differences between the two brain imaging techniques.

pain. The reader is referred to recent reviews for a more detailed description of cerebral processing associated with clinical pain conditions (e.g., Apkarian et al., 2005; Lorenz and Casey, 2005; Kupers and Kehlet, 2006).

Cerebral Processing of Muscle Pain

In a recent PET study in 10 right-handed healthy volunteers (Kupers et al., 2004), experimental muscle pain was induced by the injection of a sterile 5% solution of hypertonic saline (HS) into the right masseter muscle in accordance with previously described techniques (Svensson et al., 1998). The intensity of the muscle pain was rated on a 0–100 verbal rating scale (VRS), with 0 signifying "no pain" and 100 "most pain imaginable." Cerebral blood flow was measured with PET scans at baseline and during HS-evoked jaw muscle pain. All subjects experienced moderate to severe pain following the injection of HS. The painful condition was associated with a strong increase in regional cerebral blood flow (rCBF) in the cerebellum bilaterally (Fig. 1). Additional rCBF increases occurred in the right prefrontal cortex (Brodmann area [BA] 9, 10, 11), posterior insula (bilaterally), right anterior insula, inferior parietal cortex (BA 40), and contralateral anterior cingulate cortex (ACC) (BA 24, 32) (Fig. 1). Significant rCBF increases were also observed in the brainstem (periaqueductal gray), the caudate nucleus, and the cavernous sinus (bilaterally).

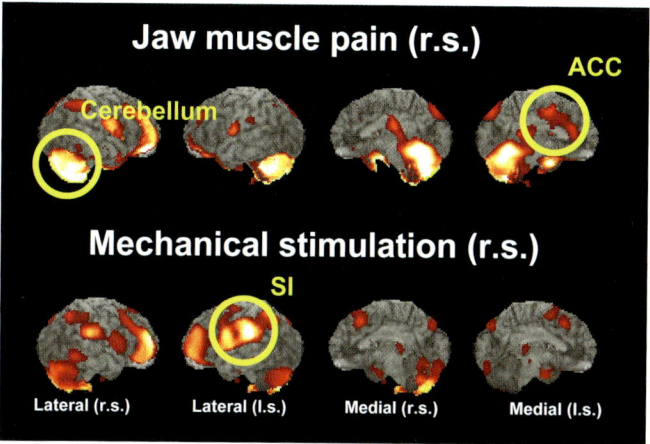

Fig. 1. Comparison of changes in regional cerebral blood flow induced by injection of hypertonic saline into the right masseter muscle or by nonpainful mechanical stimulation of the skin above the masseter muscle. Modified from Kupers et al. (2004). Note the prominent activation of the cerebellum and anterior cingulate cortex (ACC) during muscle pain and of the primary somatosensory cortex (S1) during nonpainful mechanical stimulation of the skin above the masseter muscle. Right side = r.s.; left side = l.s.

Significant rCBF decreases occurred in the subgenual and retrosplenial cingulate, the right amygdala, and the parahippocampal gyrus.

Strong cerebellar activation during experimental muscle pain has been described previously (Svensson et al., 1997). Similar activation has also been reported during thermal painful stimulation of the skin (Coghill et al., 1999; Casey et al., 2001), capsaicin-induced cutaneous pain (Iadarola et al., 1998; May et al., 1998; Witting et al., 2001), and visceral pain (Strigo et al., 2003). Cerebellar activation may represent motor planning, cognitive or affective processing, or nociceptive processing. Nociceptive information has been shown to reach the cerebellar anterior lobe (Ekerot et al., 1987), and a significant correlation has been reported between pain intensity and the blood oxygenation level-dependent (BOLD) response in the cerebellum (Helmchen et al., 2003).

No trend of primary somatosensory cortex (S1) activation was observed during HS-induced jaw muscle pain in the PET study (Kupers et al., 2004). Earlier studies using electrically induced muscle pain did, however, report increased S1 activity (Svensson et al., 1997; Niddam et al., 2002). Given that electrical stimulation activates both nociceptive and low-threshold afferents, one possibility is that S1 activation results from activation of non-nociceptive afferents. Of the relatively few nociceptive neurons in S1, only a small minority respond to input from deep tissues (Kenshalo et al., 2000), which may explain the lack of S1 activation. HS-induced muscle pain is usually diffuse and spreads over a larger area, which may contribute to the difficulty in recording distinct S1 activation in PET studies due to the relatively poor temporal and spatial resolution of this scanning technique. However, using fMRI it is possible to demonstrate significant S1 activation using experimental muscle pain stimulation. For example, Nash et al. (2007) in a preliminary report showed distinct S1 activation during HS infusion into the masseter muscle, and Henderson et al. (2007) described S1 activation during HS infusions into the leg and forearm muscles. These observations highlight the importance of methodological aspects and of the different temporal and spatial resolutions of PET and fMRI techniques in addition to differences in analysis methods (Apkarian et al. 2005). Interestingly, fMRI has shown that referred HS-induced muscle pain from the forearm and lower leg to the hand and foot is associated with a somatotopic representation in S1 from the referred pain areas in addition to local pain areas (Macefield et al., 2007). These findings illustrate the potential of brain imaging studies to better understand the pathophysiology of muscle pain and associated phenomena.

In contrast with the results of the majority of cutaneous pain studies (Apkarian et al., 2005), no rCBF increase was observed during HS-induced jaw muscle pain in the upper bank of the parietal operculum (Kupers et al. 2004). There was, however, a more posterior activation in the inferior posterior parietal cortex (BA 40). Earlier results on painful electrical intramuscular stimulation (Svensson et al., 1997; Niddam et al., 2002) did show significant activation of the secondary somatosensory cortex (S2). This discrepancy may be explained by the fact that high-threshold electrical stimulation activates both mechanoreceptive and nociceptive afferents. Studies on capsaicin-induced facial pain (May et al., 1998) and nitroglycerin-induced cluster headache (Hsieh et al., 1996) reported no S2 activation. On average, 68% of the PET studies and 81%

of the fMRI studies have described S2 activation during painful stimulation (Apkarian et al., 2005).

Jaw muscle pain was associated with a significant rCBF increase in the contralateral dorsal margin of the posterior insula (Kupers et al., 2004). When directly comparing muscle pain with nonpainful mechanical stimulation, Kupers et al. (2004) found no difference in rCBF response amplitude, suggesting that the posterior insula does not selectively encode painful or nonpainful input. This finding conforms with the proposal of a role of this region in "interoception" (Craig, 2002). Unlike nonpainful mechanical stimulation, HS-induced jaw muscle pain was associated with an additional activation in the right anterior insula, possibly subserving the limbic sensory substrate of pain (Craig, 2000). A recent study using fMRI specifically examined the somatotopic organization of the insula and provided evidence that experimental muscle pain in the leg or forearm can evoke different patterns of activity (Henderson et al., 2007). Within the posterior contralateral insula, signal increases during both muscle and skin forearm pain were located lateral and anterior to those evoked by leg pain, whereas in the ipsilateral anterior insula the pattern was reversed. There were also distinct differences in somatotopic organization related to the processing of cutaneous versus muscle pain. Thus, within the ipsilateral anterior insula, muscle pain was associated with activity in a region anterior to that activated by cutaneous pain (Henderson et al., 2007). As mentioned above, it has been suggested that the right anterior insula contains a re-representation of the dorsal posterior insula, i.e., an "interoceptive" cortex that monitors the internal state of the body (Henderson et al., 2007). Interestingly, another recent study with HS-induced pain in the low back showed a significant influence of time on cerebral processing patterns; the initial pain period was associated with activation of the ipsilateral insula but a strong bilateral deactivation of the occipitotemporal cortex. During a later stage, the muscle pain was associated with a decrease of rCBF in the left insula, inferior frontal (BA 47) and superior temporal (BA 47) cortex, right insula and temporal areas (BA 22, 38), and right ACC (BA 24, 32) and with increased rCBF in the bilateral occipital cortex (Thunberg et al., 2005). Thus, there are marked differences between the early and later stage of processing of nociceptive inputs derived from the muscles of the low back, but the somatotopic representation of the low back may differ significantly from that of other areas such as the forearm or orofacial area.

The ACC has been associated with pain unpleasantness, with attention to pain, and with the motor component of the pain response (e.g., Rainville et al., 1997; Apkarian et al., 2005). In the study by Kupers et al. (2004), HS-induced jaw muscle pain was associated with a mid-cingulate and a more rostral perigenual activation, corresponding to the cognitive and the affective divisions of the ACC, respectively (Bush et al., 2000). Svensson et al. (1997) only reported a mid-cingulate activation, which might be explained by the lower pain scores. This likelihood is confirmed by the results of Niddam et al. (2002), who also reported a rostral cingulate activation during intense muscle pain. Thus, there appears to be an intensity-dependent activation of the different subsets of the ACC.

In contrast with the results by Svensson et al. (1997), no significant thalamic activation was found during HS-induced jaw muscle pain (Kupers et al., 2004). The majority of PET studies (84%) have shown a thalamic activation by painful stimulation (Apkarian et al., 2005). The thalamic activation could be dependent on the tonic (temporal) character of the pain stimulus (Derbyshire et al., 1998). May et al. (1998) reported activation of the anterior, but not the posterior thalamus during capsaicin-induced facial pain.

In line with other pain activation studies, HS-induced jaw muscle pain was also associated with rCBF decreases in the right amygdala, the ventromedial prefrontal cortex (BA 11), and the subgenual ACC (BA 25) (Kupers et al., 2004). Experts still debate how rCBF decreases should be interpreted in brain activation studies, but Peyron et al. (2000) suggested that a reduction in rCBF reflects a depression of synaptic activity. A subgenual ACC decrease was reported during pain (Porro et al., 1998) and pain anticipation (Hsieh et al., 1999; Porro et al., 2002). This finding raises the question whether the deactivation in this area is related to pain or pain anticipation. Given that HS was injected 20 seconds before PET data acquisition (Kupers et al., 2004), it seems unlikely that anticipation effects may explain the ACC deactivation. A more likely explanation is that the ventromedial rCBF decrease reflects an attention-mediated interruption of the default state of ongoing activity in this region (Raichle et al., 2001).

Bingel et al. (2002) reported significant BOLD increases in the amygdala during laser-induced phasic cutaneous pain. Clear evidence from animal and human studies (e.g., Zubieta et al., 2001) shows that the amygdala is involved in pain processing. The amygdala receives nociceptive input (Bernard et al., 1992), and injection of morphine in the amygdala produces antinociception (Manning et al., 2001). However, it is not clear why the amygdala shows increased activity during phasic pain and decreased activity during sustained pain. A possible explanation is that the reduced activity during sustained pain reflects a coping mechanism to reduce the affective component of an inescapable pain stimulus, in this case muscle pain.

Experimental jaw muscle pain activated the dorsolateral prefrontal cortex (Kupers et al., 2004), which is less consistently activated in other PET studies (Apkarian et al., 2005). It has been suggested that activation in this region following thermal pain reflects an attentional response to sensory stimulation (Coghill et al., 1999). The fact that Kupers et al. (2004) did not find any difference in dorsolateral prefrontal activation between nonpainful and painful stimulation supports this suggestion (but see Lorenz et al., 2003 for a discussion). In line with earlier results on thermal pain (Peyron et al., 1999; Craig et al., 2000; Petrovic et al., 2000), muscle pain was also associated with an activation of the inferior prefrontal cortex. Rolls and colleagues (2003) suggested that this part of the brain is involved in processing affective aspects of sensory stimulation.

In summary, this short review, together with a recent meta-analysis of brain activation studies (Apkarian et al., 2005), show that S1 and S2, the insular cortex, the ACC, the prefrontal cortex, and the thalamus constitute an essential network for the processing of nociceptive inputs; however, there are subtle differences between experimental muscle pain and other types of experimental pain. Most notably, there appear to be differences in the activation pattern evoked by matched levels of cutaneous and muscle pain in the perigenual cingulate cortex, somatosensory cortex, motor cortex, and insula (Schreckenberger et al., 2005; Henderson et al., 2006). The implication of such differences between pain matrices for sensory, motor, autonomic, and emotional representation of both experimental and clinical pain remains to be established.

Cerebral Processing of Hyperalgesia

Very few studies have examined the cerebral correlates of muscle hyperalgesia. This is surprising because the experimental paradigms used to study PET or fMRI responses often require application of an external and time-locked somatosensory (e.g., mechanical) stimulus in order to contrast the activation patterns with a control or baseline condition. In our recent study (Kupers et al., 2004), a calibrated von Frey hair was used for mechanical punctuate stimulation. On the normal skin above the masseter muscle, this stimulus elicits a clear, sharp but nonpainful mechanical sensation (Svensson et al., 1998). However, during ongoing jaw muscle pain, the same mechanical stimulus causes increased intensity ratings, reflecting hypersensitivity (Svensson et al., 1998; Kupers et al., 2004).

Nonpainful mechanical stimulation of the skin overlying the masseter muscle causes a strong activation of the contralateral S1 corresponding to the classical face representation (Kupers et al., 2004). A significant rCBF increase was also observed in the dorsal posterior insula, the area that Craig (2002) designated as the "interoceptive" cortex. A bilateral activation was also found in the inferior parietal lobule (BA 40), which is probably the human homologue of area 7b in the monkey (Robinson and Burton, 1980). In line with earlier magnetoencephalographic (MEG) reports of a preponderance of ipsilateral activation in S2 for painful orofacial stimulation (Hari et al., 1997), the right (ipsilateral) response was stronger than the contralateral one. Finally, a significant rCBF increase was observed in the zone between the dorsal margin of the ACC (BA 32) and the medial frontal gyrus (BA 9) (Kupers et al., 2004). The stereotactic coordinates of this activation are close to those reported by Burton et al. (1999) in a tactile attention task. Therefore, this activation may reflect attentional processing of tactile stimulation.

Most of the rCBF changes observed in the jaw muscle pain condition were also observed during the mechanical hypersensitivity condition (Kupers et al., 2004). Additional rCBF increases associated with mechanical hypersensitivity were found in the contralateral S1, primary motor cortex (bilaterally), thalamus, and pulvinar. The ACC activation was more dorsal than that observed during HS-induced jaw muscle pain (Kupers et al., 2004). In addition, the activation in the inferior parietal lobule was more anterior and more ventral than that observed during experimental muscle pain. The pattern of rCBF deactivations was similar to that observed following experimental muscle pain, but there were additional rCBF decreases in the ipsilateral S1 and left hippocampal formation in the mechanical hypersensitivity condition (Kupers et al., 2004).

Further analysis of the interactions between HS-induced jaw muscle pain and mechanical stimulation revealed significant interaction effects in the subgenual cingulate and the ventrobasal thalamus (Kupers et al., 2004). Two foci could be observed in the thalamus: one in the ventroposterior-medial region (VPM) and a smaller one in the dorsomedian thalamic region. An additional rCBF increase was found in the left inferior temporal gyrus. Thus, mechanical hypersensitivity appears to be associated with a unique activity in the thalamus and anterior subgenual cingulate cortex. The main interaction effect between mechanical stimulation and HS-induced jaw muscle pain was observed in the posterior part of the thalamus, covering the VPM. This finding is consistent with results from animal studies showing that nociceptive neurons in VPM display central sensitization and reduced mechanical thresholds following nociceptive stimulation of the dental pulp (Park et al., 2006). The activation extended into the dorsomedian thalamus, which is in agreement with recent findings on heat-induced allodynia (Lorenz et al., 2002). It may underlie the increased ratings for von Frey stimulation in the presence of HS-induced jaw muscle pain. The finding of an interaction in the subgenual cingulate is in line with recent findings of an interaction in this region when subjects engaged in an attentional task during application of a painful stimulus (Bantick et al., 2002). The application of von Frey stimulation during muscle pain may have acted as an attentional distractor. This hypothesis is supported by psychophysical findings that muscle pain unpleasantness ratings were slightly lower when von Frey stimulation was simultaneously applied (Kupers et al., 2004).

Mechanical allodynia due to skin injections of capsaicin activates the prefrontal, insular, S2, and posterior parietal BA 5/7 cortices contra- or bilaterally (Iadarola et al., 1998; Witting et al., 2001). During brush-evoked allodynia, patients with peripheral nerve injury pain have significant rCBF increases in the contralateral orbitofrontal cortex, the ipsilateral insular and S2 cortices, and the cerebellum (Witting et al., 2006). These findings suggest that clinical allodynia—in contrast to acute experimental allodynia—is characterized by contralateral orbitofrontal and ipsilateral parietal cortical activation.

There is some evidence of altered processing of mechanical stimuli in fibromyalgia patients (Gracely et al., 2002). However, future brain imaging studies will be needed to outline the brain networks specifically related to muscle allodynia and hyperalgesia in different chronic muscle pain conditions.

Cerebral Processing of Modulatory Influences on Muscle Pain

A series of high-quality studies have recently addressed a number of questions specifically related to supraspinal processing of muscle pain. First, the investigators tested the importance of supraspinal antinociceptive systems involved in the regulation of experimental jaw muscle pain (Zubieta et al., 2001). They tested the function of the endogenous opioid system (including μ-opioid receptors) using PET scans and a selective μ-opioid receptor radiotracer (^{11}C-carfentanil) during ongoing HS-induced jaw muscle pain. Searches based on a priori knowledge of the endogenous opioid system revealed significant activation in the ipsilateral amygdala and in the contralateral ventrolateral portion of the thalamus. Furthermore, there were negative correlations between the sensory scores on the McGill Pain Questionnaire and the degree of μ-opioid receptor system activation in the nucleus accumbens, thalamus, and amygdala ipsilateral to the painful stimulation (Zubieta et al., 2001). Also, the unpleasantness and affective dimension of HS-induced jaw muscle pain were negatively correlated with activation of the μ-opioid receptor system in the bilateral dorsal ACC and thalamus and the ipsilateral nucleus accumbens. Overall, the study provided strong evidence in favor of a central role of the μ-opioid receptor system in the regulation of sensory and affective components of muscle pain (Zubieta et al., 2001). In a subsequent study Zubieta et al. (2002) demonstrated significant sex-related differences in the magnitude of μ-opioid receptor system activation in the anterior thalamus, ventral basal ganglia, and amygdala with less activity in women in the follicular phase than in men. Furthermore, women had reductions in the basal state of activation of the μ-opioid receptor system in the nucleus accumbens compared to men. Important aspects of these results are that the endogenous pain modulatory system seems to be activated differently in men and women when they report the same magnitude of experimental jaw muscle pain. Smith et al. (2006) recently showed that low-estradiol conditions are associated with increased pain sensitivity by a reduction in endogenous opioid receptor system function. Significant positive correlations were made between estradiol plasma concentrations and μ-opioid receptor system activation in the amygdala during sustained jaw muscle pain.

Part of the interindividual variation in activation of the endogenous pain inhibitory system during sustained jaw muscle pain appears to be linked to a functional polymorphism of the catechol-*O*-methyltransferase (COMT) gene (Zubieta et al., 2003). COMT is involved in the metabolism of catecholamines and is an important modulator of dopaminergic and adrenergic/noradrenergic neurotransmission. There were significant effects of genotype on activation of the μ-opioid receptor system in the anterior thalamus, the thalamic pulvinar ipsilateral to the painful side, and the ventral basal ganglia bilaterally, encompassing the nucleus accumbens (Zubieta et al., 2003). The level of COMT activity could also be correlated to activation of the μ-opioid receptor system in the nucleus accumbens. The authors interpreted the varying levels of catecholamine metabolism dictated by the COMT polymorphism to reflect downstream alterations of the functional responses of the μ-opioid receptor system and to implicate the dopaminergic system in the basal ganglia (Zubieta et al., 2003). These observations prompted further studies on the importance of the basal ganglia and the role of the dopaminergic system in the modulation of muscle pain. Activation of the dorsal nucleus caudate and putamen dopamine D_2 receptors was positively associated with individual variations in subjective ratings of sensory and affective qualities of HS-induced jaw muscle pain (Scott et al., 2006). However, the nucleus accumbens dopamine receptor activation, which may involve both D_2 and D_3 receptors, was exclusively associated with variations in the subject's emotional responses during sustained HS-induced jaw muscle pain. Overall, the study suggested that dopamine D_2/D_3 receptor function in the ventral basal ganglia may represent an important point of interaction between the neurobiological substrates of emotion, reward, and pain regulation (Scott et al., 2006).

In summary, the supraspinal modulation of muscle pain is beginning to be understood. Some of the important brain regions have been identified, together with key neuromodulators. The genetic contribution to individual differences in sensory and emotional aspects of muscle pain is emerging, in addition to an appreciation of sex-related effects on modulation of the endogenous pain inhibitory system. These aspects require further studies in both experimental and clinical muscle pain conditions.

Conclusions

This chapter has described the evolution of brain imaging studies from fairly simple, but important, studies on activation patterns triggered by painful stimulation of the muscles. The pain matrix related to muscle pain appears to partly overlap with that of cutaneous pain, but there are noticeable differences that may contribute to the different somatosensory, motor, autonomic, and emotional responses in these types of pain. Nonpainful somatosensory stimuli, expectations of pain, and processing of other sensory inputs may activate the pain matrix. Few studies have specifically looked at the processing of muscle allodynia or hyperalgesia, but there are clear differences in supraspinal processing of a painful or a nonpainful mechanical stimulus. Finally, the μ-opioid receptor system and the dopaminergic system appear to be strong modulators of the clinical manifestation of muscle pain. Overall, technological developments with brain imaging tools have advanced our knowledge on muscle pain. Further studies using a combination of multimodal brain imaging and genetic and neurochemistry techniques may help to test specific hypothesis on the networks related to processing of muscle pain and hyperalgesia.

References

Apkarian AV, Bushnell MC, Treede RD, Zubieta JK. Human brain mechanisms of pain perception and regulation in health and disease. Eur J Pain 2005;9:463–484.

Bantick SJ, Wise RG, Ploghaus A, Clare S, Smith SM, Tracey I. Imaging how attention modulates pain in humans using functional MRI. Brain 2002;125:310–319.

Bernard JF, Huang GF, Besson JM. Nucleus centralis of the amygdala and the globus pallidus ventralis: electrophysiological evidence for an involvement in pain processes. J Neurophysiol 1992;68:551–569.

Bingel U, Quante M, Knab R, Bromm B, Weiller C, Buchel C. Subcortical structures involved in pain processing: evidence from single-trial fMRI. Pain 2002;99:313–321.

Bush G, Luu P, Posner MI. Cognitive and emotional influences in anterior cingulate cortex. Trends Cogn Sci 2000;4:215–222.

Casey KL, Morrow TJ, Lorenz J, Minoshima S. Temporal and spatial dynamics of human forebrain activity during heat pain: analysis by positron emission tomography. J Neurophysiol 2001;85:951–959.

Coghill RC, Sang CN, Maisog JM, Iadarola MJ. Pain intensity processing within the human brain: a bilateral, distributed mechanism. J Neurophysiol 1999;82:1934–1943.

Craig AD. How do you feel? Interoception: the sense of the physiological condition of the body. Nat Rev Neurosci 2002;3:655–666.

Craig AD, Chen K, Bandy D, Reiman EM. Thermosensory activation of insular cortex. Nat Neurosci 2000;3:184–190.

Derbyshire SWG, Jones AK. Cerebral responses to a continual tonic pain stimulus measured using positron emission tomography. Pain 1998;76:127–135.

Ekerot CF, Gustavsson P, Oscarsson O, Schouenborg J. Climbing fibres projecting to cat cerebellar anterior lobe activated by cutaneous A and C fibres. J Physiol 1987;386:529–538.

Gracely RH, Petzke F, Wolf JM, Clauw DJ. Functional magnetic resonance imaging evidence of augmented pain processing in fibromyalgia. Arthritis Rheum 2002;46:1333–1343.

Hari R, Portin K, Kettenmann B, Jousmaki V, Kobal G. Right-hemisphere preponderance of responses to painful CO_2 stimulation of the human nasal mucosa. Pain 1997;72:145–151.

Helmchen C, Mohr C, Erdmann C, Petersen D, Nitschke MF. Differential cerebellar activation related to perceived pain intensity during noxious thermal stimulation in humans: a functional magnetic resonance imaging study. Neurosci Lett 2003;335:202–206.

Henderson LA, Bandler R, Gandevia SC, Macefield VG. Distinct forebrain activity patterns during deep versus superficial pain. Pain 2006;120:286–296.

Henderson LA, Gandevia SC, Macefield VG. Somatotopic organization of the processing of muscle and cutaneous pain in the left and right insula cortex: a single-trial fMRI study. Pain 2007;128:20–30.

Hsieh JC, Hannerz J, Ingvar M. Right-lateralised central processing for pain of nitroglycerin-induced cluster headache. Pain 1996;67:59–68.

Hsieh JC, Stone-Elander S, Ingvar M. Anticipatory coping of pain expressed in the human anterior cingulate cortex: a positron emission tomography study. Neurosci Lett 1999;262:61–64.

Iadarola MJ, Berman KF, Zeffiro T, Byas-Smith MG, Gracely RH, Max MB, Bennett GJ. Neural activation during acute capsaicin-evoked pain and allodynia assessed with PET. Brain 1998;121:931–947.

Kenshalo DR, Iwata K, Sholas M, Thomas DA. Response properties and organization of nociceptive neurons in area 1 of monkey primary somatosensory cortex. J Neurophysiol 2000;84:719–729.

Kupers R, Kehlet H. Brain imaging of clinical pain states: a critical review and strategies for future studies. Lancet Neurol 2006;5:1033–1044.

Kupers RC, Svensson P, Jensen TS. Central representation of muscle pain and mechanical hyperesthesia in the orofacial region: a positron emission tomography study. Pain 2004;108:284–293.

Lorenz J, Casey KL. Imaging of acute versus pathological pain in humans. Eur J Pain 2005;9:163–165.

Lorenz J, Cross D, Minoshima S, Morrow T, Paulson P, Casey K. A unique representation of heat allodynia in the human brain. Neuron 2002;35:383–393.

Lorenz J, Minoshima S, Casey KL. Keeping pain out of mind: the role of the dorsolateral prefrontal cortex in pain modulation. Brain 2003;126:1079–1091.

Manning BH, Merin NM, Meng ID, Amaral DG. Reduction in opioid- and cannabinoid-induced antinociception in rhesus monkeys after bilateral lesions of the amygdaloid complex. J Neurosci 2001;21:8238–8246.

Macefield VG, Gandevia SC, Henderson LA. Discrete changes in cortical activation during experimentally induced referred muscle pain: A single-trial fMRI study. Cereb Cortex 2007;17:2050–2059.

May A, Kaube H, Büchel C, et al. Experimental cranial pain elicited by capsaicin: a PET study. Pain 1998;74:61–66.

Nash P, Henderson L, Macefield V, Klineberg I, Murray G. Brain representation of noxious stimulation of masseter: an fMRI study. International Association for Dental Research, 2007, abstract 259.

Niddam DM, Yeh TC, Wu YT, Lee PL, Ho LT, Arendt-Nielsen L, Chen AC, Hsieh JC. Event-related functional MRI study on central representation of acute muscle pain induced by electrical stimulation. Neuroimage 2002;17:1437–1450.

Park SJ, Zhang S, Chiang CY, Hu JW, Dostrovsky JO, Sessle BJ. Central sensitization induced in thalamic nociceptive neurons by tooth pulp stimulation is dependent on the functional integrity of trigeminal brainstem subnucleus caudalis but not subnucleus oralis. Brain Res 2006;1112:134–145.

Petrovic P, Petersson KM, Ghatan PH, Stone-Elander S, Ingvar M. Pain-related cerebral activation is altered by a distracting cognitive task. Pain 2000;85:19–30.

Peyron R, Garcia-Larrea L, Gregoire MC, Costes N, Convers P, Lavenne F, Mauguiere F, Michel D, Laurent B. Haemodynamic brain responses to acute pain in humans: sensory and attentional networks. Brain 1999;122:1765–1780.

Peyron R, Laurent B, García-Larrea L. Functional imaging of brain responses to pain. A review and meta-analysis. Neurophysiol Clin 2000;30:263–288.

Porro CA, Baraldi P, Pagnoni G, Serafini M, Facchin P, Maieron M, Nichelli P. Does anticipation of pain affect cortical nociceptive systems? J Neurosci 2002;22:3206–3214.

Porro CA, Cettolo V, Francescato MP, Baraldi P. Temporal and intensity coding of pain in human cortex. J Neurophysiol 1998;80:3312–3320.

Raichle ME, MacLeod AM, Snyder AZ, Powers WJ, Gusnard DA, Shulman GL. A default mode of brain function. Proc Natl Acad Sci USA 2001;98:676–682.

Rainville P, Duncan GH, Price DD, Carrier B, Bushnell MC. Pain affect encoded in human anterior cingulate but not somatosensory cortex. Science 1997;277:968–971.

Robinson CJ, Burton H. Somatic submodality distribution within the second somatosensory (SII), 7b, retroinsular, postauditory, and granular insular cortical areas of M. fascicularis. J Comp Neurol 1980;192:93–108.

Rolls ET, O'Doherty J, Kringelbach ML, Francis S, Bowtell R, McGlone F. Representations of pleasant and painful touch in the human orbitofrontal and cingulate cortices. Cereb Cortex 2003;13:308–317.

Sarlani E, Greenspan JD. Why look in the brain for answers to temporomandibular disorder pain? Cells Tissues Organs 2005;180:69–75.

Schreckenberger M, Siessmeier T, Viertmann A, Landvogt C, Buchholz HG, Rolke R, Treede RD, Bartenstein P, Birklein F. The unpleasantness of tonic pain is encoded by the insular cortex. Neurology 2005;64:1175–1183.

Scott DJ, Heitzeg MM, Koeppe RA, Stohler CS, Zubieta JK. Variations in the human pain stress experience mediated by ventral and dorsal basal ganglia dopamine activity. J Neurosci 2006;26:10789–10795.

Smith YR, Stohler CS, Nichols TE, Bueller JA, Koeppe RA, Zubieta JK. Pronociceptive and antinociceptive effects of estradiol through endogenous opioid neurotransmission in women. J Neurosci 2006;26:5777–5785.

Strigo IA, Duncan GH, Boivin M, Bushnell MC. Differentiation of visceral and cutaneous pain in the human brain. J Neurophysiol 2003;89:3294–3303.

Svensson P, Graven-Nielsen T, Arendt-Nielsen L. Mechanical hyperesthesia of human facial skin induced by tonic painful stimulation of jaw muscles. Pain 1998;74:93–100.

Svensson P, Minoshima S, Beydoun A, Morrow TJ, Casey KL. Cerebral processing of acute skin and muscle pain in humans. J Neurophysiol 1997;78:450–460.

Thunberg J, Lyskov E, Korotkov A, Ljubisavljevic M, Pakhomov S, Katayeva G, Radovanovic S, Medvedev S, Johansson H. Brain processing of tonic muscle pain induced by infusion of hypertonic saline. Eur J Pain 2005;9:185–194.

Witting N, Kupers RC, Svensson P, Arendt-Nielsen L, Gjedde A, Jensen TS. Experimental brush-evoked allodynia activates posterior parietal cortex. Neurology 2001;57:1817–1824.

Witting N, Kupers RC, Svensson P, Jensen TS. A PET activation study of brush-evoked allodynia in patients with nerve injury pain. Pain 2006;120:145–154.

Zubieta JK, Heitzeg MM, Smith YR, Bueller JA, Xu K, Xu Y, Koeppe RA, Stohler CS, Goldman D. COMT val$_{158}$met genotype affects mu-opioid neurotransmitter responses to a pain stressor. Science 2003;299:1240–1243.

Zubieta JK, Smith YR, Bueller JA, Xu Y, Kilbourn MR, Jewett DM, Meyer CR, Koeppe RA, Stohler CS. Regional mu opioid receptor regulation of sensory and affective dimensions of pain. Science 2001;293:311–315.

Zubieta JK, Smith YR, Bueller JA, Xu Y, Kilbourn MR, Jewett DM, Meyer CR, Koeppe RA, Stohler CS. Mu-opioid receptor-mediated antinociceptive responses differ in men and women. J Neurosci 2002;22:5100–5107.

Correspondence to: Peter Svensson, DDS, PhD, Dr Odont, Department of Clinical Oral Physiology, Royal Dental College, University of Aarhus, Vennelyst Boulevard 9, DK-8000 Aarhus C, Denmark. Fax: +45 8619 5665; email: psvensson@odont.au.dk.

Part II

Key Factors Determining Muscle Pain Sensitivity

Referred Muscular Hyperalgesia from Visceral Structures

Maria Adele Giamberardino,[a] Raffaele Costantini,[b] and Giannapia Affaitati[a]

[a]Pathophysiology of Pain Laboratory, Ce.S.I., "G. D'Annunzio" Foundation, Department of Medicine and Science of Aging, "G. D'Annunzio" University of Chieti, Italy; [b]Department of General Surgery, "G. D'Annunzio" University of Chieti, Italy

Visceral pain represents a major clinical problem that motivates a vast number of medical consultations. Referral of the sensation (referred visceral pain) to somatic areas is a typical feature of pain originating from internal organs (Procacci et al., 1986; Giamberardino and Cervero, 2007), and secondary muscle hyperalgesia almost always accompanies the spontaneous symptom in the referred zone (Giamberardino et al., 2006). Although common in routine medical practice, only in relatively recent times have referred muscle symptoms from viscera been extensively investigated in both clinical and experimental studies (Giamberardino et al., 1995, 2005; Vecchiet et al., 1999; Arendt-Nielsen and Svensson, 2001; Arendt-Nielsen et al., 2004). This chapter provides an outline of the state of the art in referred muscle phenomena from internal organs in terms of both clinical characterization and pathophysiological interpretation.

Referred Muscle Pain/Hyperalgesia from Visceral Structures in the Clinical Setting

Referred pain occurs constantly in visceral nociception. In fact, after a transitory phase (lasting a few minutes or hours) in which visceral pain is perceived as a midline, poorly discriminated sensation accompanied by marked neurovegetative signs and emotional reactions ("true visceral pain"), the symptom is "transferred" to somatic areas of the body wall neuromerically connected to the involved organ (Procacci et al., 1986). The referral area most often becomes the site of secondary hyperalgesia (increased sensitivity to painful stimuli and decreased pain threshold), especially if the algogenic condition of the internal organ recurs frequently or is prolonged. This condition may involve all three somatic tissues of the body wall—skin, subcutis, and muscle—but it is most often localized at the muscle level (referred muscle pain without and with hyperalgesia) (Vecchiet et al., 1989, 1992). In myocardial infarction, for instance, referred pain typically occurs in the precordial region and upper limbs, mostly the left arm; hyperalgesia affects the pectoralis major muscle and forearm muscles. The trapezius and deltoid muscles are less frequently involved. In a low percentage of cases, pain is also referred to the subcutis and skin, within dermatomes C8–T1 on the ulnar side of the arm and forearm, and hyperalgesia is found at the same level (Procacci et al., 1986; Loeser, 2001). Fig. 1 shows patterns of referred muscle hyperalgesia from the heart.

In urinary colic from calculosis, pain is referred to the lumbar region of the affected side, radiating toward the ipsilateral flank and anteriorly toward the groin, with hyperalgesia characteristically affecting the quadratus lumborum muscle and external oblique muscle (Vecchiet et al., 1989). In biliary calculosis, pain is perceived in the upper right quadrant of the abdomen, radiating toward the back; hyperalgesia typically develops in the rectus abdominis muscle, around the cystic point area (at the level of junction of the 10th rib and the outer margin of the same muscle) (Giamberardino et al., 2005). Fig. 2 shows patterns of referred muscle hyperalgesia from the biliary tract. In dysmenorrhea, pain

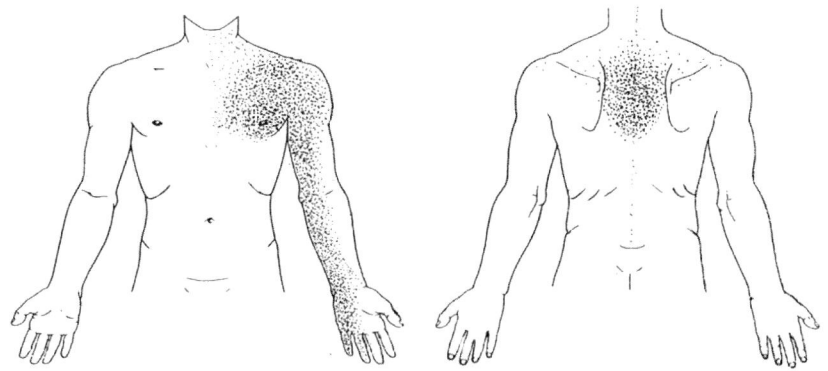

Fig. 1. Patterns of referred muscle hyperalgesia from the heart.

is referred to the lowest abdominal quadrants, radiating toward the groin and the upper part of the thighs; hyperalgesia develops in the rectus abdominis muscle and in muscles of the pelvic region (Giamberardino et al., 1997). In irritable bowel syndrome (IBS), pain is perceived in the abdomen, around the umbilical area; hyperalgesia of the rectus abdominis muscle at the same level is a typical finding (Caldarella et al., 2006). In all the previous examples, hyperalgesia may also eventually involve the subcutis and skin overlying the tender muscles in cases of repeated and/or prolonged painful episodes (Vecchiet et al., 1999).

Muscle hypersensitivity in the referred pain zones can easily be detected clinically by manual compression, the maneuver provoking an evident pain reaction by the patient. However, precise quantification of the extent of the sensory changes can only be provided by instrumental measurements. Evaluation of pain thresholds to different stimuli has been usefully employed to this purpose (Vecchiet et al., 1989; Giamberardino et al., 1997, 2005; Arendt-Nielsen and Svensson, 2001). The application of pressure, chemical, and electrical stimuli has allowed study of the development and progression of muscle hyperalgesia in referred pain areas from different internal organs. As a general rule, irrespective of the specific organ involved, researchers have found that in recurrent visceral pain conditions, such as urinary or biliary colics or dysmenorrhea, muscle hyperalgesia (evidenced by a significant decrease in pain threshold)

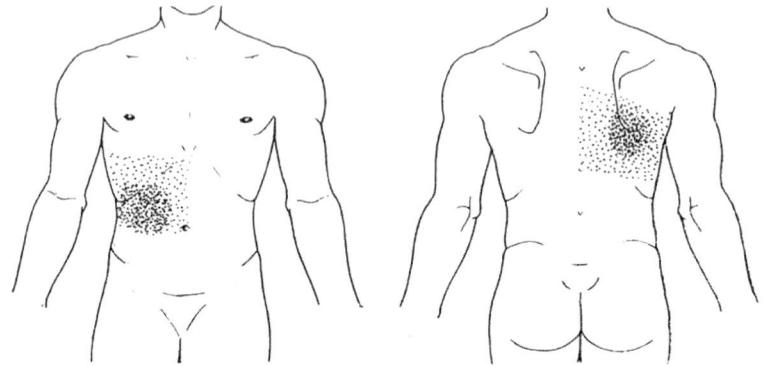

Fig. 2. Patterns of referred muscle hyperalgesia from the biliary tract.

develops early in the process of pain referral, being detectable after just a few pain episodes. It tends to be accentuated by repeated visceral pain attacks and is a prolonged phenomenon, outlasting the spontaneous pain and often even the presence of the primary source of noxious impulses in the internal organs (Giamberardino, 2000a). For example, hyperalgesia in the external oblique musculature of patients with urinary calculosis develops after the first few colic episodes, is more pronounced as they recur, and is detectable in the intervals between pain attacks, sometimes persisting even after stone elimination (Vecchiet et al., 1992; Giamberardino et al., 1994). Fig. 3 shows patterns of referred muscle hyperalgesia from the urinary tract.

In cases of acute inflammatory visceral pain, referred muscle hyperalgesia has also been documented. Patients with acute appendicitis showed lower pain thresholds to pressure stimuli in the referred abdominal pain area (McBurney's point) compared with the contralateral control area. Thresholds were also decreased in the referred pain area in patients compared with the same area in healthy control subjects (Stawowy et al., 2002).

Patients with acute cholecystitis also presented hypersensitivity to pressure stimulation in the referred pain area and in the contralateral control area of the abdomen. However, the hypersensitivity normalized after cholecystectomy (Stawowy et al., 2004). This latter finding is different from the results reported above on the persistence of some degree of hyperalgesia even after removal of the primary visceral focus. It probably indicates that repeated noxious inputs from viscera (in recurrent conditions such as colics or painful menstruation), rather than isolated acute episodes, are required to leave persistent hyperalgesic traces in the referral area.

Referred muscle hyperalgesia is most often accompanied by a dystrophic change in the tissue, as revealed by a decreased thickness and section area of muscle measured via ultrasound (Procacci et al., 1986). Like the hyperalgesia, the trophic muscle changes are set off by the noxious impulses from the internal organ. Interestingly, however, whereas the hyperalgesia tends to diminish with the reduction of the noxious potential of the visceral focus (while remaining significant), the trophic changes do not. Patients with symptomatic gallbladder calculosis presenting both muscle hyperalgesia and trophic changes in the cystic point area at their primary evaluation were re-evaluated after a period of 6 months. During that time one subgroup of patients had not complained of further colics while another subgroup had continued to have colics. The hyperalgesia was accentuated in the symptomatic subgroup but diminished in the asymptomatic subgroup; in contrast, trophic changes remained unaltered in both. Thus, whereas referred muscle hyperalgesia appears to be strictly modulated by the algogenic input from the

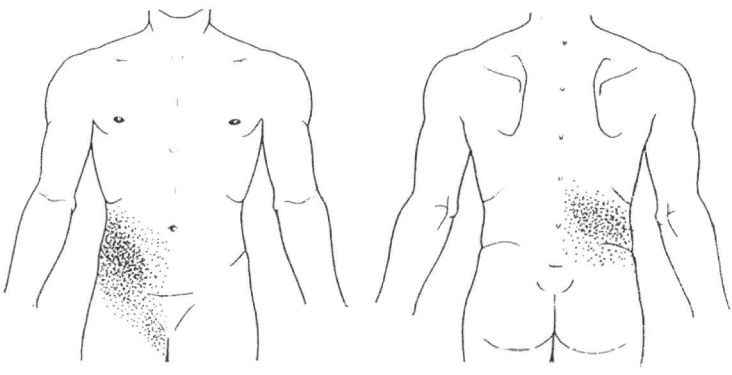

Fig. 3. Patterns of referred muscle hyperalgesia from the urinary tract.

viscera, the referred trophic changes seem to be an "on or off" phenom-enon (Giamberardino et al., 2005).

Referred Muscle Pain/Hyperalgesia in "Viscero-Visceral Hyperalgesia"

Cases in which two visceral pain conditions affect the same patient are extremely frequent in medical practice. When the two involved viscera share at least part of their central sensory projection, the phenomenon of "viscero-visceral" hyperalgesia may occur, consisting of an enhancement of typical pain symptoms from both regions (Giamberardino, 2000a). This condition involves not only the spontaneous sensation but also re-ferred muscle hyperalgesia, which is far more pronounced than in the case of a single visceral pain disease. For instance, the uterus and colon share a neuronal projection at the level of T10–L1 (Loeser, 2001). Wom-en with both dysmenorrhea and IBS frequently report more menstrual pain, intestinal pain, and somatic abdominal/pelvic hyperalgesia (in the areas of referral from the uterus and from the intestine) than women with only one of these conditions (unpublished observation). Dysmenor-rhea patients present intestinal hypersensitivity even when they do not show—or have not yet shown—obvious symptoms of IBS (Brinkert et al., 2007). This hypersensitivity is probably a result of centrally mediated vis-cero-visceral hyperalgesia due to recurrent intense menstrual pain.

Similarly, patients with dysmenorrhea or endometriosis together with urinary calculosis have increased menstrual pain, urinary colic pain, and muscle hyperalgesia of the abdominopelvic/lumbar area (in the sites of referred pain from the uterus and from the urinary tract) compared to patients with only one of these conditions (Berkley et al., 1993a,b; Giam-berardino et al., 2001). The link is a common projection between the uterus and upper urinary tract at the level of T10–L1.

The interdependence of the painful phenomena from the two viscera involved is indirectly shown by the fact that effective treatment of one condition may significantly improve typical symptoms of the other. For example, urinary pain and referred lumbar muscle hyperalgesia may decrease after hormonal treatment of dysmenorrhea, or menstrual pain and referred abdominopelvic muscle hyperalgesia may lessen after urinary stone elimination following lithotripsy (Giamberardino, 2000a, 2001).

Pathophysiology of Referred Muscle Pain and Hyperalgesia from Visceral Structures

Referred pain was initially attributed to viscerosomatic convergence occurring in primary afferent fibers, where multiple peripheral branches innervate both the viscera and somatic structures, whether in the skin or in deeper tissues (see Cervero and Laird, 2004). The number of fibers with these characteristics is, however, too limited to account for such a widespread phenomenon as referred pain, which occurs for virtually all internal organs. In contrast, there is wide experimental documentation of the convergence of both visceral and somatic afferent inputs onto the same sensory neurons in the central nervous system, thanks to extensive electrophysiological and anatomical studies in the spinal cord and higher brain centers (Cervero, 2002; Cervero and Laird, 2004). Regarding convergences between muscles and viscera at the spinal level, neurons receiving input from both internal organs and deep somatic structures (including muscles) are located in the deep layers of the dorsal horn. These neurons have a diffuse and bilateral visceral and somatic input, with large and multireceptive receptive fields, and they are subject to descending excitatory control—probably originating from the rostral medullary centers—as well as inhibitory control. A number of these neurons project to the reticular formation of the brainstem (Cervero, 2002).

Based on this phenomenon, visceral pain would be referred to muscle structures because of a "misinterpretation" of higher brain centers due to memory traces of previous experiences of muscle pain (the convergence-projection theory) (see Procacci et al., 1986; Cervero and Laird, 2004). With the repetition of the sensory input from viscera, a state of "central sensitization" would be set off in the spinal cord, with hyperactivity and hyperexcitability of viscerosomatic convergent neurons (Ji et al., 2003). In this situation, the central effect of even normal sensory inputs coming from the somatic area of referral would be facilitated (the convergence-facilitation theory) (Cervero and Laird, 2004). Sensitization of viscerosomatic convergent neurons has indeed been documented electrophysiologically in a number of studies using animal models of referred hyperalgesia from viscera, such as the model of lumbar muscle hyperalgesia in rats with experimental ureteric calculosis (Giamberardino et al., 1995, 1996, 1997; Roza et al., 1998). The persistent enhancement of nociceptive transmission, termed "central sensitization," is dependent on the activity of N-methyl-D-aspartate (NMDA) receptors (Salter 2004). These receptors are also assumed to play an important role in the generation of referred hyperalgesia from viscera (Cervero, 2002).

Central changes after noxious input can also induce the release of vasoactive peptides from fine afferents in peripheral tissues that are not affected by the original cause, via dorsal root reflexes conducted antidromically from the spinal cord (Willis, 1999). The central changes produced by the visceral input could thus not only be responsible per se for the secondary hyperalgesia (increased responsiveness of sensitized viscerosomatic convergent neurons to painful stimuli in the somatic area of referral), but also contribute to the phenomenon via dorsal root reflexes that are conducted centrifugally out to peripheral sensory endings, where they can release neurotransmitters or alter the excitability of sensory terminals related to the referral area.

Central mechanisms also can be hypothesized for referred muscle hyperalgesia in the case of concurrent algogenic conditions from two internal organs sharing at least part of their central sensory projection (viscero-visceral hyperalgesia). Along with viscerosomatic convergence, experimental evidence exists for viscero-visceral convergence in the central nervous system, such as between the colon/rectum, bladder, vagina, and uterine cervix (Berkley et al., 1993a,b; Foreman, 2000). The increase in the excitability of viscero-viscerosomatic convergent neurons, triggered by the afferent barrage from one visceral organ, could mediate the increased reactivity to impulses from the second visceral organ and the somatic area of referral (see Giamberardino et al., 2002). This hypothesis needs to be verified experimentally in reliable animal models of viscero-visceral hyperalgesia, such as the rat model of endometriosis plus ureteral calculosis, in which the animals present increased behavioral signs of pain in both the ureter (Giamberardino et al., 1995) and the pelvic area (Wesselmann et al., 1998), as well as a notable enhancement of referred lumbar muscle hyperalgesia (Giamberardino et al., 2002). This experimental condition mimics the viscero-visceral hyperalgesia in women with endometriosis and urinary calculosis.

Central changes thus seem to play a key role in the pathophysiology of referred muscle hyperalgesia from viscera; they are accentuated by the repetition of the painful visceral episodes and are reduced when they stop. The fact that some degree of hyperalgesia often persists beyond the presence of the "macroscopic" peripheral visceral focus, however, needs to be explained on a different basis. It is theoretically possible that, once established, central plastic changes persist, becoming relatively independent of the primary triggering event. At present, however, we still lack experimental evidence that central sensitization changes survive –for days or months after the cessation of the initial peripheral insult (see Cervero and Laird, 2004). It is possible that, in spite of the apparent removal of the primary focus in the internal organ, some "clinically unapparent" peripheral visceral alteration persists, thus maintaining the state of central hyperexcitability via persistence of the peripheral drive (see Giamberardino and Cervero, 1997).

In addition to central changes, a further mechanism has also been postulated to account for referred muscle hyperalgesia and its persistence. A reflex arc could be activated by increased afferent input to the spinal cord from sensory fibers innervating the internal organs. In the spinal cord, efferent output to the skeletal muscle, initiated by the increased afferent input, could produce sustained contraction, which in turn would be responsible for sensitization of nociceptors locally (Procacci et al., 1986). In a study using the previously mentioned rat model of referred lumbar muscle hyperalgesia from artificial ureteric calculosis, this theory has found experimental support.

Ultrastructural modifications of the muscle indicative of contraction have been shown ipsilateral, but not contralateral, to the affected ureter at lumbar level. These changes include (a) decreased I band length/ sarcomere length ratio; (b) increased muscle cell membrane fluidity;

(c) increased Ca^{2+}-uptake capacity (correlated linearly to the number of ureteral "crises"); and (d) decreased ryanodine binding. The severity of these ultrastructural changes is proportional to the degree of visceral pain behavior and referred hyperalgesia recorded in the animals (Giamberardino et al., 2003). In the same model, c-Fos activation was found in the spinal cord, not only in sensory neurons but also in motoneurons, significantly more on the affected side (Aloisi et al., 2004). These results suggest the presence, proportional in degree to the activity of the ureteral pain focus, of a state of skeletal muscle contraction in the oblique musculature ipsilateral to the stone, an event that could contribute to the generation of local hyperalgesia via sensitization of muscle nociceptors. This reflex arc activation could also, at least in part, account for the referred trophic changes seen in the muscle.

Referred visceral hyperalgesia from muscles. While referred muscle hyperalgesia from viscera is relatively well studied, the opposite phenomenon of referred visceral hyperalgesia from muscles has not, so far, been systematically documented in the clinical context. Some authors speculate, however, that the frequent occurrence of visceral hypersensitivity in the form of IBS, interstitial cystitis, and dysmenorrhea in patients with diffuse musculoskeletal pain (fibromyalgia), may reflect such a phenomenon. This suggestion has been put forward on the basis of the results of experimental studies in animals. Miranda and coworkers (2004), for example, documented that injections of low-pH sterile saline into the gastrocnemius muscle significantly increased the electromyographic response from the external oblique muscle to colorectal distension in rats. Bielefeldt et al. (2006) showed that inflammation of the hindpaw via injection of nerve growth factor produces increased visceromotor responses to colorectal distension in mice. These results were attributed to facilitation of visceral messages in viscerosomatic convergent neurons in the lower spinal cord due to the somatic input. However, evidence of referred visceral hyperalgesia from somatic structures is still limited compared to that supporting referred muscle hyperalgesia from viscera. The reasons why viscerosomatic convergence would preferentially cause referred hypersensitivity to muscles rather than to viscera remain to be established.

Referred Muscle Pain/Hyperalgesia from Visceral Structures as a Function of Age and Gender

Age

The progressive aging of the population, especially in developed countries, has brought to medical attention the problem of pain in the elderly, which is a complex phenomenon, especially considering that older persons often present more than one painful condition at a time. While primary musculoskeletal pain is reported to increase with advancing age, referred muscle pain/hyperalgesia from viscera tends, instead, to decrease (Giamberardino, 2005). Paradoxically, this decrease occurs while an increase is observed, with advancing age, of a number of pathological conditions that are potentially algogenic for viscera (Gibson, 2003). One example is atherosclerosis, which increases exponentially with age but is not accompanied by a parallel increase in manifestations of ischemic pain from viscera. For instance, silent myocardial ischemia and painless myocardial infarction become more frequent in older age, with approximately 35–42% of adults over the age of 65 years experiencing an apparently silent or painless heart attack (Stern et al., 2003). Another example is acute appendicitis: about 45% of older adults with this condition do not have referred lower right quadrant pain as a presenting symptom, compared to less than 5% of younger adults (Wroblewski and Mikulowski, 1991). Moreover, referred visceral pain associated with various types of malignancy is reported to be much less intense in adults of advanced age than in younger adults (Caraceni and Portenoy, 1999).

The pathophysiology of the decreased expression of referred visceral pain in older age is far from being completely elucidated, but some of the contributing mechanisms may include impaired Aδ-fiber function and a reduction of the content and turnover of neurotransmitter systems known to be involved in nociception, such as substance P and calcitonin gene-related peptide (CGRP) (Moore and Clinch, 2004). Also worth mentioning is the higher prevalence in the elderly of medical conditions such as hypertension or diabetes, which have definitely been associated with impaired pain perception (France et al., 2002; Bierhaus et al., 2004). Thus, elderly patients affected with these conditions are at a high risk of painless diseases of internal organs, a circumstance that should always be kept in mind clinically to avoid not only misdiagnosis but, more importantly, underestimation of potentially life-threatening visceral events.

Gender

Both clinical and experimental research studies suggest gender differences in referred muscle/pain hyperalgesia from internal organs (Fillingim, 2000; Arendt-Nielsen et al., 2004). Women are more subject than men to referred visceral pain/hyperalgesia from sex-specific viscera, due to the more complex nature of their reproductive function. Examples are menstrual pain and possibly labor pain, as well as several visceral "after-pains" in the postpartum period. States of chronic pelvic pain subsequent to ascending genital infections are more frequent in women than in men for anatomical reasons (a shorter urethra) (Giamberardino, 2000b).

Gender differences in referred visceral pain/hyperalgesia also exist for non-sex-specific viscera. Many painful visceral conditions display a different prevalence, while others show a different clinical profile of painful symptoms in the two sexes. Regarding prevalence, some conditions—mostly of pathological origin—predominantly affect men (e.g., coronary heart disease, with mortality rates being four times those of women before age 55), while others prevail in women (e.g., gallbladder pathologies), mainly because of differences in risk factors between the two sexes (e.g., for atherosclerosis or biliary calculosis) linked to both hormonal status and lifestyle (Caroli-Bosc et al., 1999; Kosuge et al., 2006). Other clinical entities—mostly dysfunctional—such as IBS or interstitial cystitis—are largely prevalent in women because of the supposedly higher susceptibility of the female sex to develop sensitization phenomena, which would be at least partly responsible for the pain expressed in these conditions (Chang, 2004; Evans and Sant, 2007). Concerning the clinical profile of painful symptoms for the same visceral pathology, sex differences are reported in the intensity, location, and quality of pain as well as in the nature of other accompanying symptoms. For instance, the pattern of referred muscle pain from the heart would be much more variable and unpredictable in women than in men (Procacci et al., 1986; Kosuge et al., 2006). An important role in these symptom diversities is probably played by sociocultural factors, which would affect the way women and men approach pain (Heitkemper and Jarrett, 2001).

Irrespective of the internal organ involved, referred visceral pain conditions in women appear to be exacerbated at specific periods of the menstrual cycle (often the perimenstrual phases) during the fertile years, whereas men normally experience a more stable profile of painful symptoms over comparable periods of time (see Giamberardino, 2000b).

Another important difference between the two sexes is that women appear more prone than men to present phenomena of "viscero-visceral hyperalgesia," as demonstrated by the interaction between the female reproductive organs and urinary tract, two visceral domains that are frequently the site of potentially painful conditions throughout the course of a woman's life (Giamberardino et al., 2001). These phenomena are likely to predispose women to more complex and often longer-lasting referred painful experiences from internal organs compared to men, especially in the abdominal/pelvic area. In addition, since hyperalgesia most often develops in the referred pain areas, women are more likely than men to have extended areas of somatic (especially muscle) hyperalgesia as a consequence of multiple, concurrent, and recurrent visceral pains.

Taken together, current research data suggest more frequent and persistent referred muscle pain/hyperalgesia from viscera in women, often with a more insidious clinical profile, a circumstance that may render diagnosis and treatment more difficult than in men.

Conclusion

Referred muscle pain and hyperalgesia are a constant feature of visceral pain conditions. Clinical and experimental studies have clearly shown that secondary hyperalgesia is a prominent phenomenon that, once set off, tends to persist for a long time, often accompanied by muscle dystrophic changes that can impair tissue functionality far beyond the duration of the visceral disease. The mechanisms behind referred muscle pain and hyperalgesia from internal organs have been partially elucidated, but further research studies are needed to clarify all aspects of the phenomenon, especially in complex cases such as "viscero-visceral hyperalgesia." Clarification of these mechanisms will allow progressively more effective treatment of symptoms and may prevent the long-term muscle complications—especially dystrophic changes—that so often characterize referred pain from viscera.

References

Aloisi A, Ceccarelli I, Affaitati G, Lerza R, Vecchiet L, Lapenna D, Giamberardino MA. c-Fos expression in the spinal cord of female rats with artificial ureteric calculosis. Neurosci Lett 2004;361:212–215.

Arendt-Nielsen L, Bajaj P, Drewes AM. Visceral pain: gender differences in response to experimental and clinical pain. Eur J Pain 2004;8:465–472.

Arendt-Nielsen L, Svensson P. Referred muscle pain: basic and clinical findings. Clin J Pain 2001;17:11–19.

Berkley KJ, Guilbaud G, Benoist JM, Gautron M. Responses of neurons in and near the thalamic ventrobasal complex of the rat to stimulation of uterus, cervix, vagina, colon, and skin. J Neurophysiol 1993a;69:557–568.

Berkley KJ, Hubscher CH, Wall PD. Neuronal responses to stimulation of the cervix, uterus, colon and skin in the rat spinal cord. J Neurophysiol 1993b;69:533–544.

Bielefeldt K, Lamb K, Gebhart GF. Convergence of sensory pathways in the development of somatic and visceral hypersensitivity. Am J Physiol Gastrointest Liver Physiol 2006;291:658–665.

Bierhaus A, Haslbeck KM, Humpert PM, et al. Loss of pain perception in diabetes is dependent on a receptor of the immunoglobulin superfamily. J Clin Invest 2004;114:1741–1751.

Brinkert W, Dimcevski G, Arendt-Nielsen L, Drewes AM, Wilder-Smith OH. Dysmenorrhoea is associated with hypersensitivity in the sigmoid colon and rectum. Pain 2007;132(Suppl 1):S46–51.

Caldarella MP, Giamberardino MA, Sacco F, et al. Sensitivity disturbances in patients with irritable bowel syndrome and fibromyalgia. Am J Gastroenterol 2006;101:2782–2789.

Caraceni A, Portenoy RK. An international survey of cancer pain characteristics and syndromes, IASP Task Force on Cancer Pain. Pain 1999;82:263–274.

Caroli-Bosc FX, Deveau C, Harris A, et al. General Practitioner's Group of Vidauban. Prevalence of cholelithiasis: results of an epidemiologic investigation in Vidauban, southeast France. Dig Dis Sci 1999;44:1322–1329.

Cervero F. Mechanisms of visceral pain. In: Giamberardino MA, editor. Pain 2002–An updated review: refresher course syllabus. Seattle: IASP Press; 2002. p 403–411.

Cervero F, Laird JM. Understanding the signaling and transmission of visceral nociceptive events. J Neurobiol 2004;61:45–54.

Chang L. Review article: epidemiology and quality of life in functional gastrointestinal disorders. Aliment Pharmacol Ther 2004;20:31–39.

Evans RJ, Sant GR. Current diagnosis of interstitial cystitis: an evolving paradigm. Urology 2007;69(4 Suppl):S64–72.

Fillingim RB. Sex, gender, and pain: women and men really are different. Curr Rev Pain 2000;4:24–30.

Foreman RD. Integration of viscerosomatic sensory input at the spinal level. In: Mayer EA, Saper CB, editors. The biological basis for mind body interactions. Progress in Brain Research, Vol. 122. Amsterdam: Elsevier; 2000. p 209–221.

France CR, Froese SA, Stewart JC. Altered central nervous system processing of noxious stimuli contributes to decreased nociceptive responding in individuals at risk for hypertension. Pain 2002;98:101–108.

Giamberardino MA. Visceral hyperalgesia. In: Devor M, Rowbotham MC, Wiesenfeld-Hallin Z, editors. Proceedings of the 9th World Congress on Pain. Progress in Pain Research and Management, Vol. 16. Seattle: IASP Press; 2000a. p 523–550.

Giamberardino MA. Sex-related and hormonal modulation of visceral pain. In: Fillingim RB, editor. Sex, gender, and pain. Progress in Pain Research and Management, Vol. 17. Seattle: IASP Press; 2000b. p 135–163.

Giamberardino MA. Visceral pain. Pain: Clinical Updates 2005;XIII(6).

Giamberardino MA, Affaitati G, Costantini R. Referred pain from internal organs. In: Cervero F, Jensen TS, editors. Handbook of clinical neurology. Edinburgh: Elsevier; 2006. p 343–361.

Giamberardino MA, Affaitati G, Lerza R, Fano G, Fulle S, Belia S, Lapenna D, Vecchiet L. Evaluation of indices of skeletal muscle contraction in areas of referred hyperalgesia from an artificial ureteric stone in rats. Neurosci Lett 2003;338:213–216.

Giamberardino MA, Affaitati G, Lerza R, Lapenna D, Costantini R, Vecchiet L. Relationship between pain symptoms and referred sensory and trophic changes in patients with gallbladder pathology. Pain 2005;114:239–249.

Giamberardino MA, Berkley KJ, Affaitati G, Lerza R, Centurione L, Lapenna D, Vecchiet L. Influence of endometriosis on pain behaviors and muscle hyperalgesia induced by a ureteral calculosis in female rats. Pain 2002;95:247–257.

Giamberardino MA, Berkley KJ, Iezzi S, de Bigontina P, Vecchiet L. Pain threshold variations in somatic wall tissues as a function of menstrual cycle, segmental site and tissue depth in non-dysmenorrheic women, dysmenorrheic women and men. Pain 1997;71:187–197.

Giamberardino MA, Cervero F. The neural basis of referred visceral pain. In: Pasricha J, Willis B, Gebhart GF, editors. Chronic abdominal and visceral pain: theory and practice. New York: Informa Healthcare; 2007. p. 177–192.

Giamberardino MA, Dalal A, Valente R, Vecchiet L. Changes in activity of spinal cells with muscular input in rats with referred muscular hyperalgesia from ureteral calculosis. Neurosci Lett 1996;203:89–92.

Giamberardino MA, de Bigontina P, Martegiani C, Vecchiet L. Effects of extracorporeal shock-wave lithotripsy on referred hyperalgesia from renal/ureteral calculosis. Pain 1994;56:77–83.

Giamberardino MA, De Laurentis S, Affaitati G, Lerza R, Lapenna D, Vecchiet L. Modulation of pain and hyperalgesia from the urinary tract by algogenic conditions of the reproductive organs in women. Neurosci Lett 2001;304:61–64.

Giamberardino MA, Valente R, de Bigontina P, Vecchiet L. Artificial ureteral calculosis in rats: behavioural characterization of visceral pain episodes and their relationship with referred lumbar muscle hyperalgesia. Pain 1995;61:459–469.

Giamberardino MA, Vecchiet L. Central neuronal changes in recurrent visceral pain. Int J Clin Pharmacol Res 1997;XVII:63–66.

Gibson SJ. Pain and aging: the pain experience over the adult life span. In: Dostrovsky JO, Carr DB, Koltzenburg M, editors. Proceedings of the 10th World Congress on Pain. Progress in Pain Research and Management, Vol. 24. Seattle: IASP Press; 2003. p 767–790.

Heitkemper MM, Jarrett M. Gender differences and hormonal modulation in visceral pain. Curr Pain Headache Rep 2001;5:35–43.

Ji RR, Kohno T, Moore KA, Woolf CJ. Central sensitization and LTP: do pain and memory share similar mechanisms? Trends Neurosci 2003;26:696–705.

Kosuge M, Kimura K, Ishikawa T, et al. Differences between men and women in terms of clinical features of ST-segment elevation acute myocardial infarction. Circ J 2006;70:222–226.

Loeser JD, editor. Bonica's management of pain, 3rd ed. Philadelphia: Lippincott, Williams & Wilkins; 2001.

Miranda A, Peles S, Rudolph C, Shaker R, Sengupta JN. Altered visceral sensation in response to somatic pain in the rat. Gastroenterology 2004;126:1082–1089.

Moore AR, Clinch D. Underlying mechanisms of impaired visceral pain perception in older people. J Am Geriatr Soc 2004;52:132–136.

Procacci P, Zoppi M, Maresca M. Clinical approach to visceral sensation. In: Cervero F, Morrison JFB, editors. Visceral sensation. Progress in Brain Research. Amsterdam: Elsevier; 1986. p 21–28.

Roza C, Laird JM, Cervero F. Spinal mechanisms underlying persistent pain and referred hyperalgesia in rats with an experimental ureteric stone. J Neurophysiol 1998;79:1603–1612.

Salter MW. Cellular neuroplasticity mechanisms mediating pain persistence. J Orofac Pain 2004;18:318–324.

Stawowy M, Bluhme C, Arendt-Nielsen L, Drewes AM, Funch-Jensen P. Somatosensory changes in the referred pain area in patients with acute cholecystitis before and after treatment with laparoscopic or open cholecystectomy. Scand J Gastroenterol 2004;39:988–993.

Stawowy M, Rossel P, Bluhme C, Funch-Jensen P, Arendt-Nielsen L, Drewes AM. Somatosensory changes in the referred pain area following acute inflammation of the appendix. Eur J Gastroenterol Hepatol 2002;14:1079–1084.

Stern S, Behar S, Gottlieb S. Cardiology patient pages. Aging and diseases of the heart. Circulation 2003;108:e99–101.

Vecchiet L, Giamberardino MA, de Bigontina P. Referred pain from viscera: when the symptom persists despite the extinction of the visceral focus. Adv Pain Res Ther 1992;20:101–110.

Vecchiet L, Giamberardino MA, Dragani L, Albe-Fessard D. Pain from renal/ureteral calculosis: evaluation of sensory thresholds in the lumbar area. Pain 1989;36:289–295.

Vecchiet L, Vecchiet J, Giamberardino MA. Referred muscle pain: clinical and pathophysiological aspects. Curr Rev Pain 1999;3:489–498.

Wesselmann U, Czakanki PP, Affaitati G, Giamberardino MA. Uterine inflammation as a noxious visceral stimulus: behavioral characterization in the rat. Neurosci Lett 1999;246:73–76.

Willis WD Jr. Dorsal root potentials and dorsal root reflexes: a double-edged sword. Exp Brain Res 1999;124:395–421.

Wroblewski M, Mikulowski P. Peritonitis in geriatric inpatients. Age Ageing 1991;20:90–94.

Correspondence to: Prof. Maria Adele Giamberardino, MD, via Carlo de Tocco n. 3, 66100 Chieti, Italy. Tel/Fax: +39-0871541207; email: mag@unich.it.

Sex-Related Differences in Muscle Afferent Discharge

Brian E. Cairns and Xudong Dong

Faculty of Pharmaceutical Sciences, The University of British Columbia, Vancouver, British Columbia, Canada

Women are two to five times more likely than men to seek treatment for chronic muscle pain associated with syndromes such as fibromyalgia (FM) or myofascial temporomandibular disorders (TMD) (LeResche, 2001; Rollman and Lautenbacher, 2001; Nekora-Azak, 2004). The mechanisms responsible for sex-related differences in chronic muscle pain syndromes are incompletely understood, but they probably involve both biological and psychosocial factors. Sex hormones are one biological factor associated with sex-related differences in the incidence and prevalence of muscle pain, although the levels of the neuraxis at which sex hormones may act to influence muscle pain are still being elucidated (LeResche, 2001, 2003; Rollman and Lautenbacher, 2001; Nekora-Azak, 2004). One potential site of action of biological mechanisms that result in sex-related differences in muscle pain is the muscle itself, given that chronic muscle pain syndromes such as FM and TMD are characterized by the development of specific tender points in the muscle tissue. Indeed, sex-related differences in the response properties of slowly conducting afferent fibers (Aδ or group III, as well as C or group IV fibers) that form the first link

Fundamentals of Musculoskeletal Pain
edited by Thomas Graven-Nielsen, Lars Arendt-Nielsen, and Siegfried Mense
IASP Press, Seattle, © 2008

in the neural pathway whereby noxious stimulation of the muscle is conveyed to the central nervous system might contribute to differences in the prevalence of these syndromes in men and women.

Despite more than 50 years of research investigating the response properties of slowly conducting afferent fibers that innervate skeletal muscle and the recognition of sex-related differences in the prevalence of certain chronic muscle pain conditions, few studies have specifically addressed the possibility that there may be sex-related differences in the response of skeletal muscle afferent fibers to noxious stimulation. Most studies examining mechanical and chemical responses of skeletal muscle afferent fibers have used only male animals. This chapter presents the current evidence for sex-related differences in the response properties of slowly conducting skeletal muscle afferent fibers and describes their putative mechanisms.

Sex-Related Differences in Muscle Afferent Mechanical Properties

Relatively little is known about sex-related differences in the mechanical properties of skeletal muscle afferent fibers. Findings to date appear to be limited to slowly conducting afferent fibers that innervate the masticatory muscles. Studies measuring the mechanical threshold of putative masticatory muscle nociceptors in both male and female rats have identified no significant sex-related differences in mechanical threshold (Cairns et al., 2002, 2003; Dong et al., 2006, 2007; Mann et al., 2006; Sung et al., 2008). However, recent results do suggest sex-related differences in the relationship between baseline mechanical threshold and conduction velocity as well as an influence of plasma estrogen levels on the mechanical threshold of slowly conducting masticatory muscle afferent fibers. As discussed in Chapter 2, there is an inverse relationship between baseline mechanical threshold and conduction velocity for masticatory muscle afferent fibers (Cairns et al., 2002). However, recent evidence suggests that this inverse relationship holds true for afferent fibers recorded from male rats, but not from female rats (Mann et al., 2006). Plasma estrogen levels of normally cycling female rats, but not male rats, are positively correlated with the baseline mechanical threshold of putative masticatory muscle mechanonociceptors, which implies that under normal physiological conditions, elevation of estrogen levels is associated with increased mechanical threshold for these afferent fibers in female rats (Mann et al., 2006). Such an association may provide a mechanistic basis for the observation of increased masticatory muscle pain and sensitivity at menstruation, when estrogen levels are decreased (LeResche et al., 2003).

Sex-Related Differences in Chemically Evoked Afferent Response

Hypertonic Saline

Relatively few studies have investigated the effect of algogenic chemicals on muscle afferent discharge in male and female rats. Muscle afferent discharge evoked by injection of hypertonic saline, one of the most commonly employed algogens, into the masseter muscle is similar in male and female rats (Cairns et al., 2003). Hypertonic saline (HS) is a nonspecific activator that may directly excite the afferent fibers by opening mechanosensitive cation channels or may cause the release of other excitants (Hamill and Martinac, 2001). If HS does act by opening mechanosensitive cation channels, then the absence of sex-related differences in HS-evoked afferent discharge would be consistent with the lack of overall difference in afferent mechanical threshold between male and female rats.

NMDA Receptors

Injection of the excitatory amino acid glutamate into the masseter muscle evokes greater discharge in slowly conducting afferent fibers recorded from female rats than from male rats, which suggests a sex-related difference in the peripheral mechanisms that underlie glutamate-evoked muscle afferent discharge (Fig. 1) (Cairns et al., 2001, 2002, 2003). Excitation of afferent fibers by elevated tissue glutamate levels in masticatory muscle

appears to be mediated largely through activation of peripheral *N*-methyl
D-aspartate (NMDA) receptors (Cairns et al., 2003; Ro, 2003, 2004). Indeed, recent studies indicate that intramuscular injection of NMDA excites slowly conducting afferent fibers in both the masseter and temporalis muscles. These studies show that NMDA-evoked afferent discharge
can be attenuated by the NMDA-receptor antagonist ketamine, which
indicates that it is mediated through peripheral NMDA-receptor activation (Cairns et al., 2003; Dong et al., 2006). Injection of NMDA into
the masseter muscle excites slowly conducting afferent fibers in a con-
centration-related manner in both sexes; however, NMDA-evoked afferent discharge is significantly greater in female than in male rats (Dong et
al., 2007). These results indicate that sex-related differences in peripheral
NMDA-receptor activation appear to mediate, at least in part, differences in the response of masseter afferent fibers to glutamate in male and
female rats.

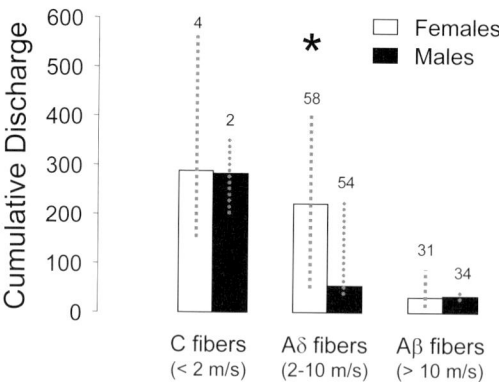

Fig. 1. The vertical bar graph illustrates the median cumulative afferent discharge
evoked after injection of glutamate (500 mM) into the masseter muscle of male and female rats. There was a significant sex-related difference in the glutamate-evoked discharge of Aδ afferent fibers but not Aβ fibers. Numbers above each bar indicate the
number of fibers examined in each sex. * $P < 0.05$, Mann-Whitney test. Dotted lines:
interquartile range.

Glutamate-evoked masseter nociceptor discharge in all stages of the estrous cycle in female rats is greater than in male rats (Cairns, 2007). Glutamate-evoked masseter afferent discharge also appears to vary through the rat estrous cycle, such that in female rats glutamate-evoked nociceptor discharge is greatest during proestrus, when serum estrogen levels are known to peak (Cairns, 2007). However, while sex-related differences in glutamate-evoked nociceptor discharge are reasonably large, estrous-cycle-related differences in glutamate-evoked nociceptor discharge in female rats are smaller and require recordings from a large population of nociceptors in order to be detected. As mentioned previously, glutamate excites masseter afferent fibers through activation of peripheral NMDA receptors. A positive correlation has also been found between serum estrogen levels and NMDA-evoked masseter afferent discharge in female rats, but not in male rats (Dong et al., 2007). Further, treatment of ovariectomized female rats with high-dose estrogen significantly increased NMDA-evoked masseter afferent discharge (Dong et al., 2007). Thus, there is an apparent interaction between estrogen levels and peripheral NMDA-receptor mechanisms.

In the central nervous system, increased estrogen levels enhance NMDA-receptor-mediated neuronal responses (Woolley et al., 1997; Foy et al., 1999). For example, the magnitude of NMDA-receptor-mediated long-term potentiation in the rat hippocampus increases with both exogenous and natural cyclic elevation of estrogen levels (Woolley et al., 1997; Foy et al., 1999; Bi et al., 2000, 2001). NMDA receptors are heteromeric complexes formed by an obligatory NR1 subunit and one or more NR2 subunits (A, B, C, or D) or NR3 subunits (A or B) (Mayer and Armstrong, 2004; Kew and Kemp, 2005). The mechanisms that contribute to this estrogen-mediated enhancement of NMDA-induced central neuronal response include increased expression of NMDA receptors and activation of Src tyrosine kinases to phosphorylate tyrosine residues on the NR2B subunit (Woolley et al., 1997; Bi et al., 2000; Cyr et al., 2001). Phosphorylation of the NR2B subunit increases the receptor's open time and its probability of opening without altering single channel conductance, resulting in increased NMDA-receptor-mediated currents (Salter and Kalia, 2004). Recent evidence indicates that trigeminal ganglion neurons that innervate the masseter muscle express NR2B (~40%) subunits and that ifenprodil, a selective NR2B-receptor antagonist (Williams, 1993; Avenet et al., 1996), can attenuate NMDA-evoked afferent discharge. Trigeminal ganglion neurons also express estrogen receptors (Bereiter et al., 2005), which suggests that estrogen and NMDA receptors are coexpressed in at least some masseter ganglion neurons (Dong et al., 2007). Indeed, the frequency of expression of NR2B subunits by masseter ganglion neurons is greater in female rats compared with male rats, and it can be further increased in ovariectomized female rats by treatment with estrogen, which suggests that increased expression of the NR2B subunit is one mechanism underlying the enhanced afferent response to injection of NMDA into the masseter muscle. On the other hand, systemic administration of the Src tyrosine kinase inhibitor PP2 did not affect NMDA-evoked afferent discharge in estrogen-treated ovariectomized female rats, which implies that this particular pathway is not involved in the effects of estrogen on peripheral NMDA receptors (Dong et al., 2007).

It has been suggested that peripheral NMDA receptors contribute to mechanical pain transduction mechanisms since activation of these receptors also leads to mechanical sensitization of masticatory muscle afferent fibers (Cairns et al., 2002, 2007; Mann et al., 2006). However, activation of peripheral NMDA receptors may play a role in modulating the transduction of innocuous mechanical stimuli, given that trigeminal mesencephalic nucleus neurons, which innervate spindle afferent fibers of masticatory muscles, also express NR2A and NR2B subunits (Turman et al., 1999). In contrast to results obtained for glutamate- and NMDA-evoked afferent discharge, there is currently no evidence for a sex-related difference in glutamate-induced afferent mechanical sensitization (Cairns et al., 2002). These findings suggest that activation of peripheral NMDA receptors may modulate the response of afferent fibers to both innocuous and noxious mechanical stimulation, but that the mechanisms underlying this effect of peripheral NMDA-receptor activation are different from those involved in direct excitation of masticatory muscle afferent fibers.

Serotonin (5-HT) Receptors

More than half of all ganglion neurons that project to the masseter and temporalis muscles express the 5-HT_3 receptor (Sung et al., 2008). The frequency of 5-HT_3-receptor expression by masticatory muscle ganglion neurons in female rats (66%) is significantly greater than in male rats (39 %). There are no obvious differences in size distribution between male and female masticatory muscle ganglion neurons, and the 5HT_3 receptor is distributed on small to medium-sized (20- to 40-μm diameter) ganglion neurons in both sexes. The 5HT_3 receptor is a nonselective cation channel, and activation of this receptor results in a rapidly desensitizing inward current in trigeminal ganglion neurons (Hu et al., 2005). Injection of 5-HT into the temporalis or masseter muscle evokes brief discharges in slowly conducting afferent fibers that are mediated, at least in part, through activation of peripheral 5HT_3 receptors (Sung et al., 2008). There are, however, no sex-related differences in the response of masticatory muscle afferent fibers to intramuscular injection of 5-HT. The lack of an apparent sex-related difference might be related to the brief duration of 5-HT evoked masticatory muscle discharge. Therefore, unlike the peripheral NMDA receptors, activation of peripheral 5-HT_3 receptors is not associated with a significant sex-related difference in masticatory muscle afferent discharge.

Calcitonin Gene-Related Peptide

Small to medium-sized trigeminal ganglion neurons that innervate the masseter muscle express calcitonin gene-related peptide (CGRP); expression of this peptide is sexually dimorphic, with 38% and 19% of masseter ganglion neurons positive for CGRP in male and female rats, respectively (Ambalavanar et al., 2003). CGRP is also expressed in roughly twice as many dorsal root ganglion (DRG) neurons in male rats as in females (Yang et al., 1998). The expression of CGRP by DRG neurons in female rats is decreased by ovariectomy, and treatment of ovariectomized female rats with estrogen increases CGRP expression to a level similar to that in intact females (Yang et al., 1998). A large percentage of

DRG neurons that express CGRP also express estrogen receptors (Yang et al., 1998). Taken together, these results suggest that as estrogen levels decrease in female rats, there could also be a decrease in the expression of CGRP by ganglion neurons that innervate skeletal muscle. Given that CGRP is a potent vasodilator of blood vessels in skeletal muscle (Arden et al., 1994), one consequence of these lower levels of CGRP might be a decrease in blood flow to skeletal muscle, which could result in more rapid onset of muscle fatigue.

The exact role of CGRP in the development and maintenance of acute or chronic muscle pain has yet to be fully elucidated, but evidence suggests that it may be involved in modulating central neuronal responses to noxious mechanical stimuli (Sun et al., 2004). CGRP may also play a role in peripheral mechanisms of mechanical sensitization, at least those induced by certain experimental models of myositis. For example, injection of complete Freund's adjuvant into the masseter muscle to produce inflammation decreases the head withdrawal thresholds in male rats in response to pressure stimuli applied to the site of injection. This inflammation-induced mechanical sensitization is attenuated by pre-administration of a CGRP antagonist (Ambalavanar et al., 2006). It is not known whether there are sex-related differences in this effect of CGRP.

Relevance for Human Muscle Pain

Human experimental pain research has shown that injection of glutamate into the masseter muscle evokes a greater pain responses in women than in men (Svensson et al., 2003). In men, glutamate-evoked muscle pain can be significantly attenuated by the NMDA-receptor antagonist ketamine, which is consistent with findings in animal studies that glutamate-evoked afferent discharge is mediated through activation of peripheral NMDA receptors (Cairns et al., 2003). However, recent results suggest that glutamate-evoked muscle pain in women is not significantly attenuated by the same concentrations of ketamine that are effective in men (Castrillon et al., 2007). In humans, skeletal muscle is innervated by slowly conducting afferent fibers (Marchettini et al., 1996), and thus it is likely that glutamate-evoked muscle pain in men and women results from the activation of the same types of slowly conducting afferent fibers as in rats (Cairns et al., 2001).

The animal data suggest that sex-related differences in glutamate-evoked muscle pain in humans could be explained by an increased expression of peripheral NMDA receptors by slowly conducting afferent fibers in the female masseter muscle. However, a higher expression of peripheral NMDA-receptors means that more receptors would need to be blocked by antagonists such as ketamine in order to significantly attenuate glutamate-evoked muscle pain, which may also explain human sex-related differences in the effect of ketamine. The lack of sex-related differences in 5-HT-evoked afferent discharge are consistent with the reported lack of sex-related differences in 5-HT-evoked masseter muscle pain in humans (Ernberg et al., 2000). Injection of CGRP into the masticatory muscles has not been reported to induce pain in humans (Pedersen-Bjergaard et al., 1991). Thus, it is not clear how a sex-related difference in the expression of CGRP by masticatory muscle afferent fibers might influence human masticatory muscle pain.

Conclusions

At this time, data regarding sex-related differences in muscle afferent discharge are limited to the effects of a small number of algogenic compounds. It seems likely that as research is expanded in this area, additional sex-related differences in peripheral receptor mechanisms will emerge. Current data, however, suggest that where sex-related differences have been identified, estrogen-related modulation of receptor expression and function plays an important mechanistic role. Whether sex-related differences in muscle afferent discharge contribute to sex-related differences in the incidence and prevalence of certain types of chronic myofascial pain remains to be determined.

Acknowledgments

The authors would like to acknowledge research support provided by a Canadian Pain Society/Astra-Zeneca Research Award, PHS grant DE15420 (NIDCR), and CIHR grant MOP-77538 (IMHA). Dr. Cairns is the recipient of a Canada Research Chair.

References

Ambalavanar R, Moritani M, Haines A, Hilton T, Dessem D. Chemical phenotypes of muscle and cutaneous afferent neurons in the rat trigeminal ganglion. J Comp Neurol 2003;460:167–179.

Ambalavanar R, Moritani M, Moutanni A, Gangula P, Yallampalli C, Dessem D. Deep tissue inflammation upregulates neuropeptides and evokes nociceptive behaviors which are modulated by a neuropeptide antagonist. Pain 2006;120:53–68.

Arden WA, Fiscus RR, Beihn LD, Derbin M, Oremus R, Gross DR. Skeletal muscle microcirculatory response to rat alpha-calcitonin gene-related peptide. Neuropeptides 1994;27:39–51.

Avenet P, Leonardon J, Besnard F, Graham D, Frost J, Depoortere H, Langer SZ, Scatton B. Antagonist properties of the stereoisomers of ifenprodil at NR1A/NR2A and NR1A/NR2B subtypes of the NMDA receptor expressed in *Xenopus* oocytes. Eur J Pharmacol 1996;296:209–213.

Bereiter DA, Cioffi JL, Bereiter DF. Oestrogen receptor-immunoreactive neurons in the trigeminal sensory system of male and cycling female rats. Arch Oral Biol 2005;50:971–979.

Bi R, Broutman G, Foy MR, Thompson RF, Baudry M. The tyrosine kinase and mitogen-activated protein kinase pathways mediate multiple effects of estrogen in hippocampus. Proc Natl Acad Sci USA 2000;97:3602–3607.

Bi R, Foy MR, Vouimba R-M, Thompson RF, Baudry M. Cyclic changes in estradiol regulate synaptic plasticity through the MAP kinase pathway. Proc Natl Acad Sci USA 2001;98:13391–13395.

Cairns BE. The influence of gender and sex steroids on craniofacial nociception. Headache 2007;47:319–324.

Cairns BE, Dong X, Mann MK, Svensson P, Sessle BJ, Arendt-Nielsen L, McErlane KM. Systemic administration of monosodium glutamate elevates intramuscular glutamate levels and sensitizes rat masseter muscle afferent fibers. Pain 2007;132:33–41.

Cairns BE, Gambarota G, Svensson P, Arendt-Nielsen L, Berde CB. Glutamate-induced sensitization of rat masseter muscle fibers. Neuroscience 2002;109:389–399.

Cairns BE, Hu JW, Arendt-Nielsen L, Sessle BJ, Svensson P. Sex-related differences in human pain perception and rat afferent discharge evoked by injection of glutamate into the masseter muscle. J Neurophysiol 2001;86:782–791.

Cairns BE, Svensson P, Wang K, Hupfeld S, Graven-Nielsen T, Sessle BJ, Berde CB, Arendt-Nielsen l. Activation of peripheral NMDA receptors contributes to human pain and rat afferent discharges evoked by injection of glutamate into the masseter muscle. J Neurophysiol 2003;90:2098–2105.

Castrillon E, Cairns BE, Ernberg M, Wang K, Sessle BJ, Arendt-Nielsen L, Svensson P. Effect of peripheral NMDA receptor blockade on glutamate-evoked masseter muscle pain and mechanical sensitization in women. J Orofac Pain 2007;21:216–224.

Cyr M, Ghribi O, Thibault C, Morissette M, Landry M, Di Paolo T. Ovarian steroids and selective estrogen receptor modulators activity on rat brain NMDA and AMPA receptors. Brain Res Rev 2001;37:153–161.

Dong XD, Mann MK, Kumar U, Svensson P, Arendt-Nielsen L, Hu JW, Sessle BJ, Cairns BE. Sex-related differences in glutamate evoked rat muscle nociceptor discharge result from estrogen-mediated modulation of peripheral NMDA receptors. Neuroscience 2007;146:822–832.

Dong XD, Mann MK, Sessle BJ, Arendt-Nielsen L, Svensson P, Cairns BE. Sensitivity of rat temporalis muscle afferent fibers to peripheral *N*-methyl-D-aspartate receptor activation. Neuroscience 2006;141:939–945.

Ernberg M, Lundeberg T, Kopp S. Effect of propranolol and granisetron on experimentally induced pain and allodynia/hyperalgesia by intramuscular injection of serotonin into the human masseter muscle. Pain 2000;84:339–346.

Foy MR, Xu J, Xie X, Brinton RD, Thompson RF, Berger TW. 17β-Estradiol enhances NMDA receptor-mediated EPSPs and long-term potentiation. J Neurophysiol 1999;81:925–929.

Hamill OP, Martinac B. Molecular basis of mechanotransduction in living cells. Physiol Rev 2001;81:685–740.

Hu WP, Li XM, Wu JL, Zheng M, Li ZW. Bradykinin potentiates 5-HT3 receptor-mediated current in rat trigeminal ganglion neurons. Acta Pharmacol Sin 2005;26:428–434.

Kew JN, Kemp JA. Ionotropic and metabotropic glutamate receptor structure and pharmacology. Psychopharmacology (Berl) 2005;179:4–29.

LeResche L. Epidemiology of orofacial pain. In: Lund JP, Lavigne GJ, Dubner R, Sessle BJ, editors. Orofacial pain: from basic science to clinical management. Chicago: Quintessence; 2001. p. 15–26.

LeResche L, Mancl L, Sherman JJ, Gandara B, Dworkin SF. Changes in temporomandibular pain and other symptoms across the menstrual cycle. Pain 2003;106:253–261.

Mann MK, Dong XD, Svensson P, Cairns BE. Influence of intramuscular nerve growth factor injection on the response properties of rat masseter muscle afferent fibers. J Orofac Pain 2006;20:325–336.

Marchettini P, Simone DA, Caputi G, Ochoa JL. Pain from excitation of identified muscle nociceptors in humans. Brain Res 1996;740:109–116.

Mayer ML, Armstrong N. Structure and function of glutamate receptor ion channels. Annu Rev Physiol 2004;66:161–181.

Nekora-Azak A. Temporomandibular disorders in relation to female reproductive hormones: a literature review. J Prosthet Dent 2004;91:491–493.

Pedersen-Bjergaard U, Nielsen LB, Jensen K, Edvinsson L, Jansen I, Olesen J. Calcitonin gene-related peptide, neurokinin A and substance P: effects on nociception and neurogenic inflammation in human skin and temporal muscle. Peptides 1991;12:333–337.

Ro JY. Contribution of peripheral NMDA receptors in craniofacial muscle nociception and edema formation. Brain Res 2003;979:78–84.

Ro JY, Capra NF, Masri R. Contribution of peripheral N-methyl-D-aspartate receptors to c-fos expression in the trigeminal spinal nucleus following acute masseteric inflammation. Neuroscience 2004;123:213–219.

Rollman GB, Lautenbacher S. Sex differences in musculoskeletal pain. Clin J Pain 2001;17:20–24.

Salter MW, Kalia LV. Src kinases: a hub for NMDA receptor regulation. Nat Rev Neurosci 2004;5:317–328.

Sun RQ, Lawand NB, Lin Q, Willis WD. Role of calcitonin gene-related peptide in the sensitization of dorsal horn neurons to mechanical stimulation after intradermal injection of capsaicin. J Neurophysiol 2004;92:320–326.

Sung D, Dong X, Ernberg M, Kumar U, Cairns BE. Serotonin (5-HT) excites rat masticatory muscle afferent fibers through activation of peripheral 5-HT3 receptors. Pain 2008;134:41–50.

Svensson P, Cairns BE, Wang K, Hu JW, Graven-Nielsen T, Arendt-Nielsen L, Sessle BJ. Glutamate-evoked pain and mechanical allodynia in the human masseter muscle. Pain 2003;101:221–227.

Turman JEJ, Ajdari J, Chandler SH. NMDA receptor NR1 and NR2A/B subunit expression in trigeminal neurons during early postnatal development. J Comp Neurol 1999;409:237–249.

Williams K. Ifenprodil discriminates subtypes of the N-methyl-D-aspartate receptor: selectivity and mechanisms at recombinant heteromeric receptors. Mol Pharmacol 1993;44:851–859.

Woolley CS, Weiland NG, McEwen BS, Schwartzkroin PA. Estradiol increases the sensitivity of hippocampal CA1 pyramidal cells to NMDA receptor-mediated synaptic input: correlation with dendritic spine density. J Neurosci 1997;17:1848–1859.

Yang Y, Ozawa H, Lu H, Yuri K, Hayashi S, Nihonyanagi K, Kawata M. Immunocytochemical analysis of sex differences in calcitonin gene-related peptide in the rat dorsal root ganglion, with special reference to estrogen and its receptor. Brain Res 1998;791:35–42.

Correspondence to: Brian E. Cairns, PhD, ACPR, RPh, Faculty of Pharmaceutical Sciences, The University of British Columbia, 2146 East Mall, Vancouver, BC, Canada V6T 1Z3. Tel: +1-604-822-7715; fax: +1-604-822-3535; email: brcairns@interchange.ubc.ca.

15

Sex-Related Differences in Clinical and Experimental Muscle Pain

Stefan Lautenbacher

Department of Physiological Psychology, University of Bamberg, Bamberg, Germany

This chapter deals with two issues: first, is there a sex difference in the presentation of muscle pain, and second, if so, how might we account for it? The first part of the chapter presents epidemiological evidence and discusses associated factors that might guide attempts to explain the evidence. However, satisfactory explanations also require evidence based on experimentally induced muscle pain, which will be reviewed in the second part of the chapter.

Epidemiological and Clinical Evidence

Epidemiological reports indicate that musculoskeletal pain is a major medical and economic problem. The pain and associated disability are linked with a significant loss of productivity and substantial health care expenditures for women. Leijon et al. (1998) observed that about 30% of all sick-leave days in Sweden are due to neck/shoulder or low back pain, which were defined as being of musculoskeletal origin. The authors determined that leave due to sickness in general, and due to musculoskeletal pain in particular, was appreciably higher among women than men.

Wijnhoven et al. (2006a) conducted a Dutch population-based study and reported a prevalence of musculoskeletal pain of 45% in women and 39% in men, based only on self-report (responses to a questionnaire). Interestingly, the degree of sex differences varied between body locations. The highest female predominance was found in this Dutch population for the hip and wrist/hand, whereas the lowest sex differences, not reaching statistical significance, were found for the lower back and knee.

Age may affect the biological and psychosocial basis of sex differences, so it is worthwhile to study musculoskeletal pain in elderly women and men. Leveille et al. (2005) investigated a major sample of women and men aged 72 years and older. Among the women, 63% reported pain in one or more regions, compared to 52% of men. Widespread pain was more prevalent among women than men (15% vs. 5%, respectively). Rekola et al. (1993) found that women aged 55 to 64 years are more likely than women of any other age group to seek medical attention for musculoskeletal problems, particularly neck and shoulder problems. In men the frequency of visits was highest in the age group between 45 and 54 years, with low back pain being the most common complaint. These findings argue against a reduction of sex differences in musculoskeletal pain with increasing age.

The evidence presented so far suggests that sex differences in musculoskeletal pain vary among different body sites. Accordingly, varying sex differences for different diagnoses of musculoskeletal pain might be expected. LeResche (2000, 2006) has made the case that musculoskeletal pain syndromes confined to one body region are moderately more prevalent in females than in males, within a range known also for chronic pain originating from other tissues (see Table I). In particular, widespread chronic pain diagnosed as fibromyalgia is associated with an extremely strong female predominance.

Do physical risk factors account for all or at least some of these sex-related effects? A number of possible explanations have been offered, including differential exposure to risks in the work environment, dif-

Table I
Sex prevalence ratios in various pain conditions
for the adult general population

Pain Site or Condition	No. Studies	Range of F:M Ratio	Median of F:M Ratio
Headache (general)	15	1.1–3.1	1.3
Migraine	14	1.6–4.0	2.5
Burning mouth	2	1.3–2.5	1.9
Knee pain	4	1.0–1.9	1.6
Abdominal pain	4	1.2–1.3	1.25
Back pain	4	0.9–1.3	1.2
Neck pain	5	1.0–3.3	1.4
Shoulder pain	5	1.0–2.2	1.3
Temporomandibular pain	10	1.2–2.6	1.5
Fibromyalgia	4	2.0–6.8	4.3

Source: Modified from LeResche (2000).

ferences in muscle strength or excess body weight, work environments designed to male norms, or differences in the way injuries in men and women are evaluated, treated, or referred for rehabilitative services. Similarly, Fredriksson et al. (1999) noted that neck, shoulder, and lower limb disorders are associated with heavy lifting, monotonous work tasks, static work postures, vibrations, repetitive jobs, and a high work pace, and found that women may be at higher risk for all such disorders. They also pointed to psychosocial risk factors such as low work content, low social support, high perceived workload, time pressure, low job control, high perceived stress, and high psychological job demands.

In a 24-year longitudinal study conducted by Nordander et al. (1999), psychosocial factors such as monotony and high mental load at work were associated with increased risk for neck and upper limb disorders in women (who had a prevalence rate about twice that of men), whereas in men more physical factors related to work were associated with an increased risk. However, the authors noted that "these two aspects of the work environment are so tightly entangled that it is not possible to estimate their separate impact on musculoskeletal disorders in this kind of work." The idea that women are vulnerable to psychosocial risk factors and men to physical risk factors would not be true. In fact, Wijnhoven et al. (2006b) observed almost the opposite tendency. Risk factors with a sex-specific association were being overweight and older age, which only had an effect in women, as well as pain catastrophizing, which was more strongly associated with chronic musculoskeletal pain among men than among women.

Not only do the predisposing factors for musculoskeletal pain differ between the two sexes, but the consequences may also vary in a sex-specific manner, although data have been scarce so far. Wijnhoven et al. (2007), who investigated a sample of 2,517 individuals from the Dutch population, observed increased health care use in women with musculoskeletal pain compared to men. Men reported more work disability, but only when suffering from low back pain.

Clearly, understanding the causes and the consequences of these epidemiological findings is much more difficult than demonstrating their existence. Men and women differ in body size and functional capacity and, perhaps, in such factors as mix of fast-twitch and slow-twitch muscle fibers, cardiovascular endurance, and other physiological variables (Punnett and Berqvist, 1999). Endocrine influences, including menstruation, oral contraceptive use, pregnancy, and hysterectomy may increase the risk of musculoskeletal disorders (Unruh, 1996). The link between musculoskeletal pain and menstruation deserves more study; certainly, the literature on temporomandibular disorder shows that the use of estrogen by postmenopausal women significantly increases their odds of having orofacial pain (LeResche et al., 1997; Wise et al., 2000). On the psychosocial side, women may experience greater stress both in and outside the job setting, less control over the work process, fewer opportunities for advancement, and different implications of reporting musculoskeletal pain and seeking or accepting compensation. Future research must isolate which of these sex-specific biological and psychosocial factors are most critical. This quest may be supported by experimental approaches.

Experimental Evidence

This section discusses experimental findings in healthy subjects and patients and presents sex differences in experimental inductions of acute musculoskeletal pain, in pressure pain sensitivity, and in temporal summation and inhibitory mechanisms relating to muscle pain (see Chapter 11, Graven-Nielsen and Arendt-Nielsen).

Experimental Induction of Acute Musculoskeletal Pain

Muscle pain can be induced by muscular overuse or misuse (see Chapter 11, Graven-Nielsen and Arendt-Nielsen). The question is whether the two sexes differ in the functional thresholds the determine the distinction between use and overuse or misuse. Karibe et al. (2003) investigated whether chewing bubble gum for 6 minutes triggers masticatory muscle pain in females and males to a similar degree. Sex differences in chewing-induced pain were found, with only women having critical levels of muscle pain. Accordingly, overuse appeared to occur in this study only in women; however, the painful effects were short-lived.

Exercise models of experimental muscle pain, which lead to longer-lasting muscle pain, are more comparable to clinical situations and thus more useful. From this perspective a phenomenon called delayed-onset muscle soreness (DOMS) has attracted interest (see Chapter 16, Dannecker). DOMS is muscle pain and soreness that is felt 12 to 48 hours after exercise, particularly after eccentric exercise (i.e., lengthening contractions) and at the beginning of a new exercise program, after a change in sports activities, or after a dramatic increase in the duration or intensity of exercise. This soreness is a normal response to unusual exertion and is part of an adaptation process that leads to greater stamina and strength as the muscles recover. DOMS can be experimentally induced very effectively by requiring the subjects to perform eccentric muscle contractions (movements that cause a muscle to forcefully contract while it lengthens). Investigations of sex differences in DOMS have produced equivocal results. Dannecker et al. (2003) found females reporting lower muscle pain intensity than males after DOMS had been induced in the elbow flexor. The decrease in pressure pain thresholds in the affected muscle, which is a regular accompaniment of DOMS, was similar in the two sexes. In a study by Nie et al. (2005b), DOMS was induced in the shoulder muscles by performing an eccentric shoulder exercise. Pain intensity, pain area, and pain ratings on the McGill Pain Questionnaire were all increased after exercise. Pressure pain threshold was significantly decreased and reached its lowest values 24 hours after exercise. However, no sex differences were found in any of the parameters used to assess the development of DOMS. Nie et al. (2007) were able to mostly replicate the results of their first study regarding the lack of sex differences in subjective pain during DOMS. A significant decrease in exerted force during exercise was only found in males, despite similar ratings of perceived exertion in both sexes. This finding was paralleled only in males by increased EMG activity during eccentric exercise. The authors concluded that women have more prominent muscle fatigue resistance compared to men.

Injection of hypertonic saline (HS) into a muscle induces pain that strongly mimics clinical forms of musculoskeletal pain. Ge et al. (2004) injected HS twice in series bilaterally into the trapezius muscle of women and men. Only the maximum pain intensity differed between the sexes, with higher ratings in women. No sex differences were observed for mean pain intensity, referred pain pattern, or pain area. The same group replicated these findings in a second study (Ge et al., 2006). There was no statistically significant difference between men and women in mean pain, maximal pain, or area under the curve of VAS ratings after either the first or second injection. Moreover, referred pain patterns were similar for men and women.

A further method for inducing muscle pain was tested by Cairns et al. (2001) by injecting glutamate into the masseter muscle. This experimental pain model led to abundant sex differences; women perceived higher levels of muscle pain overall, higher levels of peak pain, and broader areas of pain. Furthermore, the duration of pain was significantly longer in women than in men.

Despite these impressive results regarding the use of glutamate-induced pain, studies using the other experimental models, which were also designed to induce acute musculoskeletal pain similar to clinical conditions, have failed to provide evidence that they are able to reproduce the pathophysiological mechanisms responsible for the reliable sex difference in clinical musculoskeletal pain.

Testing Pressure Pain Sensitivity

Women are often found to have greater pain sensitivity than men in laboratory settings, but the effects are particularly striking when pressure pain is applied. Reviews of these sex differences are found elsewhere (Riley et al., 1998; Fillingim, 2000; Rollman et al., 2000; Rollman and Lautenbacher, 2001), so this section will focus on the evidence that the experimental use of noxious pressure is an especially sensitive test for tracking the pathology of musculoskeletal pain and its underlying mechanisms.

Abundant evidence shows that mechanical pressure is the form of noxious input that is most likely to show altered pain thresholds in musculoskeletal pain conditions. For example, changes in responsiveness to experimental pain, which is often markedly increased in patients with fibromyalgia, are particularly noteworthy when pressure pain is used as the physical stressor (Kosek et al., 1996; Sorensen et al., 1998). Lautenbacher et al. (1994) found that the effect sizes for differences between fibromyalgia patients and pain-free volunteers were 1.53 for a tender point and 1.57 for a control point when pressure pain was applied. Effect sizes decreased to 0.65 and 0.84, respectively, for heat pain and to 0.22 and 0.91, respectively, for electrocutaneous pain. Although some of the differences between patients and controls for heat and electrocutaneous pain were significant, none of them reached the size obtained for pressure pain.

Similarly, patients with myofascial pain and temporomandibular disorder are exceptionally pain sensitive when pressure pain is used for diagnosis, especially within the region where clinical pain is most strongly experienced (Arendt-Nielsen et al., 2004; Rollman and Gillespie, 2004). Consequently, the use of pressure pain seems to tie into the processes underlying musculoskeletal pain more readily than the use of other pain induction methods. This assumption is corroborated by the observation of Lautenbacher et al. (1994) that a sizeable negative relationship was found between the magnitude of concurrent pain in fibromyalgia patients and the pain threshold for pressure, but not the threshold for heat or electrical current.

The question arises as to whether musculoskeletal pain reduces the pain threshold or whether a reduced pain threshold—because of a state of increased pain sensitivity of peripheral or central origin—predisposes the individual to have musculoskeletal pain. Musculoskeletal pain does not necessarily lead to a decrease in pressure pain threshold. Babenko and coworkers (1999) induced muscle pain by various chemical agents without changing local pressure pain thresholds. Similarly, Graven-Nielsen et al. (1998a,b) failed to decrease the local pressure pain thresholds reliably by inducing muscle pain by HS infusion. Recent evidence provided by Slade et al. (2007) in a longitudinal study also suggests that increased pain sensitivity belongs to the relevant risk factors for later development of temporomandibular disorder. Accordingly, decreased pressure pain thresholds in women might be indicative of a generalized state of increased pain sensitivity that may predispose women to experience symptoms of musculoskeletal pain.

Interaction of sex with age has not yet received sufficient interest. Two studies indicate that clear sex differences in pressure pain sensitivity may exist only in young persons. Pickering et al. (2002) found significantly reduced pressure pain threshold in females in a group of young adults but not among elderly individuals. In one of our studies, the effect sizes for differences between females and males in the usual direction were 0.79 for pressure pain thresholds and 0.57 for heat pain thresholds in a group of young adults (Lautenbacher et al., 2005). In contrast, in individuals over 70 years of age these classical differences were eliminated (effect size for heat pain thresholds: −0.06) or even reversed (effect size for pressure pain threshold: −0.50). Such findings point to critical limitations of the research on sex differences conducted so far, which has been strongly based on investigations in young persons.

Temporal Summation and Inhibitory Mechanisms Relating to Muscle Pain

The indication of a reliably increased sensitivity to pressure may suggest central hyperexcitability or a lack of sufficient pain inhibition, which becomes apparent when using this type of physical stressor. The paradigms most often used to test such hypotheses are the assessment of temporal summation in pressure pain and the investigation of diffuse noxious inhibitory controls (DNICs) with pressure as the test stimulus.

Sarlani et al. (2004) investigated temporal summation by applying 10 repetitive, mildly noxious mechanical stimuli to the fingers of 25 women and 25 age-matched men. Temporal summation of pain intensity and unpleasantness ratings were more pronounced in women than in men. In addition, significant temporal summation occurred only with 2-second interstimulus interval in men but with 2- and 5-second interstimulus intervals in women. In a later study on patients with temporomandibular disorder, Sarlani et al. (2007) essentially replicated their findings.

We were interested in DNIC-like effects on temporal summation of pressure pain in females and males. For that purpose, we designed a study to examine the effects of tonic thermal stimulation of varying intensities (warmth, heat, and heat pain) used as a conditioning stimulus on the perception of single pulses of noxious pressure compared to the ratings of the last pressure stimulus of a series of five (0.5 Hz repetition frequency). Tonic heat (conditioning) and phasic pressure (test) stimuli were tailored to individual pain thresholds (thermal: −3°C, −1°C, and +1°C relative to pain threshold; pressure: 150% of pain threshold). VAS ratings for these stimuli did not differ between the sexes. As shown in Fig. 1, there was significant temporal summation, leading to much higher ratings for the last pulses of the repetitive series compared to those for single pulses (S. Lautenbacher et al., unpublished data). However, in contrast to Sarlani et al. (2004, 2007), in our study the two sexes did not differ in the amount of temporal summation of pressure pain. The DNIC-like reduction of the VAS ratings for pressure was generally weak because tonic heat pain did not have much more effect than warmth in this respect. Whereas the DNIC-like effects were at least visible in tendency in men, they were completely absent in women.

Our findings of no sex differences in temporal summation of pressure pain, which corroborate earlier results by Nie et al. (2005a), along with the data of Fillingim et al. (1998) showing a substantial sex difference in temporal summation of heat pain, suggest that temporal summation of pressure pain is not an especially sensitive test for sex differences.

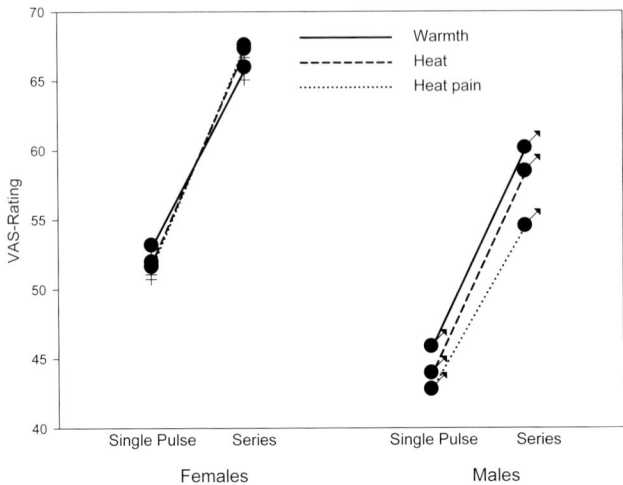

Fig. 1. Temporal summation of pressure pain in 20 women and 20 men. Mean ratings on a visual analogue scale (VAS, 0–100) of pain from single pulse stimulation were compared with those of the last stimulus in a series of five repeated stimuli with a repetition frequency of 0.5 Hz. Stimulations were applied to the fingertips of the left hand. The slopes indicate substantial temporal summation but without sex differences. Temporal summation was tested under concurrent application of tonic thermal stimuli (conditioning stimuli: warmth, heat, and heat pain) to assess diffuse noxious inhibitory controls. Only in men was there a tendency for reduced ratings when painful conditioning stimuli were applied. However, the comparison of the two sexes failed to reach significance in this respect (S. Lautenbacher et al., unpublished data).

Therefore, the studies of Sarlani et al. (2004, 2007) by themselves do not give convincing evidence of a particularly pronounced central hyperexcitability when applying repetitively noxious pressure. Furthermore, our very weak evidence for stronger DNIC-effects in men than in women when painful pressure was applied as the test stimulus discredits the hypothesis that deficient DNIC mechanisms are a critical cause of the strong sex differences in pressure pain sensitivity.

The formulation of the latter hypothesis was based in part on observations by Mense (1998, 1999). The author suggested that the descending antinociceptive systems exert a more powerful influence on the input from muscle nociceptors than on that from skin nociceptors.

Accordingly, a weakening of these antinociceptive systems should result in a lowering of pain thresholds for stimulation of muscles (because pressure stimulation activates both skin and muscle nociceptors) and in an increased likelihood of spontaneous muscle pain. Lautenbacher and Rollman (1997) and Kosek and Hansson (1997) found deficiencies in the pain inhibitory systems of fibromyalgia patients, which were especially prominent when they used pressure pain as the test stimulus compared to using heat pain.

What further evidence, other than our findings (see Fig. 1), is available for the hypothesis that sex differences in DNIC effects are especially prominent when pressure is used as the test stimulus? Ge et al. (2004) investigated sex differences in DNIC by measuring pressure pain thresholds over time in the trapezius muscles and the posterolateral neck muscles following repeated bilateral injection of hypertonic versus isotonic saline into both trapezius muscles. Significantly higher pressure pain thresholds in men than in women were shown 15 minutes after the first bilateral injection, and 7.5 and 15 minutes after the second bilateral injection. These results showed sex differences in the temporal characteristics of DNIC, with longer-lasting hypoalgesia in men than in women.

Pud et al. (2005) investigated healthy volunteers to examine the effect of tonic immersion of the fingers in ice-cold water as a conditioning stimulus on pain intensities produced by mechanical punctuate stimuli, applied both adjacent and contralateral to the cooled area. There was a significant decrease in mechanical pain intensities at both sites when stimulation was applied immediately after the cold immersion. However, the extent of pain reduction was similar for males and for females. Furthermore, there are also reports of sex differences in DNIC effects when electrical current (France and Suchowiecki, 1999) or heat (Staud et al., 2003) were used as test stimuli.

In conclusion, there is no sound empirical basis so far to assume that the descending inhibition of nociceptive input from deep tissue, i.e., from muscles, is particularly subject to sex-related factors or that it is weaker in women. However, the assessment of DNIC-like inhibition does not cover all descending inhibitory systems, and therefore sex differences in DNIC cannot be excluded by the findings to date.

Concluding Remarks

There is no doubt that there are sex differences in susceptibility to musculoskeletal pain and in pain sensitivity, with women—as a rule—being more often affected and more sensitive to pain. The question is whether such sex differences are stronger in clinical and experimental musculoskeletal pain compared to types of pain originating from other tissues. As far as the available evidence goes, at present we can be confident that chronic widespread musculoskeletal pain, specifically fibromyalgia, is outstandingly frequent in women and that sensitivity to pressure pain is more reliably increased in women compared to sensitivity for other types of noxious stressors. In regard to all other forms of clinical muscle pain and experimental methods of simulating, summating, and inhibiting muscle pain, sex differences are in the usual range known for pain in general. This evidence does not mean, however, that the experimental paradigms set up to investigate musculoskeletal pain—models such as DOMS, HS injection, temporal summation of pressure pain, and DNIC effects on muscle pain—fail to address critical aspects of muscle pain pathophysiology. It only means that they do not address those aspects that are critical for understanding the particularly strong affects seen in women in certain forms of chronic musculoskeletal pain.

Acknowledgments

Thanks to Gary B. Rollman (London, Ontario, Canada) for his input to this manuscript.

References

Arendt-Nielsen L, Graven-Nielsen T, Svensson P. Disturbances of pain perception in myofascial pain syndrome and other musculoskeletal pains. In: Lautenbacher S, Fillingim RB, editors. Pathophysiology of pain perception. New York: Kluwer Academic/Plenum Publishers; 2004. p 93–106.
Babenko V, Graven-Nielsen T, Svensson P, Drewes AM, Jensen TS, Arendt-Nielsen L. Experimental human muscle pain induced by intramuscular injections of bradykinin, serotonin, and substance P. Eur J Pain 1999;3:93–102.

Cairns BE, Hu JW, Arendt-Nielsen L, Sessle BJ, Svensson P. Sex-related differences in human pain and rat afferent discharge evoked by injection of glutamate into the masseter muscle. J Neurophysiol 2001;86:782–791.

Dannecker EA, Koltyn KF, Riley JL III, Robinson ME. Sex differences in delayed onset muscle soreness. J Sports Med Phys Fitness 2003;43:78–84.

Fillingim RB. Sex, gender, and pain: women and men really are different. Curr Rev Pain 2000;4:24–30.

Fillingim RB, Maixner W, Kincaid S, Silva S. Sex differences in temporal summation but not sensory-discriminative processing of thermal pain. Pain 1998;75:121–127.

France CR, Suchowiecki S. A comparison of diffuse noxious inhibitory controls in men and women. Pain 1999;81:77–84.

Fredriksson K, Alfredsson L, Köster M, Thorbjornsson CB, Toomingas A, Torgén M, Kilbom A. Risk factors for neck and upper limb disorders: results from 24 years of follow up. Occup Environ Med 1999;56:59–66.

Ge HY, Madeleine P, Arendt-Nielsen L. Sex differences in temporal characteristics of descending inhibitory control: an evaluation using repeated bilateral experimental induction of muscle pain. Pain 2004;110:72–78.

Ge HY, Madeleine P, Cairns BE, Arendt-Nielsen L. Hypoalgesia in the referred pain areas after bilateral injections of hypertonic saline into the trapezius muscles of men and women: a potential experimental model of gender-specific differences. Clin J Pain 2006;22:37–44.

Graven-Nielsen T, Babenko V, Svensson P, Arendt-Nielsen L. Experimentally induced muscle pain induces hypoalgesia in heterotopic deep tissues, but not in homotopic deep tissues. Brain Res 1998a;787:203–210.

Graven-Nielsen T, Fenger-Gron LS, Svensson P, Steengaard-Pedersen K, Arendt-Nielsen L, Staehelin JT. Quantification of deep and superficial sensibility in saline-induced muscle pain—a psychophysical study. Somatosens Mot Res 1998b;15:46–53.

Karibe H, Goddard G, Gear RW. Sex differences in masticatory muscle pain after chewing. J Dent Res 2003;82:112–116.

Kosek E, Ekholm J, Hansson P. Sensory dysfunction in fibromyalgia patients with implications for pathogenic mechanisms. Pain 1996;68:375–383.

Kosek E, Hansson P. Modulatory influence on somatosensory perception from vibration and heterotopic noxious conditioning stimulation (HNCS) in fibromyalgia patients and healthy subjects. Pain 1997;70:41–51.

Lautenbacher S, Kunz M, Strate P, Nielsen J, Arendt-Nielsen L. Age effects on pain thresholds, temporal summation and spatial summation of heat and pressure pain. Pain 2005;115:410–418.

Lautenbacher S, Rollman GB. Possible deficiencies of pain modulation in fibromyalgia. Clin J Pain 1997;13:189–196.

Lautenbacher S, Rollman GB, McCain GA. Multi-method assessment of experimental and clinical pain in patients with fibromyalgia. Pain 1994;59:45–53.

Leijon M, Hensing G, Alexanderson K. Gender trends in sick-listing with musculoskeletal symptoms in a Swedish county during a period of rapid increase in sickness absence. Scand J Soc Med 1998;26:204–213.

LeResche L. Epidemiologic perspectives on sex differences in pain. In: Fillingim RB, editor. Sex, gender, and pain. Seattle: IASP Press; 2000. p 233–249.

LeResche L. Gender, sex, and clinical pain. In: Flor H, Kalso E, Dostrovsky JO, editors. Proceedings of the 11th World Congress on Pain. Seattle: IASP Press; 2006. p 543–554.

LeResche L, Saunders K, Von Korff MR, Barlow W, Dworkin SF. Use of exogenous hormones and risk of temporomandibular disorder pain. Pain 1997;69:153–160.

Leveille SG, Zhang Y, McMullen W, Kelly-Hayes M, Felson DT. Sex differences in musculoskeletal pain in older adults. Pain 2005;116:332–338.

Mense S. Descending antinociception and fibromyalgia. Z Rheumatol 1998;57(Suppl 2):23–26.

Mense S. Neurobiologische Grundlagen von Muskelschmerz. Schmerz 1999;13:3–17.

Nie H, Arendt-Nielsen L, Andersen H, Graven-Nielsen T. Temporal summation of pain evoked by mechanical stimulation in deep and superficial tissue. J Pain 2005a;6:348–355.

Nie H, Arendt-Nielsen L, Kawczynski A, Madeleine P. Gender effects on trapezius surface EMG during delayed onset muscle soreness due to eccentric shoulder exercise. J Electromyogr Kinesiol 2007;17:401–409.

Nie H, Kawczynski A, Madeleine P, Arendt-Nielsen L. Delayed onset muscle soreness in neck/shoulder muscles. Eur J Pain 2005b;9:653–660.

Nordander C, Ohlsson K, Balogh I, Rylander L, Palsson B, Skerfving S. Fish processing work: the impact of two sex dependent exposure profiles on musculoskeletal health. Occup Environ Med 1999;56:256–264.

Pickering G, Jourdan D, Eschalier A, Dubray C. Impact of age, gender and cognitive functioning on pain perception. Gerontology 2002;48:112–118.

Pud D, Sprecher E, Yarnitsky D. Homotopic and heterotopic effects of endogenous analgesia in healthy volunteers. Neurosci Lett 2005;380:209–213.

Punnett L, Bergqvist U. Musculoskeletal disorders in visual display unit work: gender and work demands. Occup Med 1999;14:113–124.

Rekola KE, Keinanen-Kiukaanniemi S, Takala J. Use of primary health services in sparsely populated country districts by patients with musculoskeletal symptoms: consultations with a physician. J Epidemiol Community Health 1993;47:153–157.

Riley JL, III, Robinson ME, Wise EA, Myers CD, Fillingim RB. Sex differences in the perception of noxious experimental stimuli: a meta-analysis. Pain 1998;74:181–187.

Rollman GB, Gillespie JM. Disturbances of pain perception in temporomandibular pain syndrome. In: Lautenbacher S, Fillingim RB, editors. Pathophysiology of pain perception. New York: Kluwer Academic/Plenum Publishers; 2004. p 107–118.

Rollman GB, Lautenbacher S. Sex differences in musculoskeletal pain. Clin J Pain 2001;17:20–24.

Rollman GB, Lautenbacher S, Jones KS. Sex and gender differences in responses to experimentally induced pain in humans. In: Fillingim RB, editor. Sex, gender, and pain. Seattle: IASP Press; 2000. p 165–190.

Sarlani E, Garrett PH, Grace EG, Greenspan JD. Temporal summation of pain characterizes women but not men with temporomandibular disorders. J Orofac Pain 2007;21:309–317.

Sarlani E, Grace EG, Reynolds MA, Greenspan JD. Sex differences in temporal summation of pain and aftersensations following repetitive noxious mechanical stimulation. Pain 2004;109:115–123.

Slade GD, Diatchenko L, Bhalang K, Sigurdsson A, Fillingim RB, Belfer I, Max MB, Goldman D, Maixner W. Influence of psychological factors on risk of temporomandibular disorders. J Dent Res 2007;86:1120–1125.

Sorensen J, Graven-Nielsen T, Henriksson KG, Bengtsson M, Arendt-Nielsen L. Hyperexcitability in fibromyalgia. J Rheumatol 1998;25:152–155.

Staud R, Robinson ME, Vierck CJ Jr, Price DD. Diffuse noxious inhibitory controls (DNIC) attenuate temporal summation of second pain in normal males but not in normal females or fibromyalgia patients. Pain 2003;101:167–174.

Unruh AM. Gender variations in clinical pain experience. Pain 1996;65:123–167.

Wijnhoven HA, de Vet HC, Picavet HS. Prevalence of musculoskeletal disorders is systematically higher in women than in men. Clin J Pain 2006a;22:717–724.

Wijnhoven HA, de Vet HC, Picavet HS. Explaining sex differences in chronic musculoskeletal pain in a general population. Pain 2006b;124:158–166.

Wijnhoven HA, de Vet HC, Picavet HS. Sex differences in consequences of musculoskeletal pain. Spine 2007;32:1360–1367.

Wise EA, Riley JL III, Robinson ME. Clinical pain perception and hormone replacement therapy in postmenopausal women experiencing orofacial pain. Clin J Pain 2000;16:121–126.

Correspondence to: Prof. Stefan Lautenbacher, PhD, Physiological Psychology, University of Bamberg, Markuspl. 3, 96045 Bamberg, Germany. Tel: +49-951-8631851; fax: +49-951-8631976; email: stefan.lautenbacher@uni-bamberg.de.

Sex-Related Differences in Delayed-Onset Muscle Pain

Erin A. Dannecker

Department of Physical Therapy, University of Missouri, Columbia, Missouri, USA

A common topic of conversation during the first few days of the work week is muscle pain and soreness from unaccustomed physical activity over the weekend. Some people are surprised to develop delayed-onset muscle soreness (DOMS), while others were expecting DOMS, but are surprised by its severity, duration, and impact. This chapter describes why pain researchers are increasingly interested in DOMS. In addition, it reviews current evidence of sex differences in DOMS and outlines the methodological issues that researchers should consider when investigating sex differences in DOMS.

Delayed-Onset Muscle Soreness

Although studies of DOMS did not begin appearing in pain journals until the late 1990s, one of the earliest reports of this condition was published almost 100 years earlier (Hough, 1902). The report described soreness in finger muscles after a series of contractions against a "stiff spring." Since that early report, the term "delayed-onset muscle soreness" has appeared commonly in the exercise science literature to describe the muscle pain and soreness that develop after unusual physical activity.

Muscle pain and soreness, muscle tissue damage, and levels of inflammation and reactive oxygen species are greater after muscle contractions, in which the muscle lengthens (i.e., eccentric), than muscle contractions, in which the muscle shortens (i.e., concentric) (Pedersen et al., 1998; Gibala et al., 2005; Kon et al., 2007). Because of this finding, researchers currently believe that high strain on muscle and connective tissue causes muscle tissue damage, inflammation, and oxidative stress, which may sensitize nociceptors (Pyne, 1994). However, experts disagree whether post-exercise increases in levels of inflammation and reactive oxygen species are physiological or pathological. Indeed, some investigators have argued against a pathological relationship due to the lack of association among post-exercise muscle damage, inflammation, reactive oxygen species, and pain or soreness (Lee et al., 2002; Nosaka et al., 2002; Yu et al., 2002). Also, the effects of inhibited inflammation and oxidative stress on the signs and symptoms of muscle damage are mixed (Close et al., 2005; Peake et al., 2005).

Regardless, it is important to appreciate that muscle pain does not develop in isolation after unaccustomed exercise. Muscle damage, weakness, loss of range of motion, swelling, decreased sense of position and of force production, and altered muscle activation have all been reported after controlled lengthening muscle contractions (Hortobagyi et al., 1998; Bottas et al., 2005; Peake et al., 2005; Proske and Allen, 2005). In addition, allodynia and hyperalgesia may occur along with enhanced temporal summation (Bajaj et al., 2000; Barlas et al., 2000; Gibson et al., 2006).

The signs and symptoms induced by muscle contractions resemble those of acute soft-tissue injuries, repetitive strain injuries, and chronic myalgia. The duration of induced signs and symptoms enables researchers to investigate study participants' behaviors outside the laboratory. For example, post-exercise muscle pain interferes with participants' normal daily activities, and participants engage in self-care behaviors for their muscle pain (Dannecker et al., 2004). Therefore, the DOMS model as applied in research studies has clinical relevance.

The level and duration of post-exercise signs and symptoms vary across participants, and investigators must be conscious of the possibility of "high responders." For example, Sayers and Clarkson (2001) found that 17% of participants lost more than 70% of their strength immediately after lengthening muscle contractions and did not fully recover their strength within 26 days of follow-up assessments. Also, in rare circumstances, large amounts of swelling in a body compartment without sufficient expansion may impair neurovascular function by causing what is known as compartment syndrome, and high post-exercise levels of the muscle protein myoglobin could lead to myoglobinuria and renal failure (West, 2007). Consequently, the methodologies for inducing DOMS must be carefully developed, and study participants must be carefully screened.

Sex Differences in Post-Exercise Muscle Soreness and Pain

The literature on sex differences in response to lengthening muscle contractions has significantly progressed from anecdotal reports to controlled investigations. This chapter will focus on investigations of voluntary lengthening contractions instead of electrically stimulated lengthening contractions because these types of contractions differ in motor unit activation (Paillard et al., 2005) and muscle damage (Crameri et al., 2007). (Chapter 4 by Mizumura and Taguchi provides an excellent description of an electrically stimulated animal model.) This chapter reviews studies with human subjects because no published animal investigations of sex differences in muscle pain or soreness after voluntary muscle contractions were located.

Newham and colleagues (1987) were one of the first groups of investigators to examine sex differences in post-exercise muscle soreness. They reported "no obvious relationship" between the sex of participants and the pressure "discomfort" threshold in a sample of five women and three men. However, the authors did not describe conducting any statistical analyses of sex differences.

Two later studies examined sex differences within investigations of interventions for post-exercise muscle pain. High and colleagues (1989) randomly assigned 31 men and 31 females to stretching protocols or a control group and found no significant difference between the sexes, regardless of group assignment. Rinard and colleagues (2000) had participants complete a bout of uncontrolled lengthening contractions as part of a pharmaceutical intervention study. Of the 802 participants, 64% perceived "moderate soreness" and were randomly assigned to receive the active drug or a placebo. Among the 82 men and 82 women in the placebo group with "moderate soreness," no sex difference in muscle soreness was detected. Thus, these studies did not detect sex differences, but neither study controlled the relative intensity of the exercise stimulus for each sex, which is essential for drawing conclusions about sex differences.

The intensity of the exercise stimulus can be controlled either by treating exercise intensity as a statistical covariate or by administering the same relative intensity of exercise to all participants, both men and women. The latter approach is commonly used. For example, in a group of eight men and eight women, Evans and colleagues (1998) based the intensity of lengthening contractions upon the participants' baseline strength; they found no sex difference in the average pain rating after the lengthening contractions. However, another study, which also based the intensity of lengthening contractions upon the participants' baseline strength, found that women's (n = 35) muscle pain intensity ratings were lower than men's (n = 32) two days after exercise, when pre-exercise muscle pain intensity ratings were controlled (Dannecker et al., 2003). Unfortunately, neither of these studies examined muscle pain ratings across multiple time points after exercise.

Testing sex differences in the pattern of muscle pain ratings across time is important. For example, MacIntyre and colleagues (2000) found that post-exercise pain intensity continued to increase across 24 hours in women (n = 10) but did not change in men (n = 12). However, no statistically significant overall difference in pain intensity between the sexes was found. Thus, additional examinations of sex differences in muscle pain across time after exercise were needed.

In response to this need, seven other published studies have both controlled for exercise intensity and examined sex differences across time after exercise (Poudevigne et al., 2002; Dannecker et al., 2005, in press; Nie et al., 2005, 2007; Edwards et al., 2007; Kawczynski et al., 2007). None of these studies detected significant sex differences in muscle pain or sex differences in patterns of muscle pain across time. For example, Dannecker and colleagues (2005) observed no significant sex by time interactions for either pain intensity or pain unpleasantness (Figs. 1 and 2). Thus, a simple summary of the current literature suggests that there are no significant sex differences in post-exercise muscle pain, which contradicts the literature on sex differences in other types of muscle pain as reviewed by Lautenbacher in Chapter 15.

Methodological Issues in the Current Literature

The current literature on sex differences in post-exercise muscle pain seems to conflict with a large volume of literature on muscle pain from

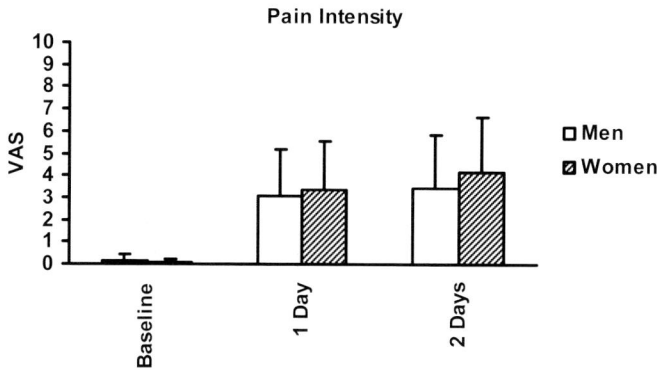

Fig. 1. Visual analogue scale (VAS) ratings of muscle pain intensity (mean ± SD) in a study of delayed-onset muscle pain in men and women (N = 95) during movement through active elbow range of motion from baseline to 2 days after lengthening contractions. Adapted from Dannecker et al. (2005), with permission.

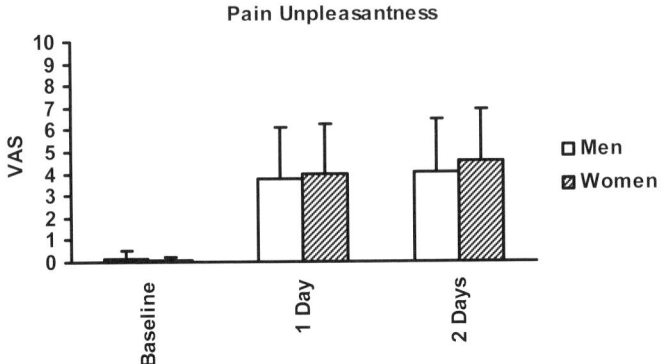

Fig. 2. VAS ratings (mean ± SD) of muscle pain unpleasantness in men and women (*N* = 95) during movement through active elbow range of motion (as in Fig. 1) from baseline to 2 days after lengthening contractions. Adapted from Dannecker et al. (2005), with permission.

mechanical pressure and algesic injections. However, simple summaries of the literature on post-exercise muscle pain often neglect important methodological issues that may affect the interpretation of research findings. The importance of controlling for exercise intensity and measuring muscle pain ratings across time have already been mentioned, but several other methodological issues are essential to consider.

Statistical power. Inadequate sample size is the most obvious methodological issue regarding the failure to detect significant sex differences in post-exercise muscle pain. A meta-analysis of pain responses to experimental stimuli such as heat and mechanical pressure concluded that women's responses were higher than men's, with an average effect size of 0.55 for pain threshold and 0.57 for pain tolerance (Riley et al., 1998). However, the estimated magnitude of sex differences in post-exercise muscle pain at a single time point (2 days after exercise) in four of the previously discussed studies suggests small to moderate sex differences (Cohen's *d* ≈ 0.39) (Dannecker et al., 2003, 2005, in press; Nie et al., 2007). Thus, tests in larger numbers of men and women would ultimately end up detecting significant sex differences, but the direction of results

from three of these five studies suggests that women's muscle pain ratings would be significantly lower than men's.

Estrogen. There is evidence that sex hormones can influence
pain response (Sherman and LeResche, 2006) and that estrogen inhibits muscle inflammation (Tiidus, 2003). None of the previously reviewed
studies of sex differences in post-exercise muscle pain have controlled for
estrogen levels. Several studies have examined the effects of estrogen levels in women who had completed lengthening contractions at controlled
exercise intensities, and the results depended on the outcome measure
(Miles and Schneider, 1993; Thompson et al., 1997; Arnett et al., 2000;
Carter et al., 2001). In general, these studies do not support relationships
between estrogen and post-exercise blood levels of the muscle protein
creatine kinase, which is used as an indirect indicator of muscle damage
(Miles and Schneider, 1993; Thompson et al., 1997; Arnett et al., 2000),
although there was one exception (Carter et al., 2001). With regard to
muscle soreness, one study found that women taking oral contraceptives
had lower ratings than normally menstruating women (Thompson et al.,
1997), but other studies found no difference between groups (Miles and
Schneider, 1993; Carter et al., 2001). Therefore, the importance of estrogen levels to sex differences in post-exercise muscle damage and pain has
not been established. Future examinations of the mediating effects of sex
hormones (e.g., estrogen, progesterone, testosterone) on the signs and
symptoms of muscle damage are needed to further clarify sex differences
in DOMS.

Exercise stimuli. The reviewed studies of sex differences in post-
exercise muscle pain vary in the types of exercise (e.g., aerobic and anaerobic) and exercise parameters (e.g., muscle length, velocity, intensity, number of repetitions, and rest periods). The importance of this
variability depends on the influence of the exercise parameters on the
mechanical strain imposed on the muscle fibers, because it is currently
believed that mechanical strain induces muscle damage (Butterfield and
Herzog, 2006). However, readers must be cautious when generalizing results across studies that have used different exercise stimuli.

Another potentially important source of variability across studies is the method used for controlling exercise intensity. Almost all of the previously reviewed studies that controlled exercise intensity did so based on participants' own baseline strength, so that relative intensity was equivalent across participants. Unfortunately, these studies measured baseline strength only during static muscle contractions and then generalized that type of strength to lengthening muscle contractions. Sex differences in the relationship between static muscle contractions and lengthening muscle contractions may exist, similar to reported sex differences in the relationship between shortening and lengthening muscle contractions (Seger and Thorstensson, 1994). The relative exercise intensity of lengthening contractions would thus be unequal between the sexes if it were based on shortening muscle contractions. However, the only study to have based the intensity of lengthening contractions on baseline strength during lengthening contractions also failed to detect significant sex differences (Dannecker et al., 2005).

A final potentially important source of variability in exercise stimuli across studies is the muscle group used in the lengthening exercise. The outcomes from lengthening exercise cannot be generalized from one muscle group to another (Jamurtas et al., 2005). One reason is that lengthening muscle contractions primarily affect fast-twitch (i.e., type II) muscle fibers (Lieber and Friden, 1988), and the fast-twitch fiber composition of different muscles may vary (Travnik et al., 1995; Klein et al., 2003). Miller and colleagues (1993) found that women had a smaller percentage of fast-twitch fibers in the vastus lateralis than men, although there was no sex difference in the percentage of fast-twitch fibers in the biceps brachii.

Pain or soreness measurement. Measurement issues within the previously reviewed literature are operational definitions of "muscle pain" and "muscle soreness" and variability in the protocols for assessing pain and soreness. Numerous studies have used the terms "muscle pain" and "muscle soreness" as synonymous constructs. None directly compared measures of muscle pain and muscle soreness, but two investigations separately measured both constructs (Arima et al., 1999, 2001). Visual examination of the patterns of muscle pain intensity and muscle soreness across time were similar (Figs. 3 and 4), with the exception that ratings of muscle soreness tended to be higher than those of muscle pain.

Arima and colleagues (1999, 2001) measured muscle pain and soreness when the muscles were in a resting state. However, delayed-onset muscle pain and soreness are typically measured during muscle contraction and with the application of mechanical pressure. There is substantial variability in the types of movement and pressure stimuli that have been administered. For example, Rinard and colleagues (2000) measured soreness during arm curls with a 1-pound (~0.45-kg) weight and during participants' palpation of their arms. In contrast, Nie and colleagues (2005) collected muscle pain intensity ratings, McGill Pain Questionnaire scores, and pressure pain thresholds after static and dynamic muscle contractions. This variability in assessment protocols across studies inhibits our ability to summarize the literature, but the thorough measurement approach of Nie and colleagues (2005) may help to establish new standards.

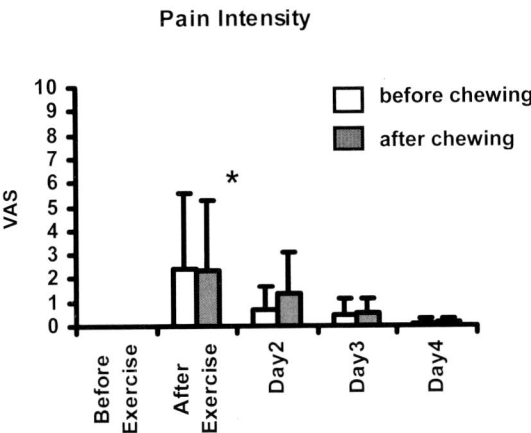

Fig. 3. Ratings of muscle pain intensity in a study of pain and soreness perception after contracting the masticatory muscles. Mean (± SE) VAS ratings in a sample of 12 men of muscle pain intensity at rest from baseline to 4 days after a tooth-grinding exercise show significant increases in pain intensity from before the exercise to immediately afterwards. Reprinted from Arima et al. (1999), with permission.

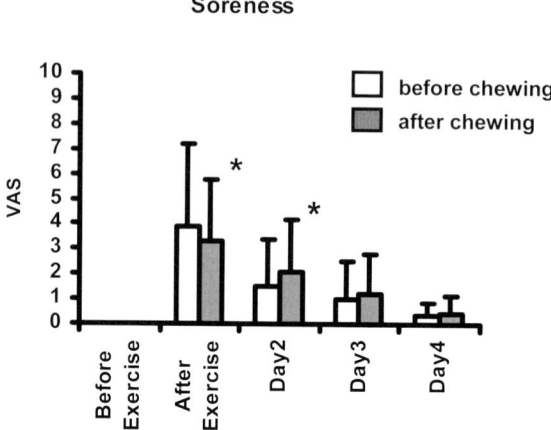

Fig. 4. Mean (± SE) VAS ratings of muscle soreness from baseline to 4 days after the grinding exercise (as in Fig. 3) show significant increases in soreness from before the exercise to immediately afterwards and 1 day later. Reprinted from Arima et al. (1999), with permission.

Conclusions

The literature does not support meaningful sex differences in DOMS. The failure to detect such sex differences is surprising, considering the literature supporting higher muscle pain responses to pressure and algesic injections in women than men. However, all types of muscle pain are not the same just because the tissue in which the pain is reported is the same, and the DOMS model does induce temporary tissue damage. Therefore, health care providers and investigators must be cautious about assuming that there are moderate to large sex differences in all types of muscle pain.

Despite clear progress in research methodologies for testing sex differences in DOMS, much work remains to be done. More investigations that control exercise stimulus intensity, measure levels of sex hormones, and assess post-exercise muscle pain with controlled contractions and pressure are clearly needed. Well-designed investigations of sex differences in DOMS may substantially contribute to our understanding of acute soft-tissue injuries, repetitive strain injuries, and chronic myalgia due to their common signs and symptoms.

References

Arima T, Arendt-Nielsen L, Svensson P. Effect of jaw muscle pain and soreness evoked by capsaicin before sleep on orofacial motor activity during sleep. J Orofac Pain 2001;15:245–256.

Arima T, Svensson P, Arendt-Nielsen L. Experimental grinding in healthy subject: a model for postexercise jaw muscle soreness? J Orofac Pain 1999;13:104–114.

Arnett MG, Hyslop R, Dennehy CA, Schneider CM. Age-related variations of serum CK and CK MB response in females. Can J Appl Physiol 2000;25:419–429.

Bajaj P, Graven-Nielsen T, Wright A, Davies LAI, Arendt-Nielsen L. Muscle hyperalgesia in postexercise muscle soreness assessed by single and repetitive ultrasound stimuli. J Pain 2000;1:111–121.

Barlas P, Walsh DM, Baxter GD, Allen JM. Delayed onset muscle soreness: Effect of an ischaemic block upon mechanical allodynia in humans. Pain 2000;87:221–225.

Bottas R, Linnamo V, Nicol C, Komi PV. Repeated maximal eccentric actions causes long-lasting disturbances in movement control. Eur J Appl Physiol 2005;94:62–69.

Butterfield TA, Herzog W. Effect of altering starting length and activation timing of muscle on fiber strain and muscle damage. J Appl Physiol 2006;100:1489–1498.

Carter A, Dobridge J, Hackney AC. Influence of estrogen on markers of muscle tissue damage following eccentric exercise. Fiziol Cheloveka 2001;27:133–137.

Close GL, Ashton T, McArdle A, Maclaren DP. The emerging role of free radicals in delayed onset muscle soreness and contraction-induced muscle injury. Comp Biochem Physiol A Mol Integr Physiol 2005;142:257–266.

Crameri RM, Aagaard P, Qvortrup K, Langberg H, Oleson J, Kjaer M. Myofibre damage in human skeletal muscle: effects of electrical stimulation versus voluntary contraction. J Physiol (London) 2007;583:365–380.

Dannecker EA, Gagnon CM, Jump RL, Brown JL, Robinson ME. Self-care behaviors for muscle pain. J Pain 2004;5:521–527.

Dannecker EA, Gormley VL, Robinson ME. Sex differences in muscle pain: self-care behaviors and effects on daily activities. J Pain 2008;9:200–209.

Dannecker EA, Koltyn KF, Riley JL, Robinson ME. Sex differences in delayed onset muscle soreness. J Sport Med Phys Fit 2003;42:458–465.

Dannecker EA, Robinson ME, Hausenblas HA, Kaminski TW. Sex differences in delayed onset muscle pain. Clin J Pain 2005;21:120–126.

Edwards KM, Burns VE, Allen LM, McPhee JS, Bosch JA, Carroll D, Drayson M, Ring C. Eccentric exercise as an adjuvant to influenza vaccination in humans. Brain Behav Immun 2007;21:209–217.

Evans GF, Haller RG, Wyrick PS, Parkey RW, Fleckenstein JL. Submaximal delayed-onset muscle soreness: correlations between MR imaging findings and clinical measures. Radiology 1998;208:815–820.

Gibala MJ, Interisano SA, Tarnopolsky MA, Roy BD, MacDonald JR, Yarasheski KE, MacDougall JD. Myofibrillar disruption following acute concentric and eccentric resistance exercise in strength-trained men. Can J Physiol Pharm 2005;78:656–661.

Gibson W, Arendt-Nielsen L, Graven-Nielsen T. Delayed-onset muscle soreness at tendon-bone junction and muscle tissue is associated with facilitated referred pain. Exp Brain Res 2006;174:351–360.

High DM, Howley ET, Franks BD. The effects of static stretching and warm-up on prevention of delayed-onset muscle soreness. Res Q Exerc Sport 1989;60:357–361.

Hortobagyi T, Houmard J, Fraser D, Dudek R, Lambert J, Tracy J. Normal forces and myofibrillar disruption after repeated eccentric exercise. J Appl Physiol 1998;84:492–498.

Hough T. Ergographic studies in muscular soreness. Am J Phys 1902;7:76–92.

Jamurtas AZ, Theocharis V, Tofas T, Tsiokanos A, Yfanti C, Paschalis V, Koutedakis Y, Nosaka K. Comparison between leg and arm eccentric exercises of the same relative intensity on indices of muscle damage. Eur J Appl Physiol 2005;95:179–185.

Kawczynski A, Nie H, Jaskolaska A, Jaskolaska A, Arendt-Nielsen L, Madeleine P. Mechanomyography and electromyography during and after fatiguing shoulder eccentric contractions in males and females. Scand J Med Sci Spor 2007;17:172–179.

Klein CS, Marsh GD, Petrella RJ, Rice CL. Muscle fiber number in the biceps brachii of young and old men. Muscle Nerve 2003;28:62–68.

Kon M, Tanabe K, Lee H, Kimura F, Akimoto T, Kono I. Eccentric muscle contractions induce greater oxidative stress than concentric contractions in skeletal muscle. Appl Physiol Nutr Metab 2007;32:273–281.

Lee J, Goldfarb AH, Rescino MH, Hedge S, Patrick S, Apperson K. Eccentric exercise effect on blood oxidative-stress markers and delayed onset of muscle soreness. Med Sci Sport Exer 2002;34:443–448.

Lieber RL, Friden J. Selective damage of fast glycolytic muscle fibers with eccentric contraction of the rabbit tibialis anterior. Acta Physiol Scand 1988;133:587–588.

MacIntyre DL, Reid WD, Lyster DM, McKenzie DC. Different effects of strenuous eccentric exercise on the accumulation of neutrophils in muscle in women and men. Eur J Appl Physiol 2000;81:47–53.

Miles MP, Schneider CM. Creatine kinase isoenzyme MB may be elevated in healthy young women after submaximal eccentric exercise. J Lab Clin Med 1993;122:197–201.

Miller AEJ, MacDougall JD, Tarnopolsky MA, Sale DG. Gender differences in strength and muscle fiber characteristics. Eur J Appl Physiol 1993;66:254–262.

Newham DJ, Jones DA, Clarkson PM. Repeated high-force eccentric exercise: Effects on muscle pain and damage. J Appl Physiol 1987;63:1381–1386.

Nie H, Arendt-Nielsen L, Kawczynski A, Madeleine P. Gender effects on trapezius surface EMG during delayed onset muscle soreness due to eccentric shoulder exercise. J Electromyogr Kinesiol 2007;17:401–409.

Nie H, Kawczynski A, Madeleine P, Arendt-Nielsen L. Delayed onset muscle soreness in neck/shoulder muscles. Eur J Pain 2005;9:653–660.

Nosaka K, Newton M, Sacco P. Delayed-onset muscle soreness does not reflect the magnitude of eccentric exercise-induced muscle damage. Scand J Med Sci Sports 2002;12:337–346.

Paillard T, Noe F, Passelergue P, Dupui P. Electrical stimulation superimposed onto voluntary muscular contraction. Sports Med 2005;35:951–966.

Peake J, Nosaka K, Suzuki K. Characterization of inflammatory responses to eccentric exercise in humans. Exerc Immunol Rev 2005;11:64–85.

Pedersen BK, Ostrowski K, Rohde T, Bruunsgaard H. The cytokine response to strenuous exercise. Can J Physiol Pharm 1998;76:505–511.

Poudevigne M, O'Connor P, Pasley J. Does sex or blood pressure affect delayed-onset muscle pain intensity? Clin J Pain 2002;18:386–393.

Proske U, Allen TJ. Damage to skeletal muscle from eccentric exercise. Exerc Sport Sci Rev 2005;33:98–104.

Pyne DB. Exercise-induced muscle damage and inflammation: a review. Aust J Sci Med Sport 1994;26:49–58.

Riley JL, Robinson ME, Wise EA, Myers CD, Fillingim RB. Sex differences in the perception of noxious experimental stimuli: a meta-analysis. Pain 1998;74:181–188.

Rinard J, Clarkson PM, Smith LL, Grossman M. Responses of males and females to high-force eccentric exercise. J Sport Sci 2000;18:229–236.

Sayers SP, Clarkson PM. Force recovery after eccentric exercise in males and females. Eur J Appl Physiol 2001;84:122–126.

Seger JY, Thorstensson A. Muscle strength and myoelectric activity in prepubertal and adult males and females. Eur J Appl Physiol 1994;69:81–87.

Sherman JJ, LeResche L. Does experimental pain response vary across the menstrual cycle? a methodological review. Am J Physiol Regul Integr Comp Physiol 2006;291:R245–R256.

Thompson HS, Hyatt JP, De Souza MJ, Clarkson PM. The effects of oral contraceptives on delayed onset muscle soreness following exercise. Contraception 1997;56:59–65.

Tiidus PM. Influence of estrogen on skeletal muscle damage, inflammation, and repair. Exerc Sport Sci Rev 2003;31:40–44.

Travnik L, Pernus F, Erzen I. Histochemical and morphometric characteristics of the normal human vastus medialis longus and vastus medialis obliquus muscles. J Anat 1995;187:403–411.

West H. Rhabdomyolysis associated with compartment syndrome resulting in acute renal failure. Eur J Emerg Med 2007;14:368–370.

Yu JG, Malm C, Thornell LE. Eccentric contractions leading to DOMS do not cause loss of desmin nor fibre necrosis in human muscle. Histochem Cell Biol 2002;118:29–34.

Correspondence to: Erin A. Dannecker, PhD, ATC, University of Missouri-Columbia, Department of Physical Therapy, 106 Lewis Hall, Columbia, MO 65211-4250, USA. Tel: 1-573-882-8698; fax: 1-573-884-8369; email: danneckere@missouri.edu.

17

Biopsychological and Genetic Risk Factors for Temporomandibular Joint Disorders and Related Conditions

William Maixner

Center for Neurosensory Disorders, School of Dentistry, University of North Carolina, Chapel Hill, North Carolina, USA

Temporomandibular joint disorder (TMJD) represents a cluster of disorders that involve the muscles of mastication and the temporomandibular joint. TMJD is a very common musculoskeletal disorder, with prevalence estimates ranging from 3% to 15% of the Western population (LeResche, 1997; Drangsholt and LeResche, 1999). It has become increasing evident that TMJD is frequently associated with a variety of other idiopathic pain disorders (IPDs); (Diatchenko et al., 2006b), including but not limited to fibromyalgia syndrome (FMS), irritable bowel syndrome, chronic headache, interstitial cystitis, chronic pelvic pain, chronic tinnitus, whiplash, and vulvar vestibulitis. Many of these conditions tend to aggregate as "comorbid" conditions that are characterized by a complaint of pain as well as a mosaic of abnormalities in motor function, autonomic balance, neuroendocrine function, and sleep. Although the mechanisms that underlie the majority of these conditions are poorly understood, substantial evidence has emerged to suggest that they are associated with a state of pain amplification and psychological distress (McBeth et al., 2001; Bradley and McKendree-Smith, 2002; Verne and Price, 2002; Gracely et al., 2004).

Fundamentals of Musculoskeletal Pain
edited by Thomas Graven-Nielsen, Lars Arendt-Nielsen, and Siegfried Mense
IASP Press, Seattle, © 2008

My colleagues and I have recently proposed (Diatchenko et al., 2006b) that pain amplification and psychological distress, which are mediated by an individual's genetic variability and exposure to environmental events, represent two primary pathways of vulnerability that underlie the development of TMJD and other highly prevalent IPDs (Fig. 1).

Evidence for a State of Pain Amplification in TMJD

The outcomes of several cross-sectional studies provide evidence that TMJD is associated with enhanced pain sensitivity and augmented capacity to temporally summate pain (Maixner et al., 1995a,b, 1998; Svens-

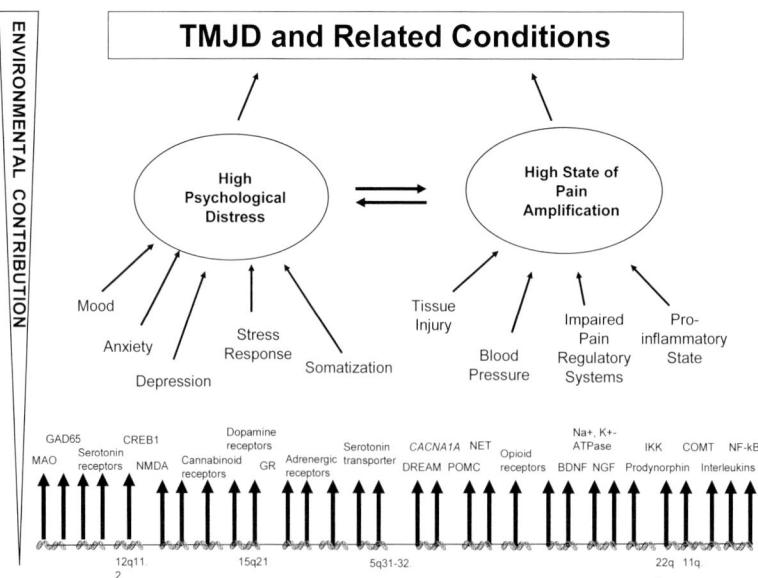

Fig. 1. A descriptive model that depicts likely determinants of the onset and maintenance of temporomandibular joint disorder (TMJD) and related idiopathic pain disorders. These factors are determined by both genetic variability and environmental events that determine an individual's psychological profile and pain amplification status. These two primary domains are interactive and influence the risk of pain onset and persistence. Likely modifiers of the interaction between genetic and environmental factors include sex and ethnicity. Adapted from Diatchenko et al. (2006b).

son et al., 2001; Sarlani and Greenspan, 2003; Maixner, 2004). TMJD patients, when compared to age- and gender-matched control subjects, have reduced pressure pain thresholds across several cranial muscles and at regions remote to sites of clinical pain report (Maixner et al., 1998). TMJD patients also show enhanced sensitivity both to noxious thermal stimuli applied to the volar forearm or face and to an aversive ischemic stimulus applied to the arm (Maixner et al., 1995a). Svensson and co-workers (2001) have also shown that TMJD patients report greater pain and larger zones of pain referral to hypertonic saline administered into the masseter muscle compared to control subjects. Consistent with the suggestion that this condition is associated with a state of pain amplification, TMJD patients also rate the magnitude of suprathreshold noxious thermal stimuli to be enhanced relative to pain-free subjects and show enhanced temporal summation of heat pain (Maixner et al., 1995a,b, 1998). These experimental observations are not specific to TMJD; similar findings have been reported for other IPDs (e.g., migraine headache, tension headache, irritable bowel syndrome, and vulvodynia) (Langemark et al., 1989; Schoenen et al., 1991; Granges and Littlejohn, 1993; McBeth et al., 2001; Bradley and McKendree-Smith, 2002; Verne and Price, 2002; Giesecke et al., 2004; Gracely et al., 2004). These findings suggest that the processing of nociceptive information is enhanced in patient populations with TMJD and associated comorbid conditions.

A handful of studies have sought to prospectively identify risk factors or risk determinants that are associated with or mediate the onset and maintenance of IPDs. A well-established predictor of IPD onset is the presence of another chronic pain condition, characterized by a state of pain amplification (Verne and Price, 2002). Additionally, widespread pain is a risk indicator for dysfunction associated with painful TMJD and for lack of response to treatment (Raphael and Marbach, 2001). Enhanced sensitivity to noxious stimuli also appears to be a risk factor for TMJD onset because individuals who are more sensitive to noxious stimuli are significantly more likely to develop painful TMJD than those who are less sensitive (incidence density ratio [IDR] = 2.7; 95% CI = 1.3–5.7) (Slade et al., 2007).

Mechanisms Supporting Pain Amplification in Patients with TMJD

The underlying neural mechanisms that contribute to enhanced pain sensitivity and summation of pain in TMJD are largely unknown. Enhanced encoding of nociceptive input is probably involved, mediated either by enhanced activity of peripheral nociceptors or by enhanced encoding of nociceptive information by central nervous system (CNS) networks (Dubner, 1995; Dubner and Basbaum, 1995; Maixner et al., 1995b). Peripheral nociceptive input and CNS regulatory systems modulate the activity of central neural networks and produce dynamic, time-dependent alterations in the excitability and response characteristics of central networks responsible for the perception of pain and mood.

Peripheral Factors

While there is substantial evidence that central mechanisms contribute to the onset and maintenance of TMJD and related conditions, a generalized and widespread increase in the sensitivity of peripheral nociceptive afferents cannot be discounted as an important etiological contributor to TMJD and other IPDs. Indeed, variations in the synthesis and release of endogenous substrates for peripheral vanilloid (TRPV) receptors, purinergic (P2X) receptors, corticotropin-releasing factor receptors, adrenergic receptors, acid-sensing ion channels, and cytokine channels—and associated transduction mechanisms—represent only a few pathways through which peripheral substrates can produce a generalized increase in cutaneous and visceral pain sensitivity (Scholz and Woolf, 2002).

Spinal Transmission

Neurotransmitters and neuromodulators released by C fibers can produce persistent excitatory effects on central neurons that respond to nociceptive and tactile input. Evidence is also emerging that cytokines released from activated glial tissues can enable persistent pain states

(Watkins and Maier, 2002; Watkins et al., 2003). Furthermore, alterations in CNS inhibitory and excitatory pathways can occur independently of peripheral afferent input, and these changes can alter the activity of central neural networks that respond to tissue damage. It thus seems plausible that an enhancement or disinhibition of CNS excitatory mechanisms, resulting from peripheral and/or central changes, could increase pain sensitivity in TMJD and related conditions. This hypothesis allows for the development of painful perceptions that appear to be disproportionate and even independent of primary afferent drive and the status of peripheral tissues. In support of this hypothesis, spinal dorsal horn neurons that respond to inputs from skeletal muscle nociceptors are normally under much greater central tonic inhibitory control than dorsal horn neurons responding to input from cutaneous nociceptors (Mense, 1990, 1993; Yu et al., 1991). The processes that enhance pain sensitivity and the temporal summation of pain may be of particular relevance to the understanding of the neural mechanisms that underlie the cranial myalgia and arthralgia associated with TMJD, given the frequent "mismatch" between the amount of pain reported by patients and the physical findings observed during examination. Individuals with less inhibitory influence on central nociceptive transmission (i.e., disinhibition) are likely to show enhanced sensitivity to noxious stimuli and a greater capacity to develop persistent pain states following either peripheral events (e.g., joint trauma or muscle trauma) or central events (e.g., psychological or emotional stress) that can serve as triggers for the development of TMJD (Dworkin, 1994; Turner et al., 2001) as well as related conditions such as FMS (Aaron et al., 1997; Alarcon and Bradley, 1998; Kersh et al., 2001).

Similarly, a plethora of spinal and supraspinal molecular processes and pathways can contribute to the onset of TMJD and related IPDs. Alterations in spinal receptors/channels (e.g., opioid, calcitonin gene-related peptide, neurokinin, glutamate, adrenergic, serotoninergic, and cytokine), transporters (e.g., serotonin), enzymatic pathways (e.g., cyclo-oxygenase, nitric oxide synthase), and transduction pathways (e.g., mitogen-activated protein kinase, protein kinases A and C) represent a few of the known pathways (Scholz and Woolf, 2002).

Impaired Diffuse Noxious Inhibitory Control

Several endogenous systems regulate pain perception and may be altered in patients with TMJD. One such system that has been extensively examined is the "diffuse noxious inhibitory control" (DNIC) system (Le Bars et al., 1979a,b; Willer et al., 1999; Millan, 2002). A general feature of this system is that a noxious conditioning stimulus applied to one body region is able to suppress the perception of pain evoked by a test noxious stimulus applied at another anatomical site. The generalized increased sensitivity of the skin, as well as of musculoskeletal tissues, to noxious thermal stimuli suggests an impairment in the processes that regulate pain perception in TMJD patients. Consistent with this view, individuals who develop TMJD show a relative impairment in DNIC compared to pain-free control subjects. Specifically, we showed that ischemic arm pain fails to recruit DNIC in TMJD patients (Maixner et al., 1995b), although the same procedure is quite able to suppress acute pain resulting from an inflammatory condition (i.e., acute pulpitis; Sigurdsson and Maixner, 1994). Kashima and coworkers (1999) have also reported that ischemic arm pain fails to increase pain thresholds on the opposite side of the body in TMJD as effectively as it does in normal subjects. Although not consistently observed (Staud et al., 2001, 2003), there is evidence that fibromyalgia syndrome is associated with impairment in DNIC (Kosek et al., 1996; Kosek and Hansson, 1997; Julien et al., 2005). The discrepancies between laboratories may result from differences in the experimental paradigms such as the temporal parameters of the noxious conditioning stimulus (Julien et al., 2005).

Impaired Baroreceptor and Vagal Afferent Function

Another process that may contribute to central disinhibition of pain regulatory systems so as to alter pain processing is related to activity of brainstem systems that receive afferent information from carotid sinus and cardiopulmonary visceral afferents (i.e., baroreceptor afferents). The peripheral activation of these pathways suppresses nociceptive reflexes and neuronal responses to noxious stimuli in several species and diminishes pain perception in humans (Randich and Maixner, 1984; Maixner, 1991, 2004; Bruehl and Chung, 2004). In contrast, TMJD patients show an impairment in baroreceptor regulation of pain because they fail to show a relationship between resting arterial blood pressure and pain perception (Maixner et al., 1997). These observations suggest that the enhanced pain sensitivity seen in TMJD patients may result, at least in part, from impairments in baroreceptor modulation of central pain regulatory systems. Whether baroreceptor function is impaired in other IPDs remains an open question, but it has been reported that FMS is associated with autonomic abnormalities that are consistent with impairments in baroreceptor function (Bou-Holaigah et al., 1997; Petzke and Clauw, 2000; Raj et al., 2000; Naschitz et al., 2001).

The central neural networks by which impairments in baroreceptor pathways affect sensory perception have not been fully elucidated, but it has been proposed that impairments in the nucleus of the solitary tract of the vasomotor center, the first relay for baroreceptor afferent input, disinhibit the ascending reticular activating system (Fig. 2) (Zanchetti et al., 1952; Bonvallet et al., 1954; Olson, 1980; Maixner et al., 1995b). This system is a nontopographic cortical projecting system that originates from a diverse number of nuclear groups in the brainstem and basal forebrain (e.g., parabrachial nucleus, locus ceruleus, raphe system, and nucleus basalis). It plays an important role in sculpturing sensory, motor, and autonomic responses, as well as hypothalamic-pituitary-adrenal (HPA) axis responses to stress and somatosensory input (Steriade 1988; Steriade and Llinas 1988; Whitsel et al. 1990; Maixner 1991).

The ascending reticular activating system is normally inhibited by baroreceptor stimulation and can be disinhibited by deafferentation of baroreceptor pathways (Steriade, 1988; Steriade and Llinas, 1988; Whitsel et al., 1990; Maixner, 1991). Disinhibition of this system, by diminishing the efficacy of baroreceptor afferent input, may contribute to the variety of chronic, maladaptive psychological, sensory, motor, autonomic, sleep, and HPA axis responses associated with TMJD and related disorders. In addition to altering the ascending reticular activating system, impairments in baroreceptor-mediated regulation of nociception may result in a suppression of diffuse inhibitory pathways that actively inhibit

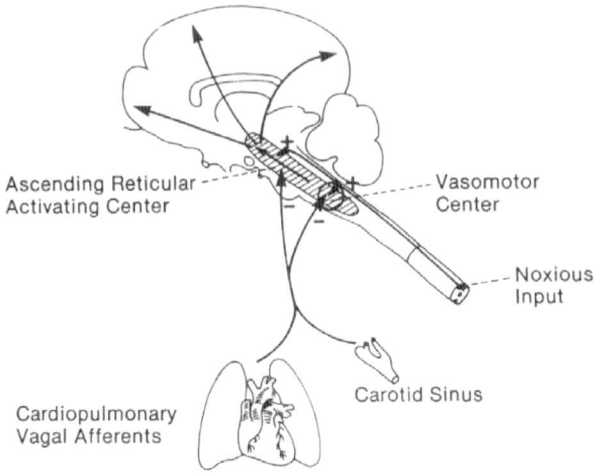

Fig. 2. Schematic diagram of the inhibitory effect of carotid sinus baroreceptors and vagal afferents on cortical arousal evoked by nociceptive input. Impairments of these visceral afferent inputs will disinhibit the ascending reticular activating system, resulting in altered cortical arousal, enhanced sensory processing, enhanced motor responses, sympathetic hyperactivity, and impaired hypothalamic-pituitary-adrenal (HPA) axis function. Adapted from Bonvallet et al. (1954).

trigeminal and dorsal horn neurons that respond to muscle and cutaneous nociceptive inputs (Steriade, 1988; Steriade and Llinas, 1988; Whitsel et al., 1990; Maixner, 1991). As noted above, impairment in DNIC may also contribute to the enhanced temporal summation of pain and pain amplification observed in IPDs.

Impairments in baroreceptor and vagal afferent pathways may also increase pain sensitivity by invoking an enhanced increase in the release of epinephrine from the adrenal medulla, resulting in a β-adrenoreceptor-mediated increase in nociceptor sensitivity (Fig. 3) (Khasar et al., 1998, 1999, 2003). Chronic increases in circulating levels of catecholamines such as epinephrine may further enhance pain sensitivity and inflammatory responses by stimulating peripheral nociceptors or suppressing the HPA axis (Kizildere et al., 2003). Recent findings by Nackley and coworkers (2007) have shown that inhibition of catechol-*O*-methyl transferase (COMT), a key enzyme that metabolizes catecholamines, induces mechanical and thermal hyperalgesia and produces proinflammatory

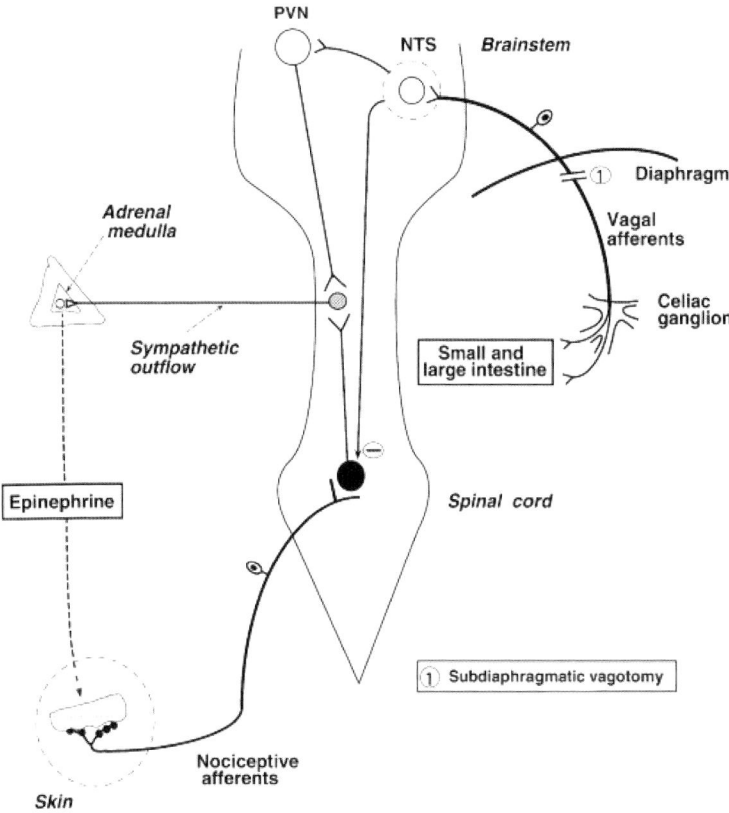

Fig. 3. Schematic diagram of proposed circuit for vagal-adrenal medullary modulation of nociception. Vagal afferents terminate in the nucleus of the solitary tract (NTS),
which in turn projects to the paraventricular nucleus (PVN). Preganglionic sympathetic
nerves from the PVN innervate the adrenal medulla. Stressful stimuli stimulate the production of corticotropin-releasing factor (CRF), a coordinator of the stress response.
Activation of the locus ceruleus by CRF is transmitted to the adrenal medulla via sympathetic fibers in the splanchnic nerve, leading to the release of epinephrine. From
Khasar et al. (2003).

cytokines in rats. These effects are sensitive to blockade with selective
β_2- and β_3-adrenoreceptor antagonists, but they are not selective to β_1-
adrenoreceptor blockade. Consistent with these observations, the blockade
of β-adrenoreceptors with the nonselective β-adrenoreceptor antagonist
propranolol diminished clinical pain report in a subpopulation of patients
with TMJD and FMS (Light and Maixner, unpublished observation). It is

also noteworthy that β-adrenoreceptor blockade reverses the suppression of the HPA axis by increasing the secretion of cortisol (Kizildere et al., 2003). These findings suggest that certain β-adrenoreceptor antagonists may prove effective in treating TMJD and IPDs by impacting both peripheral nociceptor function and enhancing HPA function.

Psychological Distress and Onset and Persistence of TMJD and Related Idiopathic Disorders

Heightened psychological distress is another domain or pathway of vulnerability that can lead to IPDs (Fig. 1). Patients with TMJD, and those with other IPDs, display a complex mosaic of depression, anxiety (Vassend et al., 1995), and perceived stress relative to pain-free controls (Beaton et al., 1991). Somatization, which is the tendency to report numerous physical symptoms in excess to what is expected from physical examination (Escobar et al., 1987), is associated with more than a twofold increase in TMJD incidence, decreased improvement in TMJD facial pain after 5 years (Ohrbach and Dworkin, 1998), and increased pain following treatment (McCreary et al., 1992). Somatization is also highly associated with widespread pain, with the number of muscle sites painful to palpation (Wilson et al., 1994), and with the progression from acute to chronic TMJD (Garofalo et al., 1998). In a recently completed prospective cohort study that recruited 244 initially TMJD-free females, we found that somatization (IDR = 6.0; 95% CI = 2.5–14.8), trait anxiety (IDR = 5.5; 95% CI = 2.2–13.4), depression (IDR = 2.1; 95% CI = 1.0–4.6), and perceived stress (IDR = 3.4; 95% CI: 1.5–7.8) represented significant risk factors for TMJD onset (Slade et al., 2007). These results suggest that somatization, negative affect/mood, and environmental stress act either independently or jointly to contribute to the risk of onset and maintenance of TMJD and other IPDs.

Genetic Variations Influencing Pain Amplification and Psychological Distress

Pain amplification and psychological distress domains are influenced by specific genetic variants that modulate the activity of physiological pathways that underlie these domains. Polymorphic variations in genes coding for key regulators of these pathways, when coupled with environmental factors such as physical or emotional stress, interact to produce a phenotype that is vulnerable to TMJD and related IPDs. Both clinical and experimental pain perception are influenced by genetic variants (Mogil, 1999; Zubieta et al., 2003; Diatchenko et al., 2005, 2007; Norbury et al., 2007; Nielsen et al., 2008). Several recent studies have also established a genetic association for a variety of psychological traits and disorders that influence the risk of developing IPDs (Exton et al., 1914; Bouchard and McGue, 1954; Eid et al., 1971; Gordon and Hen, 2004; Lesch, 2004). Within recent years, polymorphic variations in several genes associated with pain sensitivity and a variety of complex psychological disorders such as depression, anxiety, stress response, and somatization have increased exponentially. A few examples of the genes associated with these traits include catechol-O-methyltransferase (*COMT*) (Gursoy et al., 2003; Drabant et al., 2006), adrenergic receptor β_2 (*ADRB2*) (Diatchenko et al., 2006a), and serotonin transporter (*5-HTT*) (Herken et al., 2001; Caspi et al., 2003; Gordon and Hen, 2004), as well as genes that code for cyclic AMP-response element binding protein 1 (Zubenko et al., 2003), monoamine oxidase A (Deckert et al., 1999), GABA-synthetic enzyme (Smoller et al., 2001), D_2 dopamine receptor (Lawford et al., 2003), glucocorticoid receptor (Wust et al., 2004), interleukins 1β and 1α (Yu et al., 2003), Na$^+$, K$^+$-ATPase, and voltage-gated calcium channels (Estevez and Gardner, 2004).

A common single nucleotide polymorphism (SNP) in codon 158 (*val^{158}met*) of the *COMT* gene has been associated with the perception of pain in humans (Zubieta et al., 2003). Recently, three genetic variants (haplotypes) of the gene encoding COMT—designated as the low pain sensitivity (LPS), average pain sensitivity (APS), and high pain sensitivity

(HPS) haplotypes—have been identified that encompass 96% of the human population (Diatchenko et al., 2005). Five combinations of these haplotypes are strongly associated with variation in sensitivity to experimental pain. The presence of even a single LPS haplotype diminishes, by as much as 2.3 times, the risk of developing TMJD. The LPS haplotype produces much higher levels of COMT enzymatic activity compared to the APS or HPS haplotypes, and inhibition of COMT in the rat results in a profound increase in pain sensitivity (Diatchenko et al., 2005; Nackley et al., 2006). Thus, COMT activity substantially influences pain sensitivity, and the three major haplotypes determine COMT activity in humans that inversely correlates with pain sensitivity and the risk of developing TMD. Furthermore, inhibition of COMT activity results in heightened pain sensitivity and proinflammatory cytokine release in animal models via activation of $\beta_{2/3}$-adrenergic receptors (Nackley et al., 2007). Consistent with these observations, our group has also reported that three major haplotypes of the human gene *ADRB2* are strongly associated with the risk of developing a TMJD (Diatchenko et al., 2006a).

Conclusion

Growing evidence indicates that individuals who show less inhibitory influence on central nociceptive transmission are more likely to show enhanced sensitivity to noxious stimuli and a greater capacity to develop persistent pain states following either peripheral events such as joint or muscle trauma or central events such as psychological or emotional stress. The onset of TMJD and related IPDs appears to be associated with both physical and psychological triggers that initiate the enhanced temporal summation of pain and pain amplification observed in these patient populations. While there are individual differences in responses, most TMJD patients show altered responses to physiological and psychological stressors. There is frequently, if not generally, a "mismatch" between the amount of pain reported by patients and the physical findings observed upon examination. Elucidation of the biological, psychological, and genetic factors that contribute to pain amplification and psychological distress is of particular relevance to understanding the underlying mechanisms that evoke pain in individual patients with TMJD and related IPDs. By furthering our understanding of the biological, psychological, and genetic factors that contribute to individual pathways of vulnerability, we will be able to develop individually tailored treatments and therapies for TMJD and other IPDs.

Acknowledgments

I would like to thank the outstanding group of investigators and patients who have assisted me with this work over the last several years. I am much indebted and appreciative of your contributions. This work was supported by NIH grants DE07509, NS045685, DE16558, and NS41670.

References

Aaron LA, Bradley LA, Alarcon GS, Triana-Alexander M, Alexander RW, Martin MY, Alberts KR. Perceived physical and emotional trauma as precipitating events in fibromyalgia. Associations with health care seeking and disability status but not pain severity. Arthritis Rheum 1997;40:453–460.

Alarcon GS, Bradley LA. Advances in the treatment of fibromyalgia: current status and future directions. Am J Med Sci 1998;315:397–404.

Bartorelli C, Bizzi E, Libretti A, Zanchetti A. Inhibitory control of sinocarotid pressoceptive afferents on hypothalamic autonomic activity and sham rage behavior. Arch Ital Bio 1968;98:308–326.

Beaton RD, Egan KJ, Nakagawa-Kogan H, Morrison KN. Self-reported symptoms of stress with temporomandibular disorders: comparisons to healthy men and women. J Prosthet Dent 1991;65:289–293.

Bonvallet M, Dell P, Hiebel G. Tonus sympathique et activite electrique corticale. Electroencephalogr Clin Neurophysiol 1954;6:119–144.

Bouchard TJ Jr, McGue M. Genetic and environmental influences on human psychological differences. J Neurobiol 2003;54:4–45.

Bou-Holaigah I, Calkins H, Flynn JA, Tunin C, Chang HC, Kan JS, Rowe PC. Provocation of hypotension and pain during upright tilt table testing in adults with fibromyalgia. Clin Exp Rheumatol 1997;15:239–246.

Bradley LA, McKendree-Smith NL. Central nervous system mechanisms of pain in fibromyalgia and other musculoskeletal disorders: behavioral and psychologic treatment approaches. Curr Opin Rheumatol 2002;14:45–51.

Bruehl S, Chung OY. Interactions between the cardiovascular and pain regulatory systems: an updated review of mechanisms and possible alterations in chronic pain. Neurosci Biobehav Rev 2004;28:395–414.

Caspi A, Sugden K, Moffitt TE, et al. Influence of life stress on depression: moderation by a polymorphism in the 5-HT T gene. Science 2003;301:386–389.

Deckert J, Catalano M, Syagailo YV, et al. Excess of high activity monoamine oxidase A gene promoter alleles in female patients with panic disorder. Hum Mol Genet 1999;8:621–624.

Diatchenko L, Anderson AD, Slade GD, et al. Three major haplotypes of the beta2 adrenergic receptor define psychological profile, blood pressure, and the risk for development of a common musculoskeletal pain disorder. Am J Med Genet B Neuropsychiatr Genet 2006a;141:449–462.

Diatchenko L, Nackley AG, Slade GD, Fillingim RB, Maixner W. Idiopathic pain disorders—pathways of vulnerability. Pain 2006b;123:226–230.

Diatchenko L, Nackley AG, Tchivileva IE, Shabalina SA, Maixner W. Genetic architecture of human pain perception. Trends Genet 2007;23:605–613.

Diatchenko L, Slade GD, Nackley AG, et al. Genetic basis for individual variations in pain perception and the development of a chronic pain condition. Hum Mol Genet 2005;14:135–143.

Drabant EM, Hariri AR, Meyer-Lindenberg A, Munoz KE, Mattay VS, Kolachana BS, Egan MF, Weinberger DR. Catechol O-methyltransferase val158met genotype and neural mechanisms related to affective arousal and regulation. Arch Gen Psychiatry 2006;63:1396–1406.

Drangsholt MT, LeResche L. Temporomandibular disorder pain. In: Crombie IK, Croft PR, Linton SJ, LeResche L, Von Korff M, editors. Epidemiology of pain. Seattle: IASP Press; 1999. p 203–233.

Dubner R. Hyperalgesia in response to injury to cutaneous and deep tissues. In: Fricton JR, Dubner R, editors. Orofacial pain and temporomandibular disorders. New York: Raven Press; 1995. p 61–83.

Dubner R, Basbaum AI. Spinal dorsal horn plasticity following tissue or nerve damage. In: Wall PD, Melzack R, editors. Textbook of pain, Vol. 3. Edinburgh: Churchill Livingston; 1995. p 225–241.

Dworkin SF. Somatization, distress and chronic pain. Qual Life Res 1994;3(Suppl 1):S77–S83.

Eid M, Riemann R, Angleitner A, Borkenau P. Sociability and positive emotionality: genetic and environmental contributions to the covariation between different facets of extraversion. J Pers 2003;71:319–346.

Escobar JI, Burnam MA, Karno M, Forsythe A, Golding JM. Somatization in the community. Arch Gen Psychiatry 1987;44:713–718.

Estevez M, Gardner KL. Update on the genetics of migraine. Hum Genet 2004;114:225–235.

Exton MS, Artz M, Siffert W, Schedlowski M. G protein beta3 subunit 825T allele is associated with depression in young, healthy subjects. Neuroreport 2003;1914:531–533.

Garofalo JP, Gatchel RJ, Wesley AL, Ellis E. Predicting chronicity in acute temporomandibular joint disorders using the research diagnostic criteria. J Am Dent Assoc 1998;129:438–447.

Giesecke J, Reed BD, Haefner HK, Giesecke T, Clauw DJ, Gracely RH. Quantitative sensory testing in vulvodynia patients and increased peripheral pressure pain sensitivity. Obstet Gynecol 2004;104:126–133.

Gordon JA, Hen R. Genetic approaches to the study of anxiety. Annu Rev Neurosci 2004;27:193–222.

Gracely RH, Geisser ME, Giesecke T, Grant MA, Petzke F, Williams DA, Clauw DJ. Pain catastrophizing and neural responses to pain among persons with fibromyalgia. Brain 2004;127:835–843.

Granges G, Littlejohn G. Pressure pain threshold in pain-free subjects, in patients with chronic regional pain syndromes, and in patients with fibromyalgia syndrome. Arthritis Rheum 1993;36:642–646.

Gursoy S, Erdal E, Herken H, Madenci E, Alasehirli B, Erdal N. Significance of catechol-O-methyltransferase gene polymorphism in fibromyalgia syndrome. Rheumatol Int 2003;23:104–107.

Herken H, Erdal E, Mutlu N, Barlas O, Cataloluk O, Oz F, Guray E. Possible association of temporomandibular joint pain and dysfunction with a polymorphism in the serotonin transporter gene. Am J Orthod Dentofacial Orthop 2001;120:308–313.

Julien N, Goffaux P, Arsenault P, Marchand S. Widespread pain in fibromyalgia is related to a deficit of endogenous pain inhibition. Pain 2005;114:295–302.

Kashima K, Rahman OIF, Sakoda S, Shiba R. Increased pain sensitivity of the upper extremities of TMD patients with myalgia to experimentally-evoked noxious stimulation: Possibility of worsened endogenous opioid systems. Cranio 1999;17:241–246.

Kersh BC, Bradley LA, Alarcon GS, et al. Psychosocial and health status variables independently predict health care seeking in fibromyalgia. Arthritis Rheum 2001;45:362–371.

Khasar SG, Green PG, Miao FJ, Levine JD. Vagal modulation of nociception is mediated by adrenomedullary epinephrine in the rat. Eur J Neurosci 2003;17:909–915.

Khasar SG, McCarter G, Levine JD. Epinephrine produces a beta-adrenergic receptor-mediated mechanical hyperalgesia and in vitro sensitization of rat nociceptors. J Neurophysiol 1999;81:1104–1112.

Khasar SG, Miao FJ, Janig W, Levine JD. Vagotomy-induced enhancement of mechanical hyperalgesia in the rat is sympathoadrenal-mediated. J Neurosci 1998;18:3043–3049.

Kizildere S, Gluck T, Zietz B, Scholmerich J, Straub RH. During a corticotropin-releasing hormone test in healthy subjects, administration of a beta-adrenergic antagonist induced secretion of cortisol and dehydroepiandrosterone sulfate and inhibited secretion of ACTH. Eur J Endocrinol 2003;148:45–53.

Kosek E, Ekholm J, Hansson P. Modulation of pressure pain thresholds during and following isometric contraction in patients with fibromyalgia and in healthy controls. Pain 1996;64:415–423.

Kosek E, Hansson P. Modulatory influence on somatosensory perception from vibration and heterotopic noxious conditioning stimulation (HNCS) in fibromyalgia patients and healthy subjects. Pain 1997;70:41–51.

Langemark M, Jensen K, Jensen TS, Olesen J. Pressure pain thresholds and thermal nociceptive thresholds in chronic tension-type headache. Pain 1989;38:203–210.

Lawford BR, McD YR, Noble EP, Kann B, Arnold L, Rowell J, Ritchie TL. D2 dopamine receptor gene polymorphism: paroxetine and social functioning in posttraumatic stress disorder. Eur Neuropsychopharmacol 2003;13:313–320.

Le Bars D, Dickenson AH, Besson JM. Diffuse noxious inhibitory controls (DNIC). I. Effects on dorsal horn convergent neurones in the rat. Pain 1979a;6:283–304.

Le Bars D, Dickenson AH, Besson JM. Diffuse noxious inhibitory controls (DNIC). II. Lack of effect on non-convergent neurones, supraspinal involvement and theoretical implications. Pain 1979b;6:305–327.

LeResche L. Epidemiology of temporomandibular disorders: implications for the investigation of etiologic factors. Crit Rev Oral Biol Med 1997;8:291–305.

Lesch KP. Gene-environment interaction and the genetics of depression. J Psychiatry Neurosci 2004;29:174–184.

Maixner W. Interactions between cardiovascular and pain modulatory systems: physiological and pathophysiological implications. J Cardiovasc Electrophysiol 1991;(Suppl 2):S2–S12.

Maixner W. Myogenous temporomandibular disorder: a persistent pain condition associated with hyperalgesia and enhanced temporal summation of pain. In: Brune K, Handwerker HO, editors. Hyperalgesia: molecular mechanisms and clinical implications. Seattle: IASP Press; 2004. p 373–386.

Maixner W, Fillingim R, Booker D, Sigurdsson A. Sensitivity of patients with painful temporomandibular disorders to experimentally evoked pain. Pain 1995a;63:341–351.

Maixner W, Fillingim RB, Kincaid S, Sigurdsson A, Harris MB. Relationship between pain sensitivity and resting arterial blood pressure in patients with painful temporomandibular disorders. Psychosomatic Med 1997;59:503–511.

Maixner W, Fillingim R, Sigurdsson A, Kincaid S, Silva S. Sensitivity of patients with painful temporomandibular disorders to experimentally evoked pain: evidence for altered temporal summation of pain. Pain 1998;76:71–81.

Maixner W, Sigurdsson A, Fillingim R, Lundeen T, Booker D. Regulation of acute and chronic orofacial pain. In: Fricton JR, Dubner RB, editors. Orofacial pain and temporomandibular disorders. New York: Raven Press; 1995b. p 85–102.

McBeth J, Macfarlane GJ, Benjamin S, Silman AJ. Features of somatization predict the onset of chronic widespread pain: results of a large population-based study. Arthritis Rheum 2001;44:940–946.

McCreary CP, Clark GT, Oakley ME, Flack V. Predicting response to treatment for temporomandibular disorders. J Craniomandib Disord 1992;6:161–169.

Mense S. Structure-function relationships in identified afferent neurones. Anat Embryol (Berl) 1990;181:1–17.

Mense S. Nociception from skeletal muscle in relation to clinical muscle pain. Pain 1993;54:241–289.

Millan MJ. Descending control of pain. Prog Neurobiol 2002;66:355–474.

Mogil JS. The genetic mediation of individual differences in sensitivity to pain and its inhibition. Proc Natl Acad Sci 1999;96:7744–7751.

Nackley AG, Shabalina SA, Tchivileva IE, Satterfield K, Korchynskyi O, Makarov SS, Maixner W, Diatchenko L. Human catechol-O-methyltransferase haplotypes modulate protein expression by altering mRNA secondary structure. Science 2006;314:1930–1933.

Nackley AG, Tan KS, Fecho K, Flood P, Diatchenko L, Maixner W. Catechol-O-methyltransferase inhibition increases pain sensitivity through activation of both beta2- and beta3-adrenergic receptors. Pain 2007;128:199–208.

Naschitz JE, Rozenbaum M, Rosner I, et al. Cardiovascular response to upright tilt in fibromyalgia differs from that in chronic fatigue syndrome. J Rheumatol 2001;28:1356–1360.

Nielsen CS, Stubhaug A, Price DD, Vassend O, Czajkowski N, Harris JR. Individual differences in pain sensitivity: genetic and environmental contributions. Pain 2008;in press.

Norbury TA, MacGregor AJ, Urwin J, Spector TD, McMahon SB. Heritability of responses to painful stimuli in women: a classical twin study. Brain 2007;130:3041–3049.

Ohrbach R, Dworkin SF. Five-year outcomes in TMD: relationship of changes in pain to changes in physical and psychological variables. Pain 1998;74:315–326.

Olson RE. Myofascial pain-dysfunction syndrome: psychological aspects. In: Sarnat BG, Laskin DM, editors. The temporomandibular joint: a biological basis for clinical practice, Vol. 3. Springfield, IL: Thomas; 1980. p 300–314.

Petzke F, Clauw DJ. Sympathetic nervous system function in fibromyalgia. Curr Rheumatol Rep 2000;2:116–123.

Raj SR, Brouillard D, Simpson CS, Hopman WM, Abdollah H. Dysautonomia among patients with fibromyalgia: a noninvasive assessment. J Rheumatol 2000;27:2660–2665.

Randich A, Maixner W. Interactions between cardiovascular and pain regulatory systems. Neurosci Biobehav Rev 1984;8:343–367.

Raphael KG, Marbach JJ. Widespread pain and the effectiveness of oral splints in myofascial face pain. J Am Dent Assoc 2001;132:305–316.

Sarlani E, Greenspan JD. Evidence for generalized hyperalgesia in temporomandibular disorders patients. Pain 2003;102:221–226.

Schoenen J, Bottin D, Hardy F, Gerard P. Cephalic and extracephalic pressure-pain thresholds in chronic tension-type headache. Pain 1991;47:145–149.

Scholz J, Woolf CJ. Can we conquer pain? Nat Neurosci 2002;1062–1067.

Sigurdsson A, Maixner W. Effects of experimental and clinical noxious counterirritants on pain perception. Pain 1994;57:265–275.

Slade GD, Diatchenko L, Bhalang K, Sigurdsson A, Fillingim RB, Belfer I, Max MB, Goldman D, Maixner W. Influence of psychological factors on risk of temporomandibular disorders. J Dent Res 2007;86:1120–1125.

Smoller JW, Rosenbaum JF, Biederman J, et al. Genetic association analysis of behavioral inhibition using candidate loci from mouse models. Am J Med Genet 2001;105:226–235.

Staud R, Price DD, Vierck CJ, Dloughy BJ, Cannon RC, Robinson ME. Diffuse noxious inhibitory controls (DNIC) do not affect wind-up of fibromyalgia patients. Arthritis Rheum 2001;44:S69.

Staud R, Robinson ME, Vierck CJ Jr, Price DD. Diffuse noxious inhibitory controls (DNIC) attenuate temporal summation of second pain in normal males but not in normal females or fibromyalgia patients. Pain 2003;101:167–174.

Steriade M. New vistas on the morphology, chemical transmitters and physiological actions of the ascending brainstem reticular system. Arch Ital Biol 1988;126:225–238.

Steriade M, Llinas RR. The functional states of the thalamus and the associated neuronal interplay. Physiol Rev 1988;68:649–742.

Svensson P, List T, Hector G. Analysis of stimulus-evoked pain in patients with myofascial temporomandibular pain disorders. Pain 2001;92:399–409.

Turner JA, Dworkin SF, Mancl L, Huggins KH, Truelove EL. The roles of beliefs, catastrophizing, and coping in the functioning of patients with temporomandibular disorders. Pain 2001;92:41–51.

Vassend O, Krogstad BS, Dahl BL. Negative affectivity, somatic complaints, and symptoms of temporomandibular disorders. J Psychosom Res 1995;39:889–899.

Verne GN, Price DD. Irritable bowel syndrome as a common precipitant of central sensitization. Curr Rheumatol Rep 2002;4:322–328.

Watkins LR, Maier SF. Beyond neurons: evidence that immune and glial cells contribute to pathological pain states. Physiol Rev 2002;82:981–1011.

Watkins LR, Milligan ED, Maier SF. Glial proinflammatory cytokines mediate exaggerated pain states: implications for clinical pain. Adv Exp Med Biol 2003;521:1–21.

Whitsel BL, Favorov OV, Kelly DG, Tommerdahl M. Mechanisms of dynamic peri- and intra-columnar interactions in somatosensory cortex: Stimulus-specific contrast enhancement by NMDA receptor activation. In: Franzen O, Westman J, editors. Information processing in the somatosensory system. London: Macmillan Press; 1990.

Willer JC, Bouhassira D, Le Bars D. Neurophysiological bases of the counterirritation phenomenon: diffuse control inhibitors induced by nociceptive stimulation. Neurophysiol Clin 1999;29:379–400.

Wilson L, Dworkin SF, Whitney C, LeResche L. Somatization and pain dispersion in chronic temporomandibular disorder pain. Pain 1994;57:55–61.

Wust S, Van Rossum EF, Federenko IS, Koper JW, Kumsta R, Hellhammer DH. Common polymorphisms in the glucocorticoid receptor gene are associated with adrenocortical responses to psychosocial stress. J Clin Endocrinol Metab 2004;89:565–573.

Yu X, Hua M, Mense S. The effects of intracerebroventricular injection of naloxone, phentolamine, methysergide on the transmission of nociceptive signals in the rat dorsal horn neurones with convergent cutaneous-deep input. Neuroscience 1991;715–723.

Yu YW, Chen TJ, Hong CJ, Chen HM, Tsai SJ. Association study of the interleukin-1 beta (C-511T) genetic polymorphism with major depressive disorder, associated symptomatology, and antidepressant response. Neuropsychopharmacology 2003;28:1182–1185.

Zanchetti A, Wang SC, Moruzzi G. The effect of vagal afferent stimulation on the EEG pattern of the cat. Electroencephalogr Clin Neurophysiol 1952;4:357–361.

Zubenko GS, Maher B, Hughes HB III, Zubenko WN, Stiffler JS, Kaplan BB, Marazita ML. Genome-wide linkage survey for genetic loci that influence the development of depressive disorders in families with recurrent, early-onset, major depression. Am J Med Genet 2003;123B:1–18.

Zubieta JK, Heitzeg MM, Smith YR, Bueller JA, Xu K, Xu Y, Koeppe RA, Stohler CS, Goldman D. COMT *val158met* genotype affects mu-opioid neurotransmitter responses to a pain stressor. Science 2003;299:1240–1243.

Correspondence to: William Maixner, DDS, PhD, Center for Neurosensory Disorders, Room 2111, Old Dental Building, University of North Carolina, Chapel Hill, NC 27599-7455, USA. Tel: 1-919-966-0684; fax: 1-919-966-3683; email: bill_maixner@dentistry.unc.edu.

18

Genetic Aspects of Clinical Conditions of Deep Tissue Pain

Laurence A. Bradley

Division of Clinical Immunology and Rheumatology,
University of Alabama at Birmingham

Efforts to identify genetic influences on conditions involving deep tissue pain have greatly increased during the past 10 years. This chapter will focus on genetic and other family influences on the development of fibromyalgia and chronic widespread pain (CWP). It will first review the evidence concerning aggregation of pain sensitivity and psychological distress among first-degree relatives of persons with fibromyalgia and assess the validity of the affective spectrum disorder (ASD) hypothesis (Hudson and Pope, 1989). This hypothesis posits that heritable, etiological factors may be shared by several psychiatric disorders (e.g., major depressive disorder) and medical conditions (e.g., fibromyalgia, irritable bowel syndrome) that not only frequently co-occur in individuals as well as their family members but also tend to respond to the same pharmacological therapies (e.g., serotonin and norepinephrine reuptake inhibitors).

Next, this chapter will examine several prospective, population-based studies of factors that may contribute to the onset of CWP. It will conclude by reviewing current evidence concerning the relationships between specific candidate genes (i.e., the serotonin transporter gene, the dopamine D4 receptor gene, and COMT) and the onset of fibromyalgia or other affective spectrum disorders, as well as pain sensitivity among persons with these conditions.

This chapter uses the American College of Rheumatology (ACR) criteria (Wolfe et al., 1990) for classifying persons with CWP or fibromyalgia. Specifically, pain is considered chronic and widespread when (a) pain is present for at least 3 months; (b) pain is present in both the left and right sides of the body as well as above and below the waist; and (c) axial skeletal pain (in the cervical spine or anterior chest or thoracic spine or low back) is also present. The criteria for fibromyalgia include (a) the presence of chronic widespread pain and (b) pain reported in response to digital palpation of approximately 4 kg in at least 11 of 18 specific anatomic sites referred to as "tender points. These sites include: (a) *occiput:* bilateral, at the suboccipital muscle insertions; (b) *low cervical:* bilateral, at the anterior aspects of the intertransverse spaces at C5–C7; (c) *trapezius:* bilateral, at the midpoint of the upper border; (d) *supraspinatus:* bilateral, at origins, above the scapula spine near the medial border; (e) *second rib:* bilateral, at the second costochondral junctions, just lateral to the junctions on upper surfaces; (f) *lateral epicondyle:* bilateral, 2 cm distal to the epicondyles; (g) *gluteal:* bilateral, in the upper outer quadrants of the buttocks in the anterior fold of muscle; (h) *greater trochanter:* bilateral, posterior to the trochanteric prominence; (i) *knee:* bilateral, at the medial fat pad proximal to the joint line.

Family Aggregation Studies

Pellegrino and colleagues (1989) performed the first study of familial aggregation of symptoms associated with fibromyalgia. They reported that 52% of the first-degree relatives (i.e., parents and siblings) of 17 patients with fibromyalgia had findings consistent with the disorder. However, these findings were identified more frequently among the female relatives (71%), compared to the male family members (35%). Using the ACR classification criteria (Wolfe et al., 1990), Buskila and associates reported similar evidence of family aggregation of fibromyalgia (Buskila et al., 1996; Buskila and Neumann, 1997). Consistent with Pellegrino et al.'s initial report, these investigators found higher rates of fibromyalgia (26–28%) among the first-degree relatives of two groups of women with fibromyalgia compared to those of healthy comparison persons. Buskila and Neumann also reported that fibromyalgia occurred more frequently among the patients' female first-degree relatives (41%) compared to their male relatives (14%). The patients' male and female relatives, compared to those of the comparison group, displayed a significantly greater number of tender points (Buskila and Neumann, 1997).

The early studies described above were limited by relatively small samples of participants and reliance primarily upon tender point counts as measures of pain sensitivity. Tender point counts are more highly associated with individuals' reports of psychological distress than are measures of tenderness that randomly present stimuli in an unpredictable fashion (Petzke et al., 2003). Nevertheless, these investigations do suggest that the presence of persistent widespread pain among adult women who seek health care for symptoms of fibromyalgia is a risk factor for persistent widespread pain among their first-degree relatives. Indeed, Buskila and colleagues proposed that their findings indicate an autosomal dominant genetic transmission of fibromyalgia and that the underlying genetic factor may be sex-related, such that men show lower penetrance or milder expressivity (Buskila and Neumann, 1997).

Several recent investigations, using a variety of experimental designs and sampling procedures, have produced results that generally are consistent with the above interpretation. These investigations used methods similar to those of Buskila and colleagues to assess family aggregation of mood disorders or pain sensitivity in first-degree relatives of women with fibromyalgia. We will review these investigations and then examine several population-based studies and one twin registry study that provide additional support for the findings of the family studies.

Two recent family studies tested hypotheses derived from the ASD hypothesis first advanced by Hudson and Pope (1989). First, Arnold and colleagues (Arnold et al., 2004; Hudson et al., 2004) examined family aggregation of affective disorders as well as tender point counts in the first-degree relatives of 78 women with fibromyalgia, or probands, and those of 40 individuals (34 women, 6 men) with rheumatoid arthritis (RA). The term "proband" is defined as the individual through whom a family's medical history is assessed. Rheumatoid arthritis was chosen as the comparison condition because persons with RA, similar to those with fibromyalgia, experience persistent pain and higher frequencies of mood disorder compared to individuals in the general population. However, there is no evidence that mood disorders co-aggregate with RA in families (Arnold et al., 2004). Fibromyalgia was evaluated in probands by physical examination and among first-degree relatives either by direct interview or by interviews with family informants (e.g., Maxwell, 1992) and medical record review. The Structured Clinical Interview for DSM-IV (SCID; First et al., 1995) was used to diagnose psychiatric disorders among probands and family members. Tender point exams were performed on 146 first-degree relatives of the fibromyalgia probands (27%) and 72 of the relatives of those with RA (26%).

Table I shows that the relatives of the fibromyalgia probands were more likely to receive a diagnosis of fibromyalgia than were relatives of persons with RA. The estimated odds of having fibromyalgia were 8.5 times as great for relatives of a proband with fibromyalgia as they were for relatives of an individual with RA. A diagnosis of fibromyalgia was made for only 3 of 279 male relatives of the probands with fibromyalgia; thus, evidence of familial aggregation of fibromyalgia came almost entirely from female relatives.

Table I
Prevalence of fibromyalgia, lifetime diagnoses of major mood disorders, and mean tender point counts in first-degree relatives of 78 probands with fibromyalgia (FM) and 40 probands with rheumatoid arthritis (RA)

Lifetime Disorders	Relatives of FM Probands (N = 533; 254 F, 279 M)	Relatives of RA Probands (N = 272; 141 F, 131 M)
Diagnosis of FM	N = 34 (6%)	N = 3 (1%)
Major mood disorders (major depressive or bipolar disorder)	N = 171 (32%)	N = 52 (19%)
Mean tender point count	17	12

Source: These data were reported in Tables 4 and 6 of Arnold et al. (2004); reprinted with permission of Wiley-Liss, Inc.

Lifetime diagnoses of major mood disorder were made more frequently among the first-degree relatives of the fibromyalgia probands compared to those of individuals with RA. However, the difference in the frequency of major mood disorders among the two sets of relatives did not achieve significance when only relatives who were directly interviewed with the SCID were included in the analyses (46% among 146 fibromyalgia relatives, 29% among 72 RA relatives). The failure to find evidence of family aggregation of major mood disorder among the fibromyalgia proband relatives who were available for interview was probably caused by the smaller sample size (i.e., reduced power). Nevertheless, similar to findings reported by Buskila and Neumann (1997), Table I reveals that the 146 relatives of the fibromyalgia probands, compared to the 72 relatives of those with RA, displayed a significantly greater number of tender points. In accord with Buskila and Neumann's earlier report, the difference in tender point counts between the relatives of the fibromyalgia probands and those with RA was greatest among the women.

The evidence regarding the aggregation of fibromyalgia within families was independent of the co-aggregation of fibromyalgia with major mood disorder, the aggregation of major mood disorder, and the within-person co-occurrence of fibromyalgia and major mood disorder. However, tender point counts are limited as measures of pain sensitivity because they are associated with psychological distress levels (Petzke et al., 2003). Thus, one may question whether the greater number of tender points found among the relatives of the fibromyalgia probands, compared to those with RA, may be due largely to higher levels of psychological distress among the fibromyalgia family members rather than to enhanced pain sensitivity.

With respect to the issue of pain sensitivity in family members of probands with fibromyalgia, we recently reported preliminary data from a study of the brothers and sisters of 20 probands with fibromyalgia and those of 35 healthy controls who did not differ from one another on standardized measures of psychological distress (e.g., depressive symptoms, trait anxiety) (Bradley et al., 2006). We found that the siblings of the fibromyalgia probands, compared to those of the healthy controls, exhibited significantly lower pain thresholds in response to mechanical pressure and thermal or ischemic stimulation (see Fig. 1). We agree that tender point counts are not adequate measures of pain sensitivity. However, our findings, produced with appropriate quantitative sensory testing procedures using three stimulus modalities, do provide evidence of familial aggregation of enhanced pain sensitivity in fibromyalgia that cannot be attributed to elevated symptoms of depression or anxiety.

Two issues are important concerning enhanced pain sensitivity among first-degree relatives of women with fibromyalgia. First, there were twice as many sisters as brothers among the siblings of both the fibromyalgia probands and the healthy controls in our investigation. Therefore, we were unable to determine whether the enhanced levels of pain sensitivity among the fibromyalgia siblings were due primarily to the responses of the probands' sisters. Moreover, Gupta and colleagues (2007a) recently performed a prospective, population-based study that showed that mechanical pressure pain threshold levels do not contribute to the prediction of new cases of CWP. It remains to be determined whether enhanced pain sensitivity to tonic pain stimuli (e.g., those produced by ischemic pressure or the cold pressor task) that more closely

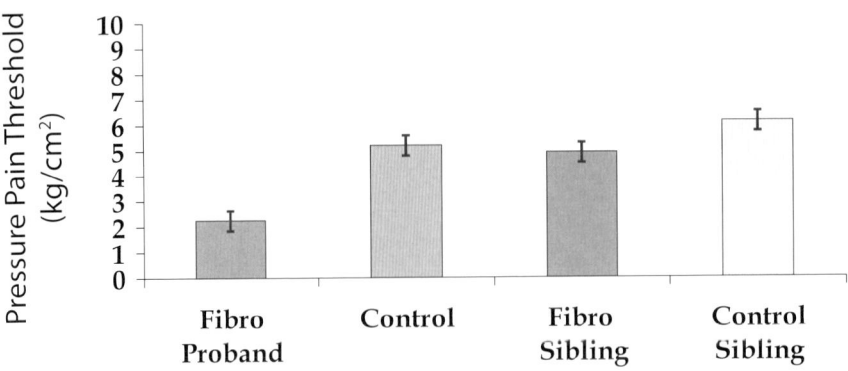

Fig. 1. Mean (± SEM) pressure pain threshold levels at 10 of 18 tender points. Fibro Probands = fibromyalgia probands (*N* = 20); Control = healthy controls (*N* = 35); Fibro Sibling = siblings of probands (*N* = 20); Control Sibling = siblings of healthy controls (*N* = 35).

resemble painful clinical symptoms may help predict the onset of CWP, fibromyalgia, or other affective spectrum disorders.

The studies reviewed above used similar experimental designs to provide support for the ASD hypothesis. Using a unique experimental design, Raphael and colleagues (2004) also found evidence of family aggregation of major depressive disorder among the first-degree relatives of female probands with fibromyalgia. These investigators examined four groups of participants. Two groups consisted of women who met criteria for fibromyalgia and were either positive or negative for major depressive disorder. The remaining two groups included women who did not meet criteria for fibromyalgia and were either positive or negative for major depressive disorder. It was hypothesized that if fibromyalgia represents an affective spectrum disorder, similar high rates of major depressive disorder would be found in the first-degree relatives of both groups of fibromyalgia probands and in those of the control subjects with histories of major depressive disorder. Indeed, the study found that the frequencies of depressive disorder in these three groups of family members were very similar (i.e., 37% to 46%); these frequencies were significantly higher than those observed in the relatives of control subjects who did not meet criteria for fibromyalgia and major depressive disorder (29%). Moreover, this pattern was particularly strong among the female first-degree relatives, indicating a sex-linked effect.

To summarize, the results of the family studies performed by Arnold, Raphael, and their colleagues provide support for the hypothesis that fibromyalgia and major mood disorders share heritable etiological factors. The relationships among these disorders appear to be sex-linked, given the especially strong findings observed among female first-degree relatives. Raphael and colleagues (2004) have suggested that individuals with fibromyalgia and major depressive disorder may have a genetic or biologically mediated vulnerability to respond to stressful or traumatic events with psychological and pain-related symptoms. This hypothesis is supported by recent findings produced by population-based studies in the United Kingdom, described below, regarding predictors of the development of CWP.

Population-Based Studies

McBeth and colleagues (2001) performed a population-based, prospective study of 825 adults who were pain-free and 833 who reported pain that did not meet criteria for CWP (Wolfe et al., 1990). At the 1-year follow-up, 2% of the individuals who initially were pain free and 8% of the individuals with pain at baseline met criteria for CWP. There were higher proportions of individuals with CWP among women and among older study participants (aged 50–64 years). However, after adjusting for age and sex, the investigators found that the most important predictors of new cases of CWP were scores in the top third of the Illness Behavior Scale, derived from the Illness Attitude Scales (Kellner et al., 1987), and reports of three or more symptoms on the Somatic Symptom Checklist (Othmer and DeSouza, 1985). These investigators reported similar findings regarding the power of a measure of sleep disturbance, in addition to the Illness Behavior Scale and the Illness Attitude Scales, in predicting the onset of CWP in a population-based, prospective study of 3,171 adults without CWP (Gupta et al., 2007b).

Although these results were intriguing, the investigators wished to determine whether examining a larger population-based sample (N = 7,784) and using psychophysiological as well as self-report measures would enhance the identification of risk factors for the development of CWP. McBeth and colleagues (2007) performed a 15-month, prospective study in which they examined baseline measures of psychological distress, sleep disturbance, and hypothalamic-pituitary-adrenal (HPA) axis function of 241 individuals, drawn from a subgroup of 768 individuals, who were classified as at "high risk" for development of CWP using the criteria established in their 2001 investigation (i.e., responses to the Somatic Symptom Checklist and the Illness Behavior subscale of the Illness Attitude Scale). Consistent with their high risk status, 28 (11.6%) of these 241 individuals did meet criteria for CWP at the end of the 15-month follow-up. After the investigators adjusted for age, sex, depressive symptoms, sleep disturbance, exposure to recent traumatic life events, and regional pain at baseline, they found that three measures of HPA axis function at baseline served as independent predictors of development of CWP among the 241 high-risk individuals. These measures were (1) low morning levels of salivary cortisol; (2) high evening levels of salivary cortisol; and (3) high plasma levels of cortisol in response to a low-dose dexamethasone suppression test. Compared to high-risk individuals who had none of the HPA axis factors described above, those who had two of these factors were twice as likely to develop CWP. Moreover, those who had three of the HPA axis factors were nearly nine times as likely to develop CWP. Overall, one or more of these three factors identified 26 of 28 cases of new-onset CWP.

To summarize, within this sample of relatively distressed, high-risk persons, HPA axis dysfunction conferred increased vulnerability to the development of CWP. It may be, then, that in accord with Raphael et al. (2004), HPA axis dysfunction may increase the vulnerability of distressed persons to develop pain-related symptoms. It remains to be determined whether HPA axis dysfunction also moderates the relationship between psychological distress and future development of mood disorders or painful symptoms associated with other affective spectrum disorders (e.g., Aaron et al., 2000; Aggarwal et al., 2006).

Genetic Influence on Chronic Widespread Pain and Fibromyalgia

The evidence reviewed above generally supports one of the main tenets of the ASD hypothesis—that heritable, etiological factors may be shared by several psychiatric and medical conditions that frequently co-occur within individuals as well as their family members. Until recently, however, there was little direct evidence of genetic influences on CWP or other conditions that may represent affective spectrum disorders. Kato and colleagues (2006) attempted to address this gap in the literature by conducting telephone interviews with 15,950 eligible twin pairs participating in the Swedish Twin Registry to ask about symptoms associated with CWP as defined by the ACR criteria (Wolfe et al., 1990). The prevalence of CWP was 4.1% among the respondents and was greater among women (6.1%) than among men (1.8%). Moreover, unspecified genetic and shared environmental factors accounted for 48–54% of the variance in CWP, and there were no significant sex differences in the importance or type of genetic influences.

Interest in genetic association studies involving CWP or fibromyalgia has increased since 1999. Limer and colleagues (2008) recently reviewed this literature and concluded that several candidate genes warrant further study, although at present, no definitive susceptibility genes have been identified. For example, there is reliable evidence that single nucleotide polymorphisms (SNPs) in the serotonin transporter (5-HTT) gene and the dopamine D4 receptor (DRD4) gene are associated with fibromyalgia (Offenbaecher et al., 1999; Cohen et al., 2002; Buskila et al., 2004). There also is substantial evidence that catechol-O-methyltransferase (COMT) gene variants are associated with the onset of temporomandibular disorder (TMD) in young women (e.g., Diatchenko et al., 2005). Given that TMD and fibromyalgia often coexist, COMT also may contribute to the onset of fibromyalgia.

Consistent findings show that patients with fibromyalgia, compared to healthy controls, are characterized by low blood serum levels of serotonin (Russell et al., 1992; Wolfe et al., 1997) and low cerebrospinal fluid (CSF) levels of the serotonin metabolite, 5-hydroxyindole acetic acid (5-HIAA) (Vaerøy et al., 1988). In addition, preliminary findings in our laboratory suggest that siblings of women with fibromyalgia, compared to siblings of healthy control women, exhibit lower serum levels of serotonin (Bradley et al., 2006).

Given these findings, several investigators have assessed the extent to which specific SNPs in the serotonin transporter gene may be associated with fibromyalgia. Offenbaecher and colleagues (1999) in Germany, as well as Cohen, Buskila, and colleagues (2002) in Israel, have reported that female patients with fibromyalgia are significantly more likely than controls to exhibit the S/S allele of the 5-HTT gene that is also associated with affective disorders, anxiety-related traits, and migraine headaches. In contrast, Gürsoy and colleagues (2002) reported that the S/S allele does not occur more frequently in patients with fibromyalgia compared to healthy controls when only fibromyalgia patients without elevated levels of psychological distress are examined. Gürsoy and colleagues, however, used substantially smaller patient and control samples than those used by previous investigators (Offenbaecher et al., 1999; Cohen et al., 2002). Therefore, the negative findings reported by Gürsoy et al. do not necessarily diminish the validity of the relationships that have been reported between fibromyalgia and the 5-HTT gene polymorphism in relatively large patient samples. Nevertheless, it remains to be determined whether large prospective studies will provide evidence that the 5-HTT gene polymorphism contributes significantly to prediction of the onset of fibromyalgia independently of the confounding effects of psychological distress.

Investigators also have begun to examine relationships between the dopamine D4 receptor (DRD4) gene and fibromyalgia. Buskila and colleagues (2004) demonstrated an association between fibromyalgia and the DRD4 exon III 7-repeat genotype and fibromyalgia using the same sample employed by Cohen et al. (2002) in their study of the 5-HTT gene polymorphism. Specifically, relative to healthy controls, the frequency of the 7-repeat genotype was significantly lower in persons with fibromyalgia. This finding is particularly intriguing given the results of a recent study indicating that women with fibromyalgia, compared to sex-matched, healthy controls, show significant reductions in presynaptic dopamine metabolism in several brain regions in which dopamine normally contributes to pain inhibition, such as the medial thalamus and the anterior cingulate cortex (Wood et al., 2007a). In addition, unlike healthy controls, patients with fibromyalgia fail to show significant release of dopamine in the basal ganglia following injection of hypertonic saline in the anterior tibialis muscle; these patients also report higher levels of pain intensity than healthy control persons following saline injection (Wood et al., 2007b).

There also is preliminary evidence that clinical symptoms that may be produced in part by altered dopamine metabolism may be reduced by pharmacological therapy. A 14-week randomized, controlled trial revealed that 4.5 mg of oral pramipexole, a dopamine agonist, compared to placebo, produced greater improvements in clinical pain, fatigue, function, and global status ratings among patients with fibromyalgia (Holman and Myers, 2005). Indeed, 42% of patients who received pramipexole, compared to 14% of those assigned to the placebo condition, achieved a decrease in pain of at least 50% at the end of the trial.

As noted recently by Buskila (2007), the evidence reviewed above suggests that altered function of both serotonergic and dopaminergic neurotransmitter pathways is involved in the development or maintenance of fibromyalgia. Thus, future studies may provide evidence that fibromyalgia patients characterized by the S/S or L/S allele of the 5-HTT gene are more likely to respond to pharmacological therapies that reduce reuptake of serotonin and norepinephrine than patients with the DRD4 exon III 7-repeat genotype. Conversely, patients in the latter group may be more likely to respond positively to pramipexole or other dopamine agonists than those with 5-HTT gene variants.

Finally, studies performed by Zubieta and colleagues at the University of Michigan and by Diatchenko and colleagues at the University of North Carolina have produced great interest in the relationship between *COMT* gene variants and reports of pain in both healthy individuals and persons with affective spectrum disorders. COMT is an enzyme that metabolizes catecholamines and has been implicated in the pathogenesis of migraine, neurodegenerative diseases, anxiety disorders, and a variety of cardiovascular diseases. However, COMT also is involved in regulating pain perception. For example, Zubieta and colleagues (2003) studied the pain and affective responses to a tonic pain challenge among healthy men and women as a function of *COMT* gene variants. They found that participants who were homozygous for the *met158* allele of the *COMT* polymorphism (*val158met*) showed diminished regional μ-opioid system responses to a tonic pain challenge compared with heterozygotes. The diminished μ-opioid system responses were associated with higher sensory and affective ratings of pain and self-reports of a more negative internal affective state.

Diatchenko and colleagues (2005, 2006) subsequently examined the relationship of several haplotypes of the *val158met* polymorphism with enhanced pain sensitivity and the onset of TMD in healthy young women. TMD is an orofacial pain syndrome that shows a high level of overlap with fibromyalgia and is associated with abnormal pain sensitivity similar to that observed in patients with fibromyalgia (Aaron et al., 2000). The haplotypes were associated with low (LPS), average (APS), or high (HPS) pain sensitivity in response to thermal, ischemic, and pressure stimuli (Diatchenko et al., 2006). Women who carry APS/APS or HPS/APS diplotypes were significantly more likely to develop TMD over a 3-year period than those who had at least one LPS haplotype (Diatchenko et al., 2005). Consistent with McBeth et al.'s reports (2001, 2007) regarding the onset of CWP, the predictive power of the *COMT* haplotypes increased significantly when combined with high baseline levels of somatization.

There is no published evidence that *COMT* variants contribute to the prediction of onset of fibromyalgia or CWP. However, Gürsoy and colleagues (2003) demonstrated that gene variants associated with relatively low levels of COMT activity are found significantly more frequently among patients with fibromyalgia compared to healthy controls. Among patients with fibromyalgia in Spain, persons with the *Met-158-Met* genotype associated with enhanced pain sensitivity, compared to those with the relatively pain-resistant *Val-158-Val* genotype, report more severe symptoms (Garcia-Fructuoso et al., 2006). Similarly, the *COMT* haplotype that is linked to relatively high pain sensitivity among healthy individuals (Diatchenko et al., 2006) was associated with reports of higher pain, fatigue, sleep disturbance, and morning stiffness among Spanish patients with fibromyalgia (Vargas-Alarcón et al., 2007). This finding, however, was not replicated among patients in Mexico.

It recently was reported that enhanced mechanical and thermal pain sensitivity associated with depressed COMT activity in Sprague-Dawley rats was completely blocked by the nonselective β-adrenergic antagonist propranolol or by the combined administration of selective β_2- and β_3-adrenergic antagonists (Nackley et al., 2007). These findings suggest that low COMT activity leads to increased pain sensitivity via a $\beta_{2/3}$-adrenergic mechanism and that chronic pain conditions associated with low COMT activity and/or elevated catecholamine levels may be treated successfully with pharmacological agents that block both β_2- and β_3-adrenergic receptors. Therefore, we anticipate that data will soon be produced regarding relationships between COMT variants and (a) the onset of CWP or fibromyalgia and (b) pain sensitivity levels among persons with these disorders.

Conclusions

Evidence produced by family studies and prospective investigations suggest that heritable etiological factors are shared by medical and psychiatric disorders that tend to co-occur within individuals and their family members. Data also support Raphael et al's (2004) suggestion that individuals with fibromyalgia and major depressive disorder may share a genetic or biologically mediated vulnerability to respond to stressful events with psychological and pain-related symptoms. One factor that may mediate this vulnerability is HPA axis dysfunction.

It still is not certain to what extent genetic factors may independently contribute to the onset of CWP and fibromyalgia, to variations in pain sensitivity, or to vulnerability to stressful events among persons with these conditions. To date, 5-HTT and DRD4 gene variants have not been studied as extensively as the COMT gene variants and haplotypes. The literature suggests, then, that it may eventually be possible to identify subgroups of persons with CWP or fibromyalgia and specific physiological abnormalities (e.g., altered function of serotonergic or dopaminergic neurotransmitter pathways) that are involved in the development or maintenance of painful symptoms. In addition, given the relatively consistent and strong relationships between COMT variants and pain sensitivity as well as the onset of TMD, it is highly likely that future investigations will reveal that variations in COMT activity are significantly associated with the onset of one or more affective spectrum disorders in addition to TMD and with alterations in painful symptoms.

Acknowledgments

This work is supported by the National Institute of Arthritis, Musculoskeletal and Skin Diseases (1 R01 AR43136, P60 AR48095), the American Fibromyalgia Syndrome Association, and by grant 5M0100032 from the National Center for Research Resources.

References

Aaron LA, Burke MM, Buchwald D. Overlapping conditions among patients with chronic fatigue syndrome, fibromyalgia, and temporomandibular disorder. Arch Intern Med 2000;160:221–227.

Aggarwal VR, McBeth J, Zakrzewska JM, Lunt M, Macfarlane GJ. The epidemiology of chronic syndromes that are frequently unexplained: do they have common associated factors? Int J Epidemiol 2006;35:468–476.

Arnold LM, Hudson JI, Hess EV, Ware AE, Fritz DA, Auchenbach MB, Starck LO, Keck PE. Family study of fibromyalgia. Arthritis Rheum 2004;50:944–952.

Bradley L, Fillingim R, Sotolongo A, Cannon R, McKendree-Smith N, Okonkwo R, McConley R, Weigent D, Alarcón G. Family aggregation of pain sensitivity in fibromyalgia (FM). J Pain 2006;7(Suppl 1):S1.

Buskila D. Genetics of chronic pain states. Best Pract Res Clin Rheumatol 2007;21:535–547.

Buskila D, Cohen H, Neumann L, Ebstein RP. An association between fibromyalgia and the dopamine D4 receptor exon III repeat polymorphism and relationship to novelty seeking personality traits. Mol Psychiatry 2004;9:730–731.

Buskila D, Neumann L. Fibromyalgia syndrome (FM) and nonarticular tenderness in relatives of patients with FM. J Rheumatol 1997;24:941–944.

Buskila D, Neumann L, Hozanov I, Carmi R. Familial aggregation in the fibromyalgia syndrome. Semin Arthritis Rheum 1996;26:605–611.

Cohen H, Buskila D, Neumann L, Ebstein RP. Confirmation of an association between fibromyalgia and serotonin transporter promoter region (5- HTTLPR) polymorphism, and relationship to anxiety-related personality traits. Arthritis Rheum 2002;46:845–847.

Diatchenko L, Nackley A, Slade GD, Bhalang K, Belfer I, Max MB, Goldman D, Maixner W. Catechol-O-methyltransferase gene polymorphisms are associated with multiple pain-evoking stimuli. Pain 2006;125:216–224.

Diatchenko L, Slade GD, Nackley AG, et al. Genetic basis for individual variations in pain perception and the development of a chronic pain condition. Hum Mol Genet 2005;14:135–143.

First MB, Spitzer RL, Gibbon M, Williams JBW. Structured clinical interview for DSM-IV seeking personality traits. Axis I disorders-patient edition (SCID-I/P), version 2.0. New York: Biometrics Research Department, New York State Psychiatric Institute, 1995.

García-Fructuoso FJ, Lao-Villadóniga JI, Beyer K, Santos C. Relationship between catechol-O-methyltransferase genotypes and fibromyalgia's severity. Reumatol Clin 2006;2:168-172.

Gupta A, McBeth J, Macfarlane GJ, Morriss R, Dickens C, Ray D, Chiu YH, Silman AJ. Pressure pain thresholds and tender point counts as predictors of new chronic widespread pain in somatising subjects. Ann Rheum Dis 2007;66:517–521.

Gupta A, Silman AJ, Ray D, Morriss R, Dickens C, MacFarlane DJ, Chiu YH, Nichol B, McBeth J. The role of psychosocial factors in predicting the onset of chronic widespread pain: results from a prospective population-based study. Rheumatology 2007b;46:666–671.

Gürsoy S. Absence of association of the serotonin transporter gene polymorphism with the mentally healthy subset of fibromyalgia patients. Clin Rheumatol 2002;21:194–197.

Gürsoy S, Erdal E, Herken H, Madensi E, Alesehirli B, Erdal N. Significance of catechol-O-methyltransferase gene polymorphism in fibromyalgia syndrome. Rheum Int 2003;23:104–107.

Holman AJ, Myers RR. A randomized, double-blind, placebo-controlled trial of pramipexole, a dopamine agonist, in patients with fibromyalgia receiving concomitant medications. Arthritis Rheum 2005;52:2495–2505.

Hudson JI, Arnold LM, Keck PE, Auchenbach MB, Pope HG Jr. Family study of fibromyalgia and affective spectrum disorder. Biol Psychiatry 2004;56:884–891.

Hudson JI, Pope HG Jr. Fibromyalgia and psychopathology: is fibromyalgia a form of "affective spectrum disorder"? J Rheumatol 1989;16(Suppl 19):15–22.

Kato K, Sullivan PF, Evengård B, Pedersen NL. Importance of genetic influences on chronic widespread pain. Arthritis Rheum 2006;54:1682–1686.

Kellner R, Abbott P, Winslow WW, Pathak D. Fears, beliefs, and attitudes in DSM-III hypochondriasis. J Nerv Ment Dis 1987;175:20–25.

Limer KL, Nicholl BI, Thomson W, McBeth J. Exploring the genetic susceptibility of chronic wide-spread pain: the tender points in genetic association studies. Rheumatology 2008; 47:572–577.

Maxwell ME. Family Interview for Genetic Studies (FIGS). Washington, DC: National Institute of Mental Health; 1992.

McBeth J, Macfarlane GJ, Benjamin S, Silman AJ. Features of somatization predict the on-set of chronic widespread pain: results of a large population-based study. Arthritis Rheum 2001;44:940–946.

McBeth J, Silman AJ, Gupta A, Chiu YH, Ray D, Morriss R, Dickens C, King Y, Macfarlane GJ. Moderation of psychosocial risk factors through dysfunction of the hypothalamic-pituitary-ad-renal stress axis in the onset of chronic widespread musculoskeletal pain: findings of a popula-tion-based prospective cohort study. Arthritis Rheum 2007;56:360–371.

Nackley AG, Tan KS, Fecho K, Flood P, Diatchenko L, Maixner W. Catechol-O-methyltransferase inhibition increases pain sensitivity through activation of both beta2- and beta3-adrenergic re-ceptors. Pain 2007;128:199–208.

Offenbaecher M, Bondy B, de Jonge S, Glatzeder K, Kruger M, Schoeps P, Ackenheil M. Possible association of fibromyalgia with a polymorphism in the serotonin transporter gene regulatory region. Arthritis Rheum 1999;42:2482–2488.

Othmer E, DeSouza C. A screening test for somatization disorder (hysteria). Am J Psychiatry 1985;142:1146–1149.

Pellegrino MJ, Waylonis GW, Sommer A. Familial occurrence of primary fibromyalgia. Arch Physi-cal Med Rehabil 1989;70:61–63.

Petzke F, Gracely RH, Park KM, Ambrose K, Clauw DJ. What do tender points measure? Influence of distress on 4 measures of tenderness. J Rheumatol 2003;30:567–574.

Raphael KG, Janal MN, Nayak S, Schwartz JE, Gallagher RM. Familial aggregation of depression in fibromyalgia: a community-based test of alternate hypotheses. Pain 2004;110:449–460.

Russell IJ, Michalek JE, Vipario GA, Fletcher EM, Javors MA, Bowden CA. Platelet 3H-imipramine uptake receptor density and serum serotonin levels in patients with fibromyalgia/fibrositis syn-drome. J Rheumatol 1992;19:104–109.

Vaerøy H, Helle R, Forre Ø, Kaåss E, Terenius L. Cerebrospinal fluid levels of beta-endorphin in pa-tients with fibromyalgia (fibrositis syndrome). J Rheumatol 1988;15:1804–1806.

Vargas-Alarcón G, Fragoso JM, Cruz-Robles D, et al. Catechol-O-methyltransferase gene haplotypes in Mexican and Spanish patients with fibromyalgia. Arthritis Res Ther 2007;9:R110.

Wolfe F, Russell IJ, Vipraio G, Ross K, Anderson J. Serotonin levels, pain threshold, and fibromyalgia symptoms in the general population. J Rheumatol 1997;24:555–559.

Wolfe F, Smythe HA, Yunus MB, et al. The American College of Rheumatology 1990 criteria for the classification of fibromyalgia. Report of the multicenter criteria committee. Arthritis Rheum 1990;33:160–172.

Wood PB, Patterson JC II, Sunderland JJ, Tainter KH, Glabus MF, Lilien DL. Reduced presynaptic dopamine activity in fibromyalgia syndrome demonstrated with positron emission tomography: a pilot study. J Pain 2007a;8:51–58.

Wood PB, Schweinhardt P, Jaeger E, Dagher A, Hakyemez H, Rabiner EA, Bushnell MC, Chizh BA. Fibromyalgia patients show an abnormal dopamine response to pain. Eur J Neurosci 2007b;25:3576–3582.

Zubieta JK, Heitzeg MM, Smith YR, Bueller JA, Xu K, Xu Y, Koeppe RA, Stohler CS, Goldman D. COMT val158 met genotype affects mu-opioid neurotransmitter responses to a pain stressor. Science 2003;299:1240–1243.

Correspondence to: Laurence A. Bradley, PhD, Division of Clinical Immunology and Rheumatology, University of Alabama at Birmingham, 178A Shelby Interdis-ciplinary, Research Building, 1825 University Boulevard, Birmingham, AL 35294, USA. Tel: 1-205-934-8550; fax: 1-205-934-1564; email: braddog@uab.edu.

19

Peripheral Opioid Analgesia in Experimental Muscle Pain

Irmgard Tegeder

Pharmazentrum Frankfurt, Institute of Clinical Pharmacology/ZAFES,
Clinic of the Johann Wolfgang Goethe University, Frankfurt am Main, Germany

Nociceptive pain activated by noxious stimulation of a highly specialized, high-threshold sensory apparatus plays an important physiological role in protecting the organism from damage, yet pain may lose this biological function and gain disease status. Central and peripheral opioid receptors constitute a major endogenous pain regulatory system that allows for immediate and long-lasting adaptation to painful conditions that are associated with actual or potential tissue damage. Peripheral opioid effects have been increasingly recognized to play an important role in pathological pain conditions, especially when the cause of pain involves inflammatory processes. This chapter summarizes the available evidence and discusses the potential implications of peripheral opioid analgesia for the treatment of muscle pain.

Molecular Mechanisms of Peripheral Opioid Antinociception

Peripheral Opioid Receptor Upregulation

Opioid receptor density in axons and nerve terminals of peripheral nociceptive neurons is normally low (Coggeshall et al., 1997), and physiological nociceptive pain is not importantly controlled by peripheral opioid
receptors. However, tissue injury or inflammation triggers transcription
of opioid receptors in nociceptive dorsal root ganglion (DRG) neurons
(Ji et al., 1995). Subsequently, an increasing number of opioid receptors
is transported along unmyelinated C fibers and thinly myelinated Aδ fibers to peripheral (Hassan et al., 1993; Ji et al., 1995) and central nerve
terminals (Coggeshall et al., 1997). This upregulation occurs similarly in
inflamed skin, muscle, or visceral tissue and can be evoked by a single
subcutaneous injection of interleukin 1β (Schafer et al., 1994). Opioid
receptor upregulation in inflamed tissue is associated with increased efficiency of G-protein coupling and subsequent inhibition of adenylyl
cyclase and voltage-gated Ca^{2+} channels. The result is a reduction in inflammation-evoked, protein kinase A- and C-mediated sensitization of
transient receptor potential vanilloid 1 (TRPV1) channels, which are upregulated together with opioid receptors in inflammation (Vetter et al.,
2006; Rau et al., 2007). The upregulation and transport are slow processes developing over a few hours (Hassan et al., 1993), and therefore probably not contributing to immediate opioid analgesia, which is likely to be
mediated by a central opioid effect.

Immune-Cell-Derived Endogenous Opioids

Extravasation of immunocytes into injured tissues, involving rolling, adhesion, and transmigration through the vessel wall, is regulated by selectins and other adhesion molecules located on opioid-containing immune
cells and in the vascular endothelium (Machelska et al., 1998). Inflam-
mation-attracted immune cells are the source of endogenous opioid pep-

tides (Machelska et al., 1998), which are secreted in response to cortico-tropin-releasing hormone or cytokines (Mousa et al., 2002). The resulting inhibition of nociceptor excitability and blocking of neuropeptide release reduces pain and accomplishes an important mechanism of endogenous peripheral pain control (Machelska et al., 1998). On the other hand, disrupting the adhesion process prevents transmigration and causes a loss of stress-evoked analgesia.

Animal Models of Peripheral Opioid Antinociception

Effects of Peripheral Opioid Treatment in Inflammatory Hyperalgesia

Agonists at the μ-opioid receptor are generally most potent at producing peripheral analgesia. However, peripherally acting κ- and δ-opioid agonists are also being developed as potential novel analgesics (Eisenach et al., 2003; Vanderah et al., 2004). For example, peripheral antinociception was demonstrated for the μ-opioid receptor agonist HS-731 after subcutaneous and oral administration in rats with carrageenan-induced hindpaw inflammation (Bileviciute-Ljungar et al., 2006). Peripheral antinociception was also demonstrated for a κ-opioid-agonistic peptide FE200041 (D-Phe-D-Phe-D-Nle-D-Arg-NH$_2$) (Vanderah et al., 2004). Muscle pain has not yet been tested with these substances, but mechanistic knowledge suggests that hyperalgesia caused or contributed to by muscle inflammation or traumatic injury may be ameliorated by these opioid receptor ligands.

Several studies have addressed peripheral opioid analgesia using direct injection of opioids into the inflamed tissue at small, systemically inactive doses (Levine and Taiwo, 1989; Stein et al., 1990; Kolesnikov et al., 1996). Naloxone-reversible antinociception occurred preferentially in inflamed tissue (Levine and Taiwo, 1989; Stein et al., 1990; Kolesnikov et al., 1996), demonstrating that the opioid receptor upregulation and axonal transport observed during inflammation determine the efficacy of peripheral opioid analgesia. Interestingly, intra-articular injection of the selective μ-opioid agonist endomorphin-1 reduced pain in a model of acute arthritis but lost its antinociceptive efficacy in a chronic model (Li et al., 2005). This finding was associated with a reduction of μ-opioid receptor expression in DRG cells ipsilateral to the chronically inflamed joint (Li et al., 2005), suggesting that a failure to maintain the adaptation of the peripheral opioid system may contribute to the development of chronic pain. The efficacy of peripheral opioids in muscle pain models is largely unknown. In a single study, injection of the μ-opioid-receptor-selective agonist DAMGO into the inflamed masseter muscle produced antinociceptive effects in rats (Nunez et al., 2007).

Loperamide is an available opioid that because of its P-glyco-protein outward transport across the blood-brain barrier does not reach effective concentrations in the brain and is therefore considered to be a peripherally acting opioid. Topical application of loperamide produced peripheral analgesia in rats after thermal injury (Nozaki-Taguchi and Yaksh, 1999). Antinociceptive effects of loperamide after subcutaneous or intraperitoneal injections have been demonstrated in inflammatory, neuropathic, and bone cancer pain models in rats and in a capsaicin-evoked thermal hyperalgesia model in primates (DeHaven-Hudkins et al., 1999; Menendez et al., 2003; Butelman et al., 2004). Its efficacy in muscle pain has not been evaluated.

Peripheral Opioids after Nerve Injury

Muscle pain may arise from peripheral or central nerve damage that causes changes in the peripheral and central opioid systems that are distinct from inflammation-evoked adaptations. Traumatic injury of the sciatic or spinal nerves results in downregulation of opioid receptors in primary afferent neurons with injured axons, whereas uninjured neighboring neurons retain their normal opioid receptor expression (Kohno et al., 2005). The loss of opioid receptors is associated with reduced axonal transport and decrease of opioid receptor density at peripheral and central terminals (Kohno et al., 2005). Patch-clamp recordings in spinal cord slices revealed that the μ-opioid agonist DAMGO elicits a much weaker inhibition of postsynaptic excitatory currents in segments receiving input of damaged afferents than in adjacent segments (Kohno et al., 2005). Consequently, spontaneous pain evoked by ectopic discharge from neuromas or damaged axons is unlikely to be prevented by peripherally acting opioids, whereas hyperalgesia caused by sensitization of uninjured adjacent neurons may be reduced. However, in contrast to inflammatory conditions, opioid receptor expression does not increase above normal levels, even in uninjured neurons. Therefore, nerve-injury-evoked hyperalgesia is less likely to respond to peripheral opioid treatment compared with inflammatory hyperalgesia.

The expression of opioid receptors in primary afferent neurons is stimulated by growth factors that are produced in the peripheral target and are retrogradely transported to the DRG neurons. During inflammation, retrograde axonal transport of nerve growth factor is increased, and disruption of this transport results in a decrease of μ-opioid receptor expression in TrkA-positive primary afferent neurons, suggesting that intact contact to the growth-factor-producing peripheral target is crucial for opioid-mediated pain control (Mousa et al., 2007). Axonal damage will offset this adaptive potential. Nevertheless, a few studies have reported a reduction of hyperalgesia with peripherally acting opioids in neuropathic pain models (Obara et al., 2007; Shinoda et al., 2007). So far, there are no well-established behavioral tests that allow for a quantitative assessment of spontaneous neuropathic pain in rodents.

Tolerance

Repeated administration of peripherally acting opioids or repeated local injection of opioids causes tolerance to peripheral-opioid-mediated antihyperalgesia (Aley and Levine, 1997). The mechanisms resemble those of central opioid tolerance. Development of tolerance to peripheral and central opioid effects can be reduced with N-methyl-D-aspartate (NMDA) receptor antagonists (Aley and Levine, 1997) and with nitric oxide synthase inhibitors (Kolesnikov et al., 1993).

Peripheral Opioid Analgesia in Humans

Peripheral Opioids in Experimental Muscle Pain and Inflammation

In the delayed-onset muscle soreness (DOMS) model, muscle pain is produced by strenuous muscle exercise including eccentric muscle contractions (Cleak and Eston, 1992; see Chapter 4 by Mizumura and Taguchi and Chapter 16 by Dannecker). The pain, which reaches its maximum between 24 and 48 hours after exercise, is thought to be due to an inflammatory response (Smith, 1991; MacIntyre et al., 1995) elicited by micro-injuries of muscle fibers (Cleak and Eston, 1992). Levels of cytokines, prostaglandins, and glutamate are increased in painful muscles (Tegeder et al., 2002). Further, plasma levels of pro-inflammatory cytokines such as IL-6 increase during DOMS (Croisier et al., 1999). Intravenously administered morphine-6-β-glucuronide (M6G), a metabolite of morphine with potent opioid agonist activity, which penetrates the central nervous system only very slowly, reduced muscle pain in the DOMS model and abolished mechanical hyperalgesia in the freeze lesion model of mild local skin inflammation (Tegeder et al., 2003) (Fig. 1). The peripheral localization of this effect was confirmed by the absence of any effects on pupil size, indicating that M6G had not penetrated the brain in relevant amounts when peripheral analgesia was observed (Fig. 2). In contrast to its effects in these inflammatory models, M6G did not increase pain threshold and tolerance to electrically evoked pain caused predominantly by activation of C fibers without hyperalgesia or inflammatory reactions. The positive control morphine, however, reduced pain in all models and decreased pupil diameter, indicating that it had acted centrally (Tegeder et al., 2003). Target tissue and plasma concentrations of morphine and M6G were confirmed by microdialysis. M6G target concentrations were achieved that are known to be devoid of central effects (Fig. 3).

Regional intravenous 0.01% morphine infusion reduced thermal, but not mechanical, hyperalgesia exclusively in inflamed skin areas (Koppert et al., 1999). Central analgesic effects were excluded by the absence of measurable plasma concentrations of morphine and its metabolites.

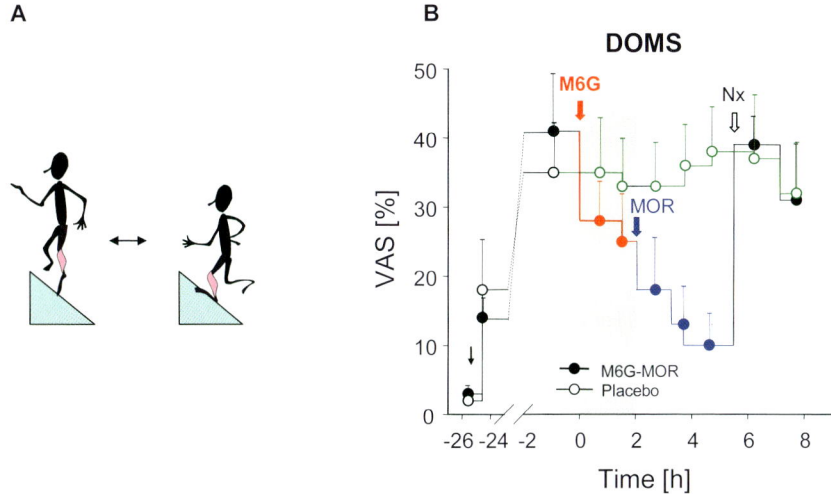

Fig. 1. (A) Illustration of the delayed-onset muscle soreness (DOMS) exercise, which consisted of two sets of 50 lifts to tiptoes on a sloped platform with a rest of 5 minutes between sets. (B) Effects of M6G and morphine on muscle hyperalgesia in the DOMS model. DOMS was induced by concentric and eccentric muscle contractions of the calf muscles of one leg. The DOMS exercise was performed 22–26 hours before starting medication. The intensity of muscle hyperalgesia while standing on tiptoes for 30 seconds was estimated with the help of a 10-cm visual analogue scale (VAS). The broad arrows indicate the start of the respective infusions. The shadowed area additionally highlights the time of M6G infusion. The thin arrow indicates the time of the DOMS exercise. Data represent the average of 10 subjects. Nx, naloxone (black); MOR, morphine (blue); M6G, morphine-6-glucuronide (red). Source: Tegeder et al. (2003).

Both of these experimental pain studies support the idea that peripheral opioids reduce inflammatory hyperalgesia but do not affect acute pain. The peripheral antihyperalgesic efficacy of opioids depends on the degree of inflammation, provided that adequate doses are used. The usefulness of peripheral opioids for control of pain that is not primarily caused by inflammation is not supported by experimental or clinical studies.

Peripheral Opioids in Clinical Pain

Analgesic efficacy of locally injected or topically applied opioids has been demonstrated in various clinical settings, including orbital or topical wound application and infiltration, and intra-articular injection after knee surgery or in chronic arthritis.

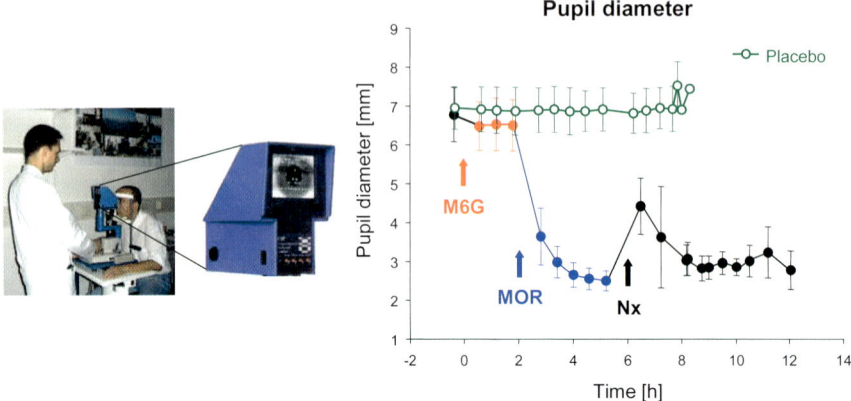

Fig. 2. Effects of M6G and morphine on pupil size as assessed with a pupillograph (illustration at left). Data represent the mean and SD for 10 subjects. Pupil diameter was determined as the mean of five measurements (separated by a 30-second rest period). The resolution of the device was 0.05 mm. Measurements took place in a dark room (light intensity <14 Lux). The broad arrows indicate the start of the respective infusions. M6G, morphine-6-glucuronide infusion (red), MOR, morphine (blue); Nx, naloxone (black). Source: Tegeder et al. (2003).

The injection of opioids into knee joints after open or arthroscopic knee surgery prolonged postoperative analgesia or reduced the need for intravenous opioid and non-opioid analgesics (Stein et al., 1991), but it failed to produce additional analgesia after arthroscopy under epidural anesthesia (Raja et al., 1992). Intra-articular morphine in addition to bupivacaine produced stronger or longer-lasting analgesia after knee surgery compared with bupivacaine alone (Joshi et al., 1993; McSwiney et al., 1993). Regional intravenous diamorphine (heroin) failed, however, to reduce postoperative pain scores after orthopedic foot surgery (Serpell et al., 2000).

In patients with chronic ostearthritis, intra-articular injection of morphine provided long-lasting analgesia (Likar et al., 1997) and reduced synovial leukocyte counts, suggesting that a possible anti-inflammatory effect may contribute to the relief of pain (Wilson et al., 1996). In patients with osteoarthritis of the temporomandibular joint, a single intra-articular injection of morphine into the joint provided some functional improvement (List et al., 2001). Local infiltration of low doses of morphine added to a local anesthetic significantly improved postoperative analgesia

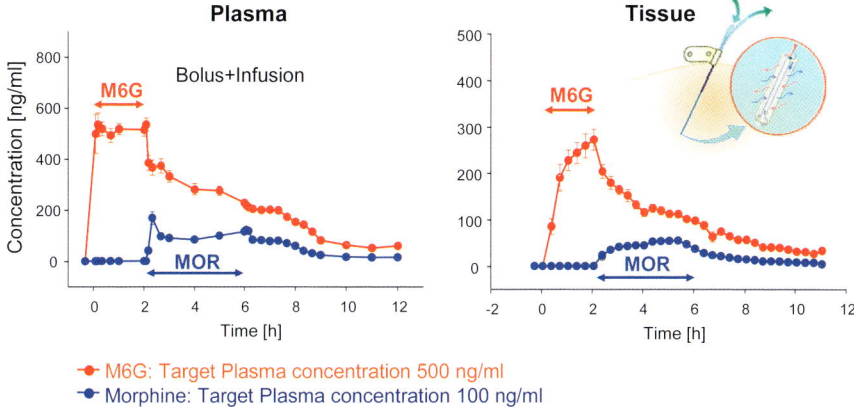

Fig. 3. Plasma and tissue concentration time course of morphine-6-glucuronide (M6G) and morphine. M6G was administered as a bolus and a subsequent continuous intravenous infusion. The arrow indicates the time of M6G infusion. Morphine treatment (bolus and infusion) was started when the infusion of M6G was stopped. The dosages of M6G and morphine were aimed at reaching plasma concentrations of 500 and 100 ng/mL, respectively. After the morphine infusion was stopped, naloxone was administered as a short 30-minute infusion. Concentrations of morphine and its metabolite were determined with high-performance liquid chromatography coupled with mass spectrometry. Subcutaneous tissue concentrations of M6G and morphine were assessed by microdialysis. Source: Tegeder et al. (2003).

after dental surgery (Likar et al., 1998). Similarly, surgical wound infiltrations with tramadol reduced acute postoperative pain in children after herniotomy (Demiraran et al., 2006). Case reports and pilot clinical studies have reported pain relief with topically applied morphine or diamorphine gel in patients with malignant or nonmalignant skin ulcers (Krajnik et al., 1999; Twillman et al., 1999). Methadone powder sprinkled onto exudative wounds also significantly reduced pain (Gallagher et al., 2005), and morphine added to silver sulfadiazine cream provided relief of burn pain (Long et al., 2001). Morphine mouthwashes reduced pain in patients with chemotherapy-induced stomatitis but caused mild itching and burning sensations as side effects (Cerchietti et al., 2003). Eye drops containing morphine reduced pain caused by corneal abrasions (Peyman et al., 1994). Although large clinical trials have not yet taken place, the available results point to a clinically relevant effect of peripheral opioids on pain evoked by inflammation.

Clinical Muscle Pain and Peripheral Opioids?

The potential benefit of locally injected or topically applied opioids for treatment of clinical muscle pain syndromes has not yet been investigated. Local injection into trigger points or systemic subcutaneous or intravenous loperamide may reduce muscle pain caused or contributed to by inflammation. Injectable formulations of loperamide are not, however, approved for clinical use. Novel peripherally acting μ- and κ-opioid agonists show efficacy in preclinical studies but have not been tested in humans. Topical application of opioid gels or cream to the skin may also be effective for local muscle pain. The efficacy of this route of administration is hampered, however, by the long diffusion distance between skin and deep muscles and by the diffusion barrier of intact skin. Moreover, no studies have investigated how peripheral opioids compare with non-opioid treatments of muscle pain with respect to efficacy and side effects.

It is also unknown whether peripherally acting opioids may reduce muscle pain in syndromes that may be caused by malfunctions of central pain control systems, such as fibromyalgia (Gracely et al., 2002; Petzke et al., 2003). Rhythmic exercise can activate central opioid systems by triggering an increased discharge from mechanosensitive afferent nerve fibers arising from contracting skeletal muscles (Thoren et al., 1990). Such exercise normally decreases thermal or mechanical pain sensitivity in local as well as remote body areas (Staud et al., 2005). In contrast, widespread hyperalgesia occurred in fibromyalgia and chronic fatigue patients (Whiteside et al., 2004; Staud et al., 2005), suggesting that the endogenous opioid systems may not respond adequately in these patients, thus facilitating sensitization. It is unknown whether these exercise effects in fibromyalgia patients result from abnormal descending inhibition or from excessive activation of muscle nociceptive afferents. In the latter case, peripherally acting opioids might help to adjust the system and may provide pain relief in fibromyalgia patients. This effect, however, is likely to be subject to tolerance.

Conclusion

Accumulating experimental and clinical evidence indicates that locally injected or peripherally acting opioids reduce inflammatory hyperalgesia and postoperative pain. The peripherally mediated pain relief depends on upregulation of opioid receptor expression in primary afferent nociceptive neurons and on transport of newly synthesized receptors to peripheral and central nerve terminals. Loss of contact between axon and peripheral target or disruption of axonal transport prevents the upregulation and reduces the efficacy of peripheral pain inhibition with endogenous and exogenous opioids.

The antihyperalgesic efficacy of peripherally acting opioids has been demonstrated in inflammatory muscle pain in rats and in experimental DOMS in humans. However, the use of peripheral opioid analgesia to treat clinical muscle pain has not yet been investigated. Peripheral opioid antinociception is most effective in inflammatory processes. By sharing some molecular characteristics with inflammatory conditions, muscle pain may be also sensitive to opioids, and patients might benefit from antihyperalgesic effects without central nervous system side effects. Establishing this therapeutic approach is a promising subject for future clinical research.

References

Aley KO, Levine JD. Different mechanisms mediate development and expression of tolerance and dependence for peripheral mu-opioid antinociception in rat. J Neurosci 1997;17:8018–8023.

Bileviciute-Ljungar I, Spetea M, Guo Y, Schutz J, Windisch P, Schmidhammer H. Peripherally mediated antinociception of the mu-opioid receptor agonist 2-[(4,5alpha-epoxy-3-hydroxy-14beta-methoxy-17-methylmorphinan-6beta-yl)amino]acetic acid (HS-731) after subcutaneous and oral administration in rats with carrageenan-induced hindpaw inflammation. J Pharmacol Exp Ther 2006;317:220–227.

Butelman ER, Harris TJ, Kreek MJ. Antiallodynic effects of loperamide and fentanyl against topical capsaicin-induced allodynia in unanesthetized primates. J Pharmacol Exp Ther 2004;311:155–163.

Cerchietti LC, Navigante AH, Korte MW, Cohen AM, Quiroga PN, Villaamil EC, Bonomi MR, Roth BM. Potential utility of the peripheral analgesic properties of morphine in stomatitis-related pain: a pilot study. Pain 2003;105:265–273.

Cleak MJ, Eston RG. Delayed onset muscle soreness: mechanisms and management. J Sports Sci 1992;10:325–341.

Coggeshall RE, Zhou S, Carlton SM. Opioid receptors on peripheral sensory axons. Brain Res 1997;764:126–132.

Croisier JL, Camus G, Venneman I, Deby-Dupont G, Juchmes-Ferir A, Lamy M, Crielaard JM, Deby C, Duchateau J. Effects of training on exercise-induced muscle damage and interleukin 6 production. Muscle Nerve 1999;22:208–212.

DeHaven-Hudkins DL, Burgos LC, Cassel JA, Daubert JD, DeHaven RN, Mansson E, Nagasaka H, Yu G, Yaksh T. Loperamide (ADL 2-1294), an opioid antihyperalgesic agent with peripheral selectivity. J Pharmacol Exp Ther 1999;289:494–502.

Demiraran Y, Ilce Z, Kocaman B, Bozkurt P. Does tramadol wound infiltration offer an advantage over bupivacaine for postoperative analgesia in children following herniotomy? Paediatr Anaesth 2006;16:1047–1050.

Eisenach JC, Carpenter R, Curry R. Analgesia from a peripherally active kappa-opioid receptor agonist in patients with chronic pancreatitis. Pain 2003;101:89–95.

Gallagher RE, Arndt DR, Hunt KL. Analgesic effects of topical methadone: a report of four cases. Clin J Pain 2005;21:190–192.

Gracely RH, Petzke F, Wolf JM, Clauw DJ. Functional magnetic resonance imaging evidence of augmented pain processing in fibromyalgia. Arthritis Rheum 2002;46:1333–1343.

Hassan AH, Ableitner A, Stein C, Herz A. Inflammation of the rat paw enhances axonal transport of opioid receptors in the sciatic nerve and increases their density in the inflamed tissue. Neuroscience 1993;55:185–195.

Ji RR, Zhang Q, Law PY, Low HH, Elde R, Hokfelt T. Expression of mu-, delta-, and kappa-opioid receptor-like immunoreactivities in rat dorsal root ganglia after carrageenan-induced inflammation. J Neurosci 1995;15:8156–8166.

Joshi GP, McCarroll SM, Brady OH, Hurson BJ, Walsh G. Intra-articular morphine for pain relief after anterior cruciate ligament repair. Br J Anaesth 1993;70:87–88.

Kohno T, Ji RR, Ito N, Allchorne AJ, Befort K, Karchewski LA, Woolf CJ. Peripheral axonal injury results in reduced mu opioid receptor pre- and post-synaptic action in the spinal cord. Pain 2005;117:77–87.

Kolesnikov YA, Jain S, Wilson R, Pasternak GW. Peripheral morphine analgesia: synergy with central sites and a target of morphine tolerance. J Pharmacol Exp Ther 1996;279:502–506.

Kolesnikov YA, Pick CG, Ciszewska G, Pasternak GW. Blockade of tolerance to morphine but not to kappa opioids by a nitric oxide synthase inhibitor. Proc Natl Acad Sci USA 1993;90:5162–5166.

Koppert W, Likar R, Geisslinger G, Zeck S, Schmelz M, Sittl R. Peripheral antihyperalgesic effect of morphine to heat, but not mechanical, stimulation in healthy volunteers after ultraviolet-B irradiation. Anesth Analg 1999;88:117–122.

Krajnik M, Zylicz Z, Finlay I, Luczak J, van Sorge AA. Potential uses of topical opioids in palliative care—report of 6 cases. Pain 1999;80:121–125.

Levine JD, Taiwo YO. Involvement of the mu-opiate receptor in peripheral analgesia. Neuroscience 1989;32:571–575.

Li Z, Proud D, Zhang C, Wiehler S, McDougall JJ. Chronic arthritis down-regulates peripheral mu-opioid receptor expression with concomitant loss of endomorphin 1 antinociception. Arthritis Rheum 2005;52:3210–3219.

Likar R, Schafer M, Paulak F, Sittl R, Pipam W, Schalk H, Geissler D, Bernatzky G. Intraarticular morphine analgesia in chronic pain patients with osteoarthritis. Anesth Analg 1997;84:1313–1317.

Likar R, Sittl R, Gragger K, Pipam W, Blatnig H, Breschan C, Schalk HV, Stein C, Schafer M. Peripheral morphine analgesia in dental surgery. Pain 1998;76:145–150.

List T, Tegelberg A, Haraldson T, Isacsson G. Intra-articular morphine as analgesic in temporomandibular joint arthralgia/osteoarthritis. Pain 2001;94:275–282.

Long TD, Cathers TA, Twillman R, O'Donnell T, Garrigues N, Jones T. Morphine-Infused silver sulfadiazine (MISS) cream for burn analgesia: a pilot study. J Burn Care Rehabil 2001;22:118–123.

Machelska H, Cabot PJ, Mousa SA, Zhang Q, Stein C. Pain control in inflammation governed by selectins. Nat Med 1998;4:1425–1428.

MacIntyre DL, Reid WD, McKenzie DC. Delayed muscle soreness. The inflammatory response to muscle injury and its clinical implications. Sports Med 1995;20:24–40.

McSwiney MM, Joshi GP, Kenny P, McCarroll SM. Analgesia following arthroscopic knee surgery. A controlled study of intra-articular morphine, bupivacaine or both combined. Anaesth Intensive Care 1993;21:201–203.

Menendez L, Lastra A, Hidalgo A, Meana A, Garcia E, Baamonde A. Peripheral opioids act as analgesics in bone cancer pain in mice. Neuroreport 2003;14:867–869.

Mousa SA, Cheppudira BP, Shaqura M, Fischer O, Hofmann J, Hellweg R, Schafer M. Nerve growth factor governs the enhanced ability of opioids to suppress inflammatory pain. Brain 2007;130:502–513.

Mousa SA, Machelska H, Schafer M, Stein C. Immunohistochemical localization of endomorphin-1 and endomorphin-2 in immune cells and spinal cord in a model of inflammatory pain. J Neuroimmunol 2002;126:5–15.

Nozaki-Taguchi N, Yaksh TL. Characterization of the antihyperalgesic action of a novel peripheral mu-opioid receptor agonist--loperamide. Anesthesiology 1999;90:225–234.

Nunez S, Lee JS, Zhang Y, Bai G, Ro JY. Role of peripheral mu-opioid receptors in inflammatory orofacial muscle pain. Neuroscience 2007;146:1346–1354.

Obara I, Makuch W, Spetea M, Schutz J, Schmidhammer H, Przewlocki R, Przewlocka B. Local peripheral antinociceptive effects of 14-O-methyloxymorphone derivatives in inflammatory and neuropathic pain in the rat. Eur J Pharmacol 2007;558:60–67.

Petzke F, Clauw DJ, Ambrose K, Khine A, Gracely RH. Increased pain sensitivity in fibromyalgia: effects of stimulus type and mode of presentation. Pain 2003;105:403–413.

Peyman GA, Rahimy MH, Fernandes ML. Effects of morphine on corneal sensitivity and epithelial wound healing: implications for topical ophthalmic analgesia. Br J Ophthalmol 1994;78:138–141.

Raja SN, Dickstein RE, Johnson CA. Comparison of postoperative analgesic effects of intraarticular bupivacaine and morphine following arthroscopic knee surgery. Anesthesiology 1992;77:1143–1147.

Rau KK, Jiang N, Johnson RD, Cooper BY. Heat sensitization in skin and muscle nociceptors expressing distinct combinations of TRPV1 and TRPV2 protein. J Neurophysiol 2007;97:2651–2662.

Schafer M, Carter L, Stein C. Interleukin 1 beta and corticotropin-releasing factor inhibit pain by releasing opioids from immune cells in inflamed tissue. Proc Natl Acad Sci USA 1994;91:4219–4223.

Serpell MG, Anderson E, Wilson D, Dawson N. I.v. regional diamorphine for analgesia after foot surgery. Br J Anaesth 2000;84:95–96.

Shinoda K, Hruby VJ, Porreca F. Antihyperalgesic effects of loperamide in a model of rat neuropathic pain are mediated by peripheral delta-opioid receptors. Neurosci Lett 2007;411:143–146.

Smith LL. Acute inflammation: the underlying mechanism in delayed onset muscle soreness? Med Sci Sports Exerc 1991;23:542–551.

Staud R, Robinson ME, Price DD. Isometric exercise has opposite effects on central pain mechanisms in fibromyalgia patients compared to normal controls. Pain 2005;118:176–184.

Stein C, Comisel K, Haimerl E, Yassouridis A, Lehrberger K, Herz A, Peter K. Analgesic effect of intraarticular morphine after arthroscopic knee surgery. N Engl J Med 1991;325:1123–1126.

Stein C, Gramsch C, Herz A. Intrinsic mechanisms of antinociception in inflammation: local opioid receptors and beta-endorphin. J Neurosci 1990;10:1292–1298.

Tegeder I, Meier S, Burian M, Schmidt H, Geisslinger G, Lotsch J. Peripheral opioid analgesia in experimental human pain models. Brain 2003;126:1092–1102.

Tegeder I, Zimmermann J, Meller ST, Geisslinger G. Metabolic functions and release of prostaglandins and nitric oxide in experimental human muscle pain. Inflamm Res 2002;51:393–402.

Thoren P, Floras JS, Hoffmann P, Seals DR. Endorphins and exercise: physiological mechanisms and clinical implications. Med Sci Sports Exerc 1990;22:417–428.

Twillman RK, Long TD, Cathers TA, Mueller DW. Treatment of painful skin ulcers with topical opioids. J Pain Symptom Manage 1999;17:288–292.

Vanderah TW, Schteingart CD, Trojnar J, Junien JL, Lai J, Riviere PJ. FE200041 (D-Phe-D-Phe-D-Nle-D-Arg-NH$_2$): a peripheral efficacious kappa opioid agonist with unprecedented selectivity. J Pharmacol Exp Ther 2004;310:326–333.

Vetter I, Wyse BD, Monteith GR, Roberts-Thomson SJ, Cabot PJ. The mu opioid agonist morphine modulates potentiation of capsaicin-evoked TRPV1 responses through a cyclic AMP-dependent protein kinase A pathway. Mol Pain 2006;2:22.

Whiteside A, Hansen S, Chaudhuri A. Exercise lowers pain threshold in chronic fatigue syndrome. Pain 2004;109:497–499.

Wilson JL, Nayanar V, Walker JS. The site of anti-arthritic action of the kappa-opioid, U-50, 488H, in adjuvant arthritis: importance of local administration. Br J Pharmacol 1996;118:1754–1760.

Correspondence to: Prof. Dr. med Irmgard Tegeder, Pharmazentrum Frankfurt, Institut für Klinische Pharmakologie/ZAFES, Klinikum der Johann Wolfgang Goethe-Universität Frankfurt, Theodor Stern Kai 7, Haus 74, Rm. 437, 60590 Frankfurt am Main, Germany. Tel: 49 69 6301 7621; fax: 49 69 6301 7636; email: tegeder@em.uni-frankfurt.de.

Augmented Central Pain Processing in Fibromyalgia Patients

Richard H. Gracely

Departments of Medicine-Rheumatology and Neurology,
University of Michigan Health System, Ann Arbor, Michigan, USA

Pressure Pain Sensitivity in Fibromyalgia

The 1990 American College of Rheumatology (ACR) research diagnostic criteria define fibromyalgia (FM) in terms of both widespread pain and tenderness to blunt pressure applied to 18 defined tender point sites (Wolfe et al., 1990). To satisfy the tenderness criteria, manual pressure of 4 kg must evoke a pain sensation in at least 11 of these 18 sites. This clinical examination using manual pressure does not contain standard controls for rating bias that are routinely applied in psychophysical investigations. Probably on the basis of this vulnerability to bias, Wolfe was one of the first to note that the tender point count measures some combination of tenderness and distress. This influence of distress has been confirmed by subsequent studies and acknowledged by those who still support the clinical utility of the method (Gracely et al., 2003; Gupta et al., 2007; Harth and Nielsen, 2007).

Pressure algometry is widely used and clinically expedient. It has provided a wealth of reliable data about pressure sensitivity throughout the body (see Chapter 11, Graven-Nielsen and Arendt-Nielsen). However, for diagnosis of FM, the ramp nature of the pressure pain threshold (PPT) test, applying a continuously increasing pressure, lacks experimental controls present in most psychophysical methods. Patients can appear to be reliable by timing their response, for example indicating sensitivity by short response latencies, and indicating an analgesic intervention by subsequent prolonged response latencies. These effects can be obtained without attending to the stimulus; for example, reliable data of this type could be obtained with pressure applied to a prosthetic thumb. In response to a perceived need to avoid this source of bias, our laboratory developed a device that applies discrete blunt pressure to the thumbnail. Pneumatic and hydraulic versions of this device have provided empirical evidence for the theoretical vulnerability of clinical measures to external biases. In separate studies of 47 control and FM patients, or 97 FM patients, we found a significant influence of distress on the tender point count and on an ascending method similar to the PPT, whereas psychophysical methods delivering randomly varying discrete stimuli were only minimally influenced by distress (Petzke et al., 2003b).

The results of these studies are not surprising; the more elaborate and time-consuming psychophysical methods were developed to control for the influence of rating biases, and the results suggest that they do. These effects were most pronounced with the tender point count. It is important to note that the degree to which factors such as distress adversely influence the PPT is unknown. A large body of consistent and informative evidence has been collected by dolorimeter assessment, supporting the validity of this method, especially under controlled, experimental conditions. Even the controversial tender point count receives support for clinical use by those who acknowledge that it most likely assesses an unknown combination of tenderness and psychological distress in each individual that has both predictive and clinical value (Gracely et al., 2003; Gupta et al., 2007; Harth and Nielson, 2007).

Increased Pain Sensitivity in Fibromyalgia Is Not Confined to Muscles

Given the role of distress, are patients still significantly tender when assessed by more controlled methods? Petzke et al. (2003) addressed this important question by assessing tenderness using both controlled and uncontrolled methods in 43 patients with FM and 28 control subjects. FM patients were significantly more sensitive according to both ascending and random direct scaling methods, supporting previous findings. This study also found increased sensitivity to contact heat using a random staircase technique, consistent with similar results using direct scaling (Geisser et al. 2003) and threshold assessment (Lautenbacher et al., 1994; Gibson et al., 1995) of reactions to painful heat. These studies indicate that increased pain sensitivity is not confined to muscles, as was also demonstrated by increased pressure sensitivity at a region of the thumb that is devoid of muscle (Petzke et al., 2003). All of the studies using heat applied the painful stimulus to the skin, which probably activated Aδ and C-fiber cutaneous nociceptors. The mechanism of pain augmentation in FM is not limited to muscles and may involve nociceptors in deep soft tissue, periosteum, and bone. The "myalgia" component of fibromyalgia reflects the historical origins of the taxonomy (e.g., fibromyositis) used to describe this disorder, but fibromyalgia may be a misnomer in describing the underlying mechanism.

Petzke et al. (2003) administered both heat and pressure to the same 43 FM patients and observed correlations of 0.41 for ascending and 0.36 for random methods, indicating that only 0.13–0.17 of the variance in sensitivity to heat can be explained by sensitivity to pressure. This modest association provides supporting evidence for the validity of the subjective responses in the sense that the augmentation does not represent a reporting style that would be assumed to influence responses to any painful stimulus modality. The modest correlations also suggest that the augmented pain sensitivity in FM may not result from a simple unitary mechanism but rather may represent the combined effect of multiple mechanisms. One possible source of variability may relate to primary afferents. The heat stimuli in the Petzke et al. study were applied sequentially to adjacent skin sites with a long interval (7 minutes) between repeated stimulations of the same site. The evoked sensation is predominately a pricking pain mediated by Aδ heat nociceptors. In contrast, the pressure stimuli applied to the thumb most likely activated deep C-fiber receptors (Treede et al., 2002). The pain sensitivity of Aδ and C-fiber nociceptors, as well as the modulation of this sensitivity by opioids, has been shown in the same individuals to correlate poorly between these two classes of nociceptors (Gracely and Hostetter, 1996).

The augmented pain sensitivity in FM extends beyond the modalities of pressure and heat to include painful cold, pain evoked by electrical stimulation, tourniquet-induced ischemic dysesthesias, and intramuscular injection of hypertonic saline. The sensitivity to cold includes both painful and nonpainful cold and also changes in sensory quality, including sensations of heat and both paresthetic and dysesthetic sensations (Lautenbacher et al., 1994; Berglund et al., 2002). Augmented sensitivity to electrical stimuli applied to the skin has been observed over painful tender points, but sensitivity was found to be normal at other locations (Arroyo and Cohen, 1993; Lautenbacher et al., 1994; Lautenbacher and Rollman, 1997). FM patients and controls rated the pain evoked by tourniquet ischemia similarly, but the pain following tourniquet ischemia was prolonged in the FM group (Kosek and Hansson, 1997).

Beyond Augmented Pain Magnitude: Temporal Summation, Spread, Persistence, and Spinal Reflexes

The augmented pain sensitivity is not confined to the intensity of evoked pain sensations, but also includes increased slow temporal summation (Price et al., 1977; Wolfe et al., 1995; Sorensen et al., 1998; Graven-Nielsen et al., 2000), increased spread of evoked and referred pain sensations (Sorensen et al., 1998; Graven-Nielsen et al., 2000), persistence of pain after stimulus termination (Staud et al., 2001, 2003), and enhanced nociceptive reflexes (Desmeules et al., 2003). The pain evoked by a single intramuscular electrical stimulation does not distinguish between FM and control subjects, but repeated stimulation produces a temporal summation that is greater in patients than in controls and is attenuated in patients after administration of the *N*-methyl-D-aspartate (NMDA) antagonist ketamine (Sorensen et al., 1998; Graven-Nielsen et al., 2000). Repeated painful heat stimuli delivered by a contact thermode evoke temporal summation in healthy control subjects at frequencies of 0.33 Hz or greater, and the magnitude of this temporal summation has been found to be greater in FM (Price et al., 1977; Staud et al., 2006). Intramuscular injections of hypertonic saline evoke more extensive pain and expanded areas of referred pain (Sorensen et al., 1998). This referred pain may occur proximally to the injection site in the tibialis anterior muscle, a locus that is never observed to be painful following injections in healthy control subjects (Graven-Nielsen et al., 2000). The sensation of evoked pain often persists after termination of a noxious stimulus. Pain evoked by heat and pressure has been found to last longer in FM patients in comparison to control subjects (Staud et al., 2001, 2003).

Response to Pharmacological Interventions

The results of several studies suggest that the effects of pharmacological interventions can be used to identify underlying mechanisms. As noted above, intravenous administration of 0.3 mg/kg ketamine attenuated several measures of evoked pain, although administration was limited to a subset of patients identified as "responders" after administration of the same dose in a previous session. The two criteria for identifying a responder were (1) two consecutive 50% reductions in visual analogue scores of widespread clinical pain after administration of ketamine and (2) no such effect after administration of placebo. In this study, 17 of 29 patients were classified as ketamine responders (Sorensen et al., 1997; Graven-Nielsen et al., 2000). In this group of responders, ketamine attenuated the intensity of pain evoked by intramuscular injection of hypertonic saline into the tibialis anterior muscle. Ketamine also reduced both the area of pain localized to the injection and the area of referred pain. Finally, ketamine reduced pain evoked by repeated intramuscular electrical stimulation and had no effect on pain evoked by single electrical stimuli, indicating an effect on temporal summation. Given that ketamine is a potent NMDA antagonist, and NMDA mechanisms are known to mediate spinal hyperexcitability, these results provide further support for the presence of spinal hyperexcitability in FM. One caveat with this reasoning is that ketamine's effects are not purely central, but include peripheral pain-suppressing effects (Warncke et al., 1997). A peripheral action could also explain the reduction of the intensity and (local) area of pain evoked by hypertonic saline, and also on the attenuation of pain produced by repeated electrical stimulation. However, co-injection of ketamine together with hypertonic saline had no significant effect on the saline-induced muscle pain intensity, indicating that the peripheral effects of ketamine on saline-induced muscle pain are limited (Cairns et al., 2003). A peripheral mechanism would be less likely to be involved in the presence of referred pain or in the reduction of the area of referred pain in FM.

In addition to basic information on underlying mechanisms, the fact that only 17 of 29 FM patients were classified as ketamine responders suggests that the response to pharmacological agents may serve as a discriminating phenotyping variable that classifies patients into functionally relevant subgroups (Henriksson and Sorensen 2002). Studies employing both ketamine and additional agents such as morphine and lidocaine (Sorensen et al., 1995, 1998) have identified patients with FM who respond to particular drugs and not others, suggesting both multiple maintaining mechanisms and a direct means of identifying these mechanisms. This preliminary evidence supports the inclusion of pharmacological challenges in genotyping and phenotyping characterization studies, with the obvious constraints of the time it takes to perform these challenges in these large-enrollment studies.

Supraspinal Processing: Functional Brain Imaging Evidence of Augmented Pain Processing

The evidence above suggests that increased sensitivity to painful stimuli in FM can be observed at the spinal level. This facilitation and additional modulation can also be evaluated by methods that assess brain processing to experimental painful stimulation, including the modulation of this processing. The first study of this type used functional magnetic resonance imaging (fMRI) to assess the pain sensitivity to blunt pressure in FM and healthy control subjects (Gracely et al., 2002). This study used a 1-cm^2 hard rubber probe to apply blunt pressure to the left thumbnail of 16 patients with FM and 16 matched healthy control subjects (all right-handed). In preliminary sessions, the amount of pressure required to evoke a subjective level of moderate to slightly intense pain was determined for both FM patients and control subjects. During the fMRI scanning sessions (1.5-Tesla system), this pressure was delivered in a 30-second block alternating with a 30-second block of nonpainful light pressure stimulation (usually 0.5 kg). Control subjects received the same functional scan as the FM patients, receiving moderate to slightly intense painful pressure alternating with nonpainful pressure. In addition, these control subjects also participated in a second functional scan in which they received much lower stimulus pressures, similar to those delivered to the patients, that evoked only a slightly intense pain sensation. This design allowed the results from the patients to be compared to two types of control conditions. In the "Equal Subjective Pain Condition" (higher stimulus intensity in controls), similar activations in each group are consistent with augmented pain sensitivity in FM (Fig. 1). The "Equal Stimulus Pressure Condition" (lower pain intensity in controls) evaluated the effects produced by the same stimulus levels in the two groups, with greater activation in the FM group also suggesting augmentation of pain sensitivity in FM (Fig. 2). This result provides fMRI evidence consistent with the verbal reports of pressure pain in each group. It suggests augmented processing in FM in a number of brain regions commonly

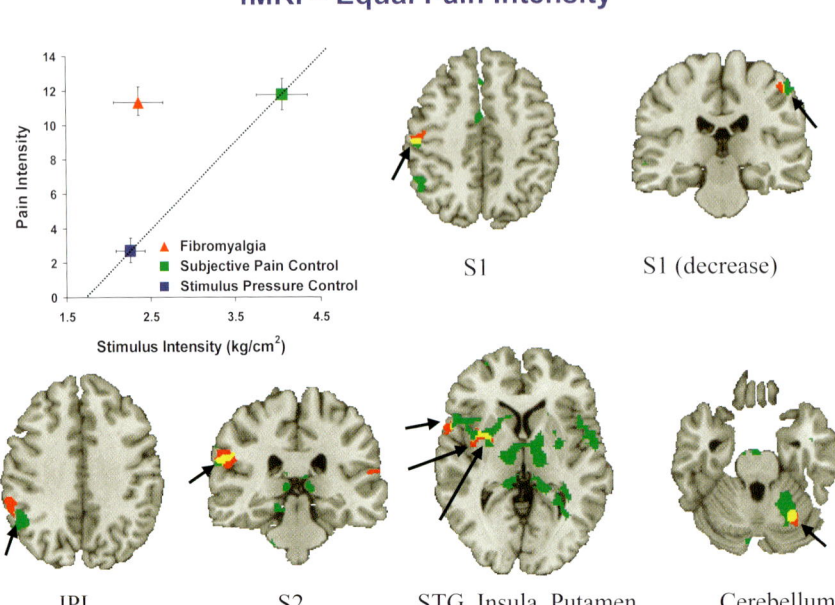

Fig. 1. Results of pressure applied to the left thumbnail in patients and controls. Stimuli adjusted to evoke a subjective level of 11 (moderate) in the patients (red) resulted in significant activations in multiple regions of the pain matrix, including the contralateral primary somatosensory cortex (S1); inferior parietal lobule (IPL); secondary somatosensory cortex (S2); superior temporal gyrus (STG), insula, and putamen; and in the ipsilateral cerebellum. The images are in radiological view, with the right brain shown on the left. Increasing the stimulus pressures to evoke the same subjective level of pain in the control subjects (green) resulted in activations in the same regions, with overlapping regions shown in yellow. Both patients and controls also showed a region of significant decreased activity in the ipsilateral S1. The statistical tests were between the effects of painful and nonpainful pressure and were corrected for multiple comparisons and displayed in standard space superimposed on an anatomical image of a standard brain. Results of the analysis of similar stimulus pressures in the patients (red) and healthy controls (blue) are shown in Fig. 2. Based on data from Gracely et al. (2002). Reprinted with permission.

activated in pain neuroimaging studies. The regions with augmented processing in FM shown in Fig. 2 include the contralateral primary somatosensory cortex (S1), inferior parietal lobule (IPL), insular cortex, anterior cingulate cortex (ACC), posterior cingulate cortex (PCC), ipsilateral secondary somatosensory cortex (S2), and bilateral superior temporal gyrus and cerebellum. This initial fMRI study was partially replicated in a second study that also included patients with idiopathic chronic low

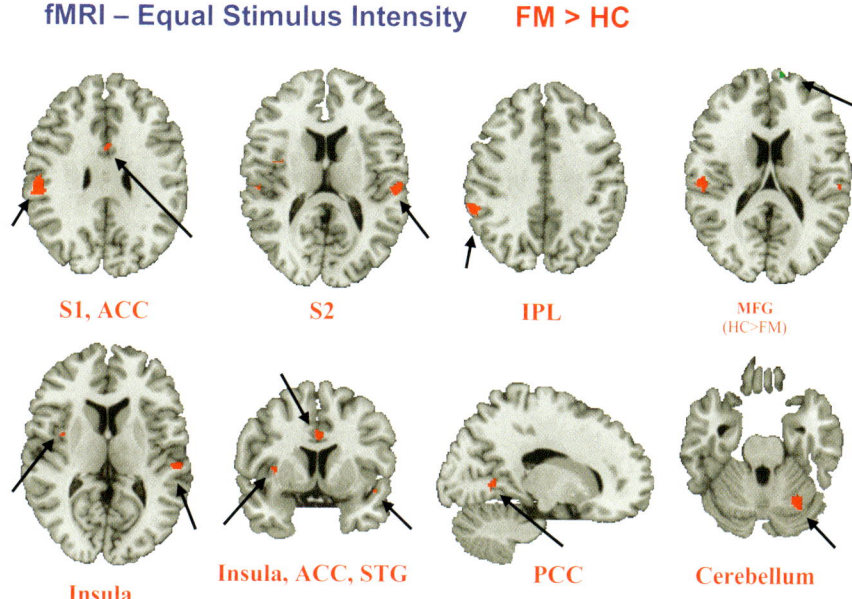

fMRI – Equal Stimulus Intensity   FM > HC

S1, ACC   S2   IPL   MFG (HC>FM)

Insula   Insula, ACC, STG   PCC   Cerebellum

Fig. 2. Evaluation of the effects of similar stimulus pressures in patients and healthy control subjects. This analysis directly compared the effect of pressure stimulation in comparison to nonpainful stimulation between the patients and control subjects using a random effects model. The regions in red are regions in which the effect in patients is significantly greater than in control subjects, showing an augmentation in many of the regions shown in Fig. 1, including S1, IPL, insula, S2, and cerebellum. The results also show significant differences in the anterior cingulate cortex (ACC) and posterior cingulate cortex (PCC). Control subjects showed one region of significantly greater activity (green), located in the medial frontal gyrus (MFG). See Fig. 1 for details and definitions. Based on data from Gracely et al. (2002). Reprinted with permission.

back pain (Giesecke et al., 2004). In this sample of 16 FM patients and 11 healthy control subjects, a constant stimulus pressure of 2 kg produced significantly greater activations in the in the patients in ipsilateral S2 and cerebellum, and in the contralateral S1 and IPL. When each group received a pressure calibrated to produce slightly intense pain, common activations were observed in the contralateral S1, S2, IPL, insular cortex, and ACC, and in the ipsilateral S2 and cerebellum.

Cooke et al. (2004) used a similar design in a fMRI study of heat pain in 9 FM patients and 9 control subjects. Equal stimulus intensities resulted in significantly increased activation in the contralateral insular cortex in the FM patient group. A similar analysis of nonpainful warm stimulation showed enhanced responses in the FM group in the bilateral prefrontal cortex, in supplemental motor areas, and in the contralateral ACC.

Supraspinal Processing: Basal Differences in Neural Activity Inferred from Differences in Regional Cerebral Blood Flow

The very first studies to apply functional brain imaging to FM used the method of single photon emission computed tomography (SPECT) to assess differences between FM and healthy controls in neural activity at rest (in the absence of painful stimulation). As with most functional brain imaging methods, neural activity is inferred from regional cerebral blood flow (rCBF). The first study was by Mountz et al. (1995), who evaluated rCBF in the bilateral thalamus and the head of the caudate nucleus in 10 patients with FM and in 7 healthy control subjects over a 32-minute period as the participants rested quietly. Infusion of 25 mCi of a radioactive tracer provided a semiquantitative measure of rCBF during this period, with a resolution of about 8.5 mm. The results showed lower rCBF in patients in all four regions, suggesting that FM was associated with decreased neural activity in the bilateral thalamus and bilateral caudate nucleus. This initial study was followed by a similar investigation by Kwiatek et al. (2000), who also used SPECT to assess baseline brain activity in the thalamus and caudate nucleus and in additional brain regions. These investigators compared brain activity a larger group of 17 patients with FM and in 22 healthy control subjects, finding decreased rCBF in the right thalamus but no other changes in either the left thalamus or the bilateral caudate nuclei. However, decreased rCBF was also found in the inferior pontine tegmentum and in a region close to the right lentiform nucleus. The observation of hypoperfusion in the right thalamus by both Mountz et al. (1995) and Kwiatek et al. (2000) was replicated by Mountz et al. (1998). The idea of reduced activity in the thalamus was supported by an interesting SPECT study that evaluated differences in basal rCBF after 3 months of amitriptyline therapy in 14 patients with FM (Adiguzel et al., 2004). Treatment was associated with decreased activity in several regions including the bilateral temporal cortex, but more importantly also with increased activity in the bilateral thalamus and bilateral basal ganglia. Together, these results suggest a hypothesis in which FM is associated with reduced thalamic activity that is normalized by treatment.

At least two studies using positron emission tomography (PET) have also assessed basal activity in FM. Like SPECT, PET infuses a radioactive tracer to assess rCBF, but with increased temporal and spatial resolution. Wik et al. (2003) assessed rCBF in 8 FM patients and 8 healthy control subjects. FM was associated with decreased rCBF in the left frontal, temporal, parietal, and occipital cortex and with regions of increased rCBF in the bilateral retrosplenial cortex. Yunus et al. (2004) used a PET method that does not infer activity from rCBF, but directly assesses regional glucose metabolism by infusing 18F-fluorodesoxyglucose (FDG). Analysis of 12 FM patients and 7 healthy controls found no difference between groups, a result that may represent either a lack of power or a discordant finding to be addressed by future experiments.

Locus of Observations of Augmented Processing and the Locus of Augmentation

The numerous observations at the spinal level of enhanced temporal summation, increased spread and persistence of sensation in FM, and attenuation of these effects by the NMDA antagonist ketamine collectively implicate central processes of hyperexcitability. This body of evidence is consistent with a model of generalized spinal sensitization that results in both the chronic widespread pain observed in FM and in the augmented sensitivity to evoked painful stimulation.

These studies of augmented supraspinal pain processing to pressure and heat stimulation in FM suggest that the augmentation that is observed spinally and reflected in psychophysical reports is also reflected in enhanced processing in a number of supraspinal regions. These results also suggest that observed augmentation could include supraspinal processes that augment particular or multiple features of the painful experience.

Arendt-Nielsen and Henriksson (2007) have described two types of FM patients—those with a previous peripheral pain disorder that has become centralized by putative spinal mechanisms (bottom-up model) and those in which the disorder originates in the central nervous system (top-down model). A spinal mechanism could conceivably be involved in either model, while supraspinal mechanisms would be more parsimoniously associated with a top-down model.

Peripheral Locus

The accumulating evidence that demonstrates augmentation at and beyond the first spinal synapse does not specify the locus of the augmentation. These results are consistent with generalized and widespread receptor sensitization that would be mediated by efferent neural processing, circulating substances, or other mechanisms that result in a generalized augmented nociceptor barrage. This augmentation could also occur in the dorsal root ganglion (DRG) or be modified further in the DRG. This peripheral mechanism could lead directly to widespread spontaneous pain and also increased pain sensitivity to evoked stimulation. Furthermore, persistent and/or augmented input could drive spinal and supraspinal mechanisms that further augment pain sensitivity. In this peripheral scenario, spinal and supraspinal measures assess the consequences of increased peripheral pain sensitivity. This scenario would represent the bottom-up model of Arendt-Nielsen and Henriksson (2007) and is consistent with proposals from other investigators (Gracely et al., 2003; Staud et al., 2003, 2006; Vierck, 2006).

Spinal Locus

Multiple lines of evidence suggest that increased sensitivity to painful stimuli in FM may originate at the spinal level, including facilitation of the nociceptive reflex, augmented temporal summation, and greater referred pain. Attenuation of both temporal summation and referred pain by the NMDA antagonist ketamine provides additional evidence consistent with the concept that this facilitation is mediated in part by spinal mechanisms. In this spinal scenario, normal input in primary afferents is augmented by spinal processes that include NMDA-mediated central sensitization. These processes would be expected to be different than those observed after peripheral injury because they would not be dependent on peripheral input and would not exhibit characteristic sensory signatures of mechanical dynamic allodynia and pinprick hyperalgesia. The lack of dependence on a maintaining input (Gracely et al., 1992) suggests spinal sensitization mechanisms that are distinctly different from classical spinal central sensitization. Alternatively, if the pain augmentation in FM represents classical spinal central sensitization, this sensitization would also be consistent with a peripheral mechanism in which a large number of deep nociceptors provide the maintaining peripheral input. The regions of altered pain sensitivity (possibly the whole body) would comprise a large primary zone with the characteristic signs of static mechanical allodynia and heat hyperalgesia (Gracely et al., 2003).

Supraspinal Locus

Functional MRI studies suggest that the response of a number of brain regions usually activated by painful stimuli is augmented in FM in comparison to the response of healthy control subjects. This augmented response may simply reflect the increased activity of supraspinal inputs that have been augmented at peripheral and/or spinal levels. Alternatively, this augmented response could reflect supraspinal processes similar to the "top-down" model proposed by Arendt-Nielsen and Henriksson (2007). If supraspinal mechanisms are the sole source of augmentation, these mechanisms must also account for the multiple findings of augmentation observed at spinal levels. These effects could be mediated by some combination of increased descending excitation and impaired descending inhibition. There is growing evidence for impaired descending inhibition in FM. In healthy individuals, noxious stimulation applied anywhere on the body evokes generalized widespread analgesia referred to as diffuse noxious inhibitory controls (DNIC) (Le Bars et al., 1979a,b, 1986). Several studies have failed to demonstrate DNIC in patients with FM (Kosek and Hansson, 1997; Lautenbacher and Rollman, 1997; Julien et al., 2005), suggesting that the pain symptoms in FM may result from a defect in this intrinsic analgesic system. These results support a parsimonious mechanism in which widespread pain and widespread evoked-pain sensitivity result from a defect in equally widespread tonic inhibition. Under normal circumstances, these descending inhibitory systems are active to some degree, attenuating painful inputs that would otherwise be felt in a widespread distribution as experienced in FM. FM is associated with dysfunction in these systems, resulting in chronic widespread pain. However, a more parsimonious explanation is that these descending systems, which are activated by externally painful stimuli, are activated robustly by the severe and widespread pain of FM. The absence of a DNIC or other inhibitory effect is not due to a dysfunction in these systems, but rather results from the fact that these systems are already maximally activated due to FM pain, and cannot be activated further by noxious stimulation (Gracely et al., 2003).

Summary

There is considerable evidence for augmented pain processing at spinal and supraspinal levels in FM. However, this evidence does not specify the locus of the augmentation, which could occur at supraspinal, spinal, or peripheral levels, or at a combination of these loci. The future challenge is to distinguish between these alternatives, evaluating primary afferent activity and the function of positive and negative feedback systems between the spinal dorsal horn and supraspinal sources of facilitatory and inhibitory systems. These studies should address whether spinal augmentation originates in the periphery or the spinal cord and whether FM leads to decreased or tonic descending inhibition.

References

Adiguzel O, Kaptanoglu E, Turgut B, Nacitarhan V. The possible effect of clinical recovery on regional cerebral blood flow deficits in fibromyalgia: a prospective study with semiquantitative SPECT. South Med J 2004;97:651–655.
Arroyo JF, Cohen ML. Abnormal responses to electrocutaneous stimulation in fibromyalgia. J Rheumatol 1993;20:1925–1931.

Berglund B, Harju EL, Kosek E, Lindblom U. Quantitative and qualitative perceptual analysis of cold dysesthesia and hyperalgesia in fibromyalgia. Pain 2002;96:177–187.

Cairns BE, Svensson P, Wang K, Hupfeld S, Graven-Nielsen T, Sessle BJ, Berde CB, Arendt-Nielsen L. Activation of peripheral NMDA receptors contributes to human pain and rat afferent discharges evoked by injection of glutamate into the masseter muscle. J Neurophysiol. 2003;90:2098–2105.

Cook DB, Lange G, Ciccone DS, Liu WC, Steffener J, Natelson BH. Functional imaging of pain in patients with primary fibromyalgia. J Rheumatol 2004;31:364–378.

Desmeules JA, Cedraschi C, Rapiti E, et al. Neurophysiologic evidence for a central sensitization in patients with fibromyalgia. Arthritis Rheum; 2003;48:1420–1429.

Geisser ME, Casey KL, Brucksch CB, Ribbens CM, Appleton BB, Crofford LJ. Perception of noxious and innocuous heat stimulation among healthy women and women with fibromyalgia: association with mood, somatic focus, and catastrophizing. Pain 2003;102:243–250.

Gibson SJ, Granges G, Littlejohn GO, Helme RD. Increased thermal pain sensitivity in patients with fibromyalgia syndrome. In: Bromm B, Desmedt JE, editors. Pain and the brain, 22nd ed. New York: Raven Press; 1995. p. 401–411.

Giesecke T, Gracely RH, Grant M, et al. Evidence of augmented central pain processing in idiopathic chronic low back pain. Arthritis Rheum 2004;50:613–623.

Gracely R, Hostetter MP. Fentanyl reduces both A-delta and C-fiber mediated thermal pain sensations. 15th Annual Scientific Meeting of the American Pain Society 1996; A-62.

Gracely RH, Grant MA, Giesecke T. Evoked pain measures in fibromyalgia. Best Pract Res Clin Rheumatol 2003;17:593–609.

Gracely RH, Lynch SA, Bennett GJ. Painful neuropathy: altered central processing maintained dynamically by peripheral input. Pain 1992;51:175–194.

Gracely RH, Petzke F, Wolf JM, Clauw DJ. Functional magnetic resonance imaging evidence of augmented pain processing in fibromyalgia. Arthritis Rheum 2002;46:1333–1343.

Graven-Nielsen T, Aspegren KS, Henriksson KG, et al. Ketamine reduces muscle pain, temporal summation, and referred pain in fibromyalgia patients. Pain 2000;85:483–491.

Gupta A, Silman AJ, Ray D, et al. The role of psychosocial factors in predicting the onset of chronic widespread pain: results from a prospective population-based study. Rheumatology (Oxford) 2007;46:666–671.

Harth M, Nielson WR. The fibromyalgia tender points: use them or lose them? A brief review of the controversy. J Rheumatol 2007;34:914–922.

Henriksson KG, Sorensen J. The promise of N-methyl-D-aspartate receptor antagonists in fibromyalgia. Rheum Dis Clin North Am 2002;28343–28351.

Julien N, Goffaux P, Arsenault P, Marchand S. Widespread pain in fibromyalgia is related to a deficit of endogenous pain inhibition. Pain 2005;114:295–302.

Kosek E, Hansson P. Modulatory influence on somatosensory perception from vibration and heterotopic noxious conditioning stimulation (HNCS) in fibromyalgia patients and healthy subjects. Pain 1997; 70:41–51.

Kwiatek R, Barnden L, Tedman R, et al. Regional cerebral blood flow in fibromyalgia: single-photon-emission computed tomography evidence of reduction in the pontine tegmentum and thalami. Arthritis Rheum 2000;43:2823–2833.

Lautenbacher S, Rollman GB. Possible deficiencies of pain modulation in fibromyalgia. Clin J Pain 1997;13:189–196.

Lautenbacher S, Rollman GB, McCain GA. Multi-method assessment of experimental and clinical pain in patients with fibromyalgia. Pain 1994;59:45–53.

Le Bars D, Dickenson AH, Besson JM. Diffuse noxious inhibitory controls (DNIC). II. Lack of effect on non-convergent neurones, supraspinal involvement and theoretical implications. Pain 1979a;6:305–327.

Le Bars D, Dickenson AH, Besson JM. Diffuse noxious inhibitory controls (DNIC). I. Effects on dorsal horn convergent neurones in the rat. Pain 1979b;6:283–304.

Le Bars D, Dickenson AH, Besson JM, Villanueva L. Aspects of sensory processing through convergent neurons. In: Yaksh TL, editor. Spinal afferent processing. New York: Plenum; 1986. p. 467–504.

Mountz JM, Bradley LA, Alarcon GS. Abnormal functional activity of the central nervous system in fibromyalgia syndrome. Am J Med Sci 1998;315:385–396.

Mountz JM, Bradley LA, Modell JG, et al. Fibromyalgia in women. Abnormalities of regional cerebral blood flow in the thalamus and the caudate nucleus are associated with low pain threshold levels. Arthritis Rheum 1995;38:926–938.

Arendt-Nielsen L, Henriksson KG. Pathophysiological mechanisms in chronic musculoskeletal pain (fibromyalgia): the role of central and peripheral sensitization and pain disinhibition. Best Pract Res Clin Rheumatol 2007;21:465–480.

Petzke F, Clauw DJ, Ambrose K, Khine A, Gracely RH. Increased pain sensitivity in fibromyalgia: effects of stimulus type and mode of presentation. Pain 2003a;105:403–413.

Petzke F, Gracely RH, Park KM, Ambrose K, Clauw DJ. What do tender points measure? Influence of distress on 4 measures of tenderness. J Rheumatol 2003b;30:567–574.

Price DD, Hu J, Dubner R, Gracely RH. Peripheral suppression of first pain and central summation of second pain evoked by noxious heat pulses. Pain 1977;3:57–68.

Sorensen J, Bengtsson A, Ahlner J, Henriksson KG, Ekselius L, Bengtsson M. Fibromyalgia: are there different mechanisms in the processing of pain? A double blind crossover comparison of analgesic drugs. J Rheumatol 1997;24:1615–1621.

Sorensen J, Bengtsson A, Backman E, Henriksson KG, Bengtsson M. Pain analysis in patients with fibromyalgia. Effects of intravenous morphine, lidocaine, and ketamine. Scandinavian Journal of Rheumatology 1995;24:360–365.

Sorensen J, Graven-Nielsen T, Henriksson KG, Bengtsson M, Arendt-Nielsen L. Hyperexcitability in fibromyalgia. J Rheumatol 1998;25:152–155.

Staud R, Robinson ME, Vierck CJ Jr, Price DD. Diffuse noxious inhibitory controls (DNIC) attenuate temporal summation of second pain in normal males but not in normal females or fibromyalgia patients. Pain 2003;101:167–174.

Staud R, Vierck CJ, Cannon RL, Mauderli AP, Price DD. Abnormal sensitization and temporal summation of second pain (wind-up) in patients with fibromyalgia syndrome. Pain 2001;91:165–175.

Staud R, Vierck CJ, Robinson ME, Price DD. Overall fibromyalgia pain is predicted by ratings of local pain and pain-related negative affect: possible role of peripheral tissues. Rheumatology (Oxford) 2006;45:1409–1415.

Treede RD, Rolke R, Andrews K, Magerl W. Pain elicited by blunt pressure: neurobiological basis and clinical relevance. Pain 2002;98:235–240.

Vierck CJ Jr. Mechanisms underlying development of spatially distributed chronic pain (fibromyalgia). Pain 2006;124:242–263.

Warncke T, Jorum E, Stubhaug A. Local treatment with the N-methyl-D-aspartate receptor antagonist ketamine, inhibit development of secondary hyperalgesia in man by a peripheral action. Neurosci Lett 1997;227:1–4.

Wik G, Fischer H, Bragee B, Kristianson M, Fredrikson M. Retrosplenial cortical activation in the fibromyalgia syndrome. Neuroreport 2003;14:619–621.

Wolfe F, Ross K, Anderson J, Russell IJ. Aspects of fibromyalgia in the general population: Sex, pain threshold, and fibromyalgia symptoms. J Rheumatol 1995;22:151–156.

Wolfe F, Smythe HA, Yunus MB, Bennett RM, Bombardier C, Goldenberg DL, Tugwell P, Campbell SM, Abeles M, Clark P. The American College of Rheumatology 1990 criteria for the classification of fibromyalgia. Report of the Multicenter Criteria Committee. Arthritis Rheum 1990;33:160–172.

Yunus MB, Young CS, Saeed SA, Mountz JM, Aldag JC. Positron emission tomography in patients with fibromyalgia syndrome and healthy controls. Arthritis Rheum 2004;51:513–518.

Correspondence to: Richard H. Gracely, PhD, 24 Frank Lloyd Wright Drive, PO Box 385, Lobby M, Ann Arbor, MI 48106, USA. Email: rgracely@umich.edu.

Clinical Manifestations of Muscle and Joint Pain

Henning Bliddal[a] and Michele Curatolo[b,c]

[a]*The Parker Institute, Frederiksberg Hospital, Frederiksberg, Denmark;*
[b]*Department of Anesthesiology, University of Bern;* [c]*Department of Anesthesiology,*
Division of Pain Therapy, Inselspital, Bern, Switzerland

Muscle pain is a natural accompaniment to physical activity. Its meaning is not always negative. In sports, for example, a few days of pain after exertion might even bring a certain sense of satisfaction as a sign of good performance. The individual will know from experience that such pain is a temporary reaction that will pass in a few days.

In contrast, muscle pain in association with disease may not be self-limiting, can produce substantial physical suffering, and is typically associated with psychological distress. According to a recent survey, 19% of adults in Europe have experienced significant long-lasting pain (Breivik et al., 2006). Chronic pain has a major impact on both patients and their health care professionals.

It may be impossible to distinguish between pain originating in the joints and pain from the adjacent muscles. Inflammatory changes within a joint affect the surrounding soft tissues, including muscles. Referred pain is a further confounding factor to be considered when diagnosing regional pain. Finally, widespread pain is a complication of rheumatological joint diseases and is typically seen in 20–25% of patients with rheumatoid arthritis or systemic lupus. The considerable overlap in the clinical manifestations of muscle and joint pain in different pain conditions frequently complicates diagnosis. However, experimental researchers have recently provided valuable findings that can help clinicians recognize patterns of pain originating from muscles and joints, thereby improving current knowledge of the manifestations of these pain conditions (see Chapter 22, Arendt-Nielsen and Graven-Nielsen).

The aim of this chapter is to highlight typical clinical manifestations of pain from muscle and joints. Particular attention will be given to the pathophysiological mechanisms responsible for symptoms and signs, and to their relationship with the diagnostic process in terms of identifying the source of pain. A thorough review of the clinical manifestations of the different painful muscle and joint diseases is beyond the scope of this chapter.

Causative Factors

Simple muscle pain may arise in all muscles after strenuous work, especially after either strenuous or unaccustomed work. Some muscle areas are especially prone to this reaction, and some types of industrial work are regularly associated with chronic problems in well-defined muscles. Sewing machine operation and assembly work typically involve neck and shoulder muscle pain (Andersen and Gaardboe, 1993), and in the fish- and meat-processing industry, elbow pain problems are frequently reported (Shiri et al., 2006).

A definite association has been demonstrated between exposure and muscle pain after industrial strain (Andersen and Gaardboe, 1993). Single events, such as whiplash injuries, may cause permanent changes in the muscles in a given area. The causal relationships in these conditions have not been clarified; only phenomenological descriptions are available. It has been suggested that trauma, such as a whiplash injury, may lead to chronification at least in part by causing central changes in the perception of sensory impulses, known as central sensitization (Curatolo et al., 2004).

Very commonly, joint disease, whether degenerative or inflammatory, is accompanied by some degree of dysfunction and pain in the adjacent muscles (Kidd, 2006; Bliddal and Danneskiold-Samsoe, 2007). Such pain is due to a combination of factors, most certainly including biomechanical changes in the joint. Noxious substances such as bradykinin, serotonin, and prostaglandin are released during inflammation, and they all have an important role in muscle pain (Graven-Nielsen and Mense, 2001). Also of importance are more specific inflammatory products released from the joint, such as interleukin-6, which may activate trigger points in the muscles (Shah et al., 2008).

Trauma to the joints may lead to changes in the loading of the muscles and thus may cause localized muscle pain (Buckwalter 2003). For example, trauma to the medial compartment of the tibiofemoral knee joint may lead to pain in the myotendinous part of the muscles, the pes anserinus, which is typical of osteoarthritis of the knee.

Pain Patterns from Muscles

Muscle pain may be perceived:
- locally in the muscle;
- diffusely spread in the area of the muscle, presumably due to secondary strain of the adjacent muscle tissue;
- in an area remote from the affected part (referred pain);
- generalized to different body sites.

Pain sensation is unpleasant by definition; it may be experienced as harmful or may even evoke a reaction of fear. Descriptions of experimental muscle pain use words such as "aching," "cramping," "boring," "drilling," "taut," "tight," "spreading," and "radiating" (Chapter 11, Graven-Nielsen and Arendt-Nielsen). If a single structure is painful in an area of the body, the surrounding tissues are likely to be affected as well and may not function normally. There is a certain predictability in the involvement of surrounding structures, which has led to the description of a number of syndromes, often due to combined joint and muscle problems. For example, in stiff-toe syndrome, walking problems caused by a stiff big toe lead to pain in the gluteal region, and denervation of the thoracicus longus nerve causes paralysis of the serratus anterior muscle and elicits pain in more or less all the other shoulder muscles.

This spread of pain should be distinguished from referred pain arising from trigger points, whose activation elicits pain in other regions, usually distal to the trigger points. Some patterns of referred pain are very regular and have been described in detail by Simons et al. (1999). These patterns are particularly predictable in the upper extremity. Fig. 1 shows typical examples of pain referred from the shoulder to the arm and hand.

Muscle pain in a given area is most pronounced during use of the muscle from which the pain originates. Further pain may be felt when the muscle is used after a period of rest. Such pain is often accompanied by stiffness in the morning, in which case a warm-up period is necessary before the painful area can be used properly. More complex conditions are characterized by pain at rest and/or by deterioration after exercise (exercise intolerance). The latter phenomenon is associated with major problems in fibromyalgia, in which post-exercise problems may last for days and can lead to a negative effect of training.

Muscle tenderness is not constant, but varies according to the type and position of the muscle. For a demonstration, the reader might test the tenderness of the quadriceps muscle on the middle of the thigh and compare it to similar pressure exerted on the trapezius or supraspinatus. The latter are almost inevitably sore, whereas the former seldom reacts with significant tenderness. This observation is supported by experimental evidence showing that muscle sensitivity is higher in the trapezius than in the anterior tibial region, particularly when stimuli that elicit central summation mechanisms are applied (Ashina et al., 2003). The probable explanation is that much more tenderness occurs in the postural muscles responsible for our continuous joint positioning, including holding an upright position; an example of these "static" muscles is the supraspinatus in the shoulder girdle. In contrast to the static postural muscles, the "phasic" muscles, such as the quadriceps, are used only for dynamic work. The higher sensitivity of the neck muscles to pain may partly explain the high prevalence of chronic pain arising in the neck and shoulder.

The neurologist and muscle specialist V. Janda clarified the distribution of these types of muscles using EMG and found that the static muscles are associated with the most frequent complaints in clinical

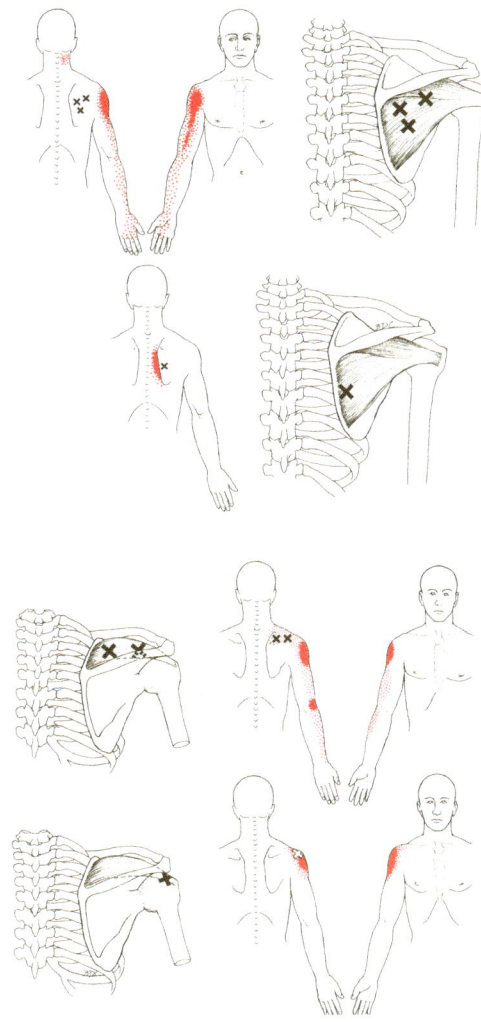

Fig. 1. Trigger points in muscles, with the area of pain referral. Trigger points are observed mainly in the static muscles, such as those of the scapula, and are relatively less frequent in phasic muscles, such as the quadriceps, corresponding to fewer changes in these muscles (top panel: infraspinatus, lower panel: supraspinatus). Reproduced with permission from Simons et al. (1999).

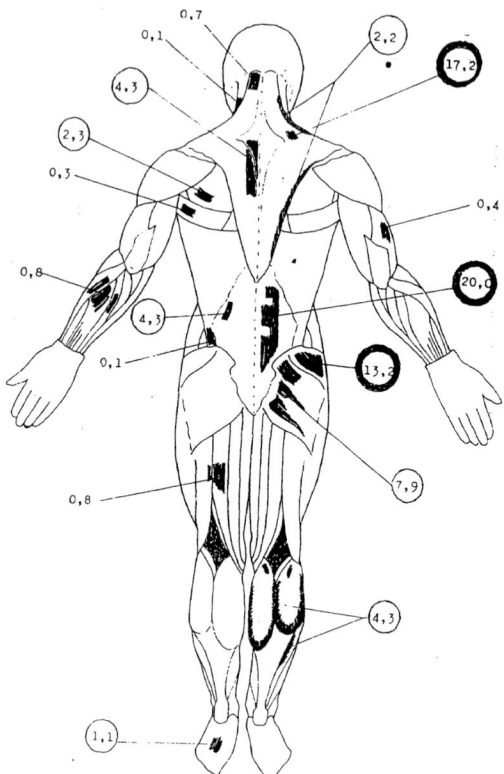

Fig. 2. Palpable defined, hard areas in muscles of individuals without muscle complaints (Clemmesen and Kalbak, 1938).

practice (Janda, 1968). Healthy persons without muscle complaints still have palpable muscle soreness at some locations, with a higher frequency of soreness in the static muscles (Fig. 2) (Clemmesen and Kalbak, 1938; Croft et al., 1994).

Pain Patterns from Joints

Patterns of pain originating from the joints have been studied mostly by stimulating the joints and recording the referred pain areas. For instance, the patterns of pain from the cervical zygapophysial joints have been studied by distending the joint capsule in healthy volunteers with injections of contrast medium under fluoroscopic control (Dwyer et al., 1990). Fig. 3 shows the resulting referred pain areas at the different zygapophysial joints. Recently, referred pain areas were determined in patients with zygapophysial joint pain as diagnosed by selective nerve blocks (Cooper et al., 2007). These data show that pain located at areas typically considered to be regions of myofascial pain syndromes can stem primarily from joints, rather than from muscles. This complication represents a diagnostic challenge for the identification of the source of pain.

Similar methods were used to study the referred pain pattern from the atlanto-axial and atlanto-occipital joints and the thoracic and lumbar zygapophysial joints, among others (Dreyfuss et al., 1994a,b; Fukui et al., 1997). A detailed description of these pain patterns is beyond the scope of this chapter. Interestingly, pain referral patterns consistently showed considerable overlap among adjacent joints, which in clinical practice precludes the identification of the symptomatic joint based only on the localization of pain.

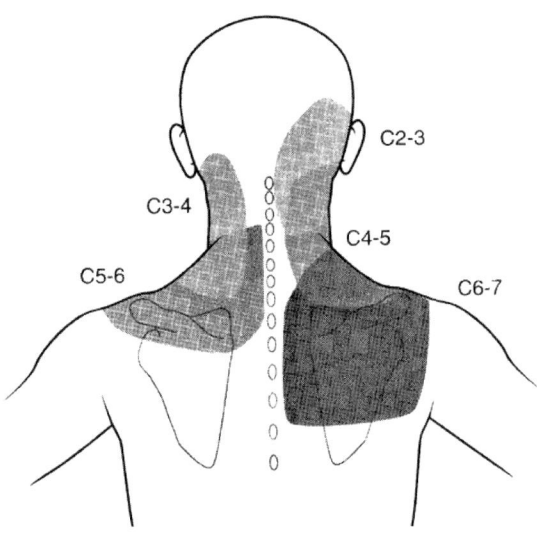

Fig. 3. Referred pain areas after distension of the zygapophysial joint capsule.

An important issue in chronic musculoskeletal disorders is diskogenic pain. Heat stimulation of lumbar intervertebral disks in patients with diskogenic pain produced pain at different areas, from the low back to the buttocks, the hip, and the distal regions of the leg (O'Neill et al., 2002). In that study, pain was evoked initially in the back and progressed distally with increasing stimulation temperature. This finding is consistent with the common experience that patients with low back pain frequently feel pain all the way down to their feet, particularly when the pain reaches high intensities.

Joint inflammation causes pain in the joint and the surrounding soft tissues, which are also under attack by inflammatory processes (Ostergaard and Szkudlarek 2001). The pain in and around the inflamed joint cannot be distinguished with certainty from muscle pain in the area. This is especially the case for pain in the shoulder region, where pain may be elicited in a number of diseases with an almost identical distribution of pain (Table I). In the shoulder, inflammatory vascular disease, i.e., polymyalgia and/or temporal arteritis, is a further confounder, and the shoulder represents a differential diagnostic challenge to the clinician (Ceccato et al., 2006). Soft tissue involvement is also seen to some extent in degenerative joint diseases, which are accompanied by varying degrees of pain.

Table I

Location	Type	Pain and Other Clinical Symptoms
Shoulder	Rotator cuff degeneration	Pain referred to the lateral aspects of upper arm, reduced active abduction
	Arthritis	As above plus resting pain and local signs of inflammation (dolor, rubor, calor, tumor)
	Polymyalgia rheumatica	Typical pain located to the trapezius from the shoulder toward the neck and lateral aspects of upper arm; reduced active abduction
Knee	Osteoarthritis, light	Pain after exercise
	Osteoarthritis, moderate	Pain triad: pain at the onset of exercise, relative relief with ambulation, and pain again with continued activity
	Osteoarthritis, severe	Pain on movement, resting pain
	Arthritis	Pain at rest and on movement; stiffness after rest, e.g., morning stiffness

In osteoarthritis, there is an intriguing lack of correlation between the local pain and the radiographic joint changes (Bagge et al., 1991); significant soft tissue problems may offer a greater chance of relief by nonsurgical disease modification, even in the presence of joint cartilage and bone degeneration (Abramson et al., 2006). Table I shows the most common joint disorders associated with muscle pain in the shoulder and knee.

Diagnostic Criteria

Muscle pain can be *localized* in a relatively confined area, typically to the elbow or shoulder, or it may be *generalized*, with involvement of extensive parts of the muscles, exemplified by the muscle pain in viral diseases such as influenza (Table II). Both the diagnostic considerations and treatment options are different in these two kinds of disease. It is of great importance for the choice of therapy and the chances of success to have a basic diagnostic differentiation between the various syndromes. There are no pathognomonic laboratory findings, and diagnostic tests remain semi-objective in the sense that the diagnosis is based on clinical examination, which requires collaboration between the patient and the clinician.

A *myofascial pain syndrome* is defined as a localized muscle pain, possibly accompanied by referred pain to another region. The extent of the pain in this case can be reliably provoked by palpatory stimulation of the trigger points of this muscle. Some of these syndromes are

Table II
Examples of primary and secondary muscle pain,
either localized or generalized

Examples	Primary (No Known Eliciting Factor)	Secondary
Localized	Unspecific low back pain	Myalgia (tender points) in extensor carpi-radialis brevis by epicondylitis lateralis humeri
Generalized, widespread	Fibromyalgia	Polymyalgia rheumatica

Note: Any patient should be characterized in this way during the diagnostic process.

very common, especially in work-related diseases such as rotator-cuff syndrome.

For the classification of *fibromyalgia* (FM), the American College of Rheumatology (Wolfe et al., 1990) has defined a standardized set of criteria, depending on duration and spread of painful symptoms and number of tender points (Fig. 4). However, a general examination of muscles both within and outside these areas should be performed. The diagnosis of FM remains clinical and cannot be restricted to patients fulfilling the classification criteria. There have been no longitudinal studies to demonstrate fluctuations in the intensity or number of tender points, although there are some indications that the prognosis is related to both of these factors (Carli et al., 2002; Gupta et al., 2007). Tender point examination follows the guidelines in the ACR criteria by application of 4 kg pressure to an area of about the size of a fingertip. For screening

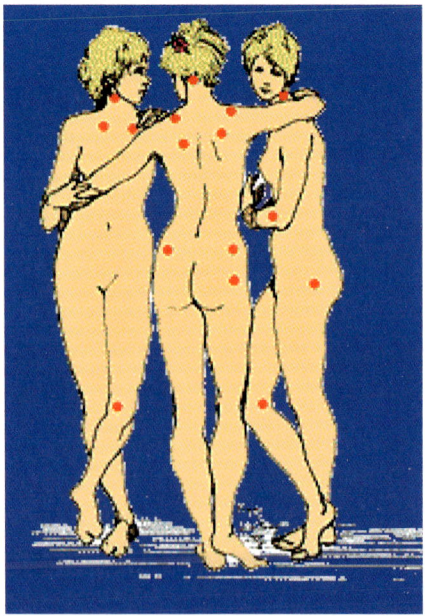

Fig. 4. Standardized 18 points to be examined in the screening for fibromyalgia. The classification requires 11 of 18 points to be significantly tender to a pressure of 4 kg/cm^2 corresponding to a fingertip pressure causing a white nail bed.

purposes this is quite enough, while in a research setting more elaborate measurements including thresholds for the pain sensation may be determined by pressure algometry (see Chapter 11, Graven-Nielsen and Arendt-Nielsen). While in the classifications criteria no exclusion diagnoses are given, the clinical practice of FM must screen for other medical diseases, which may be precipitate similar reactions.

A major problem is the identification of muscles as the primary source of pain, particularly when the currently available diagnostic tools are unable to detect evident pathology. In this respect, it is frequently difficult to ascertain whether pain felt in the muscles is the result of a pathology (or dysfunction) of those muscles or whether it represents referred pain. In the latter case, the origin of pain would be in another anatomical structure, such as a joint. Clinical examination cannot distinguish between the two conditions. For instance, tenderness at palpation can be the result of both primary muscle pain (peripheral sensitization) and referred pain (central sensitization).

For a diagnostic test to be valid, it should have acceptable sensitivity and specificity when tested against a gold standard. Such a standard is not available for the diagnosis of primary muscle pain. Consequently, we lack validated diagnostic tools for distinguishing between primary and referred muscle pain.

Conversely, certain types of joint pain can be reliably diagnosed. In particular, pain originating from the zygapophysial joints can be diagnosed by double-blind controlled blocks of the nerves that supply the joints. This method has both face validity and construct validity (Barnsley and Bogduk, 1993; Barnsley et al., 1993; Dreyfuss et al., 1997). This paradigm is based on the ability to selectively block the nerves that supply joints. Complete pain relief after injection of a local anesthetic, but not of a placebo, is an acceptable gold standard to which further tests can be compared. Unfortunately, there is lack of research on diagnostic blocks other than nerve blocks of the zygapophysial joints.

Differential Diagnosis

Given the high frequency of muscular pain syndromes, all cases should be subject to a careful clinical examination, as muscle pain may be a sign of serious medical conditions and possibly even a symptom of malignancy. A screening procedure may be performed, both clinically and biochemically, that is relatively complete and not lengthy or costly.

Suggested examples could involve:
- Determining whether the muscle pain is local, regional or widespread.
- In local cases: is the pain confined to the muscle or is it secondary to a joint problem or a tendinous change, or (if it is difficult to relate to a given structure) could it be referred from viscera? (Chapter 13, Giamberardino)
- Is the muscle or joint pain part of a generalized pain problem?
- Is there suspicion of a systemic medical disease? (For example, thyroid abnormalities may cause both local and widespread muscle pain.)

Table III
Medical diseases with muscle pain as possible symptom

Syndrome	Muscle Pain	Suggested Further Examination
Inflammatory muscle disease, vasculitis	Most often neck/shoulder	Blood tests: erythrocyte sedimentation rate and/or C-reactive protein
Heart disease	Neck/shoulder/arm	Heart auscultation, EKG
Diaphragmatic disease (e.g., pneumonia, gallstone)	Neck/shoulder	Heart auscultation, palpation of the abdomen
Intra-abdominal disease (e.g., duodenal ulceration, cancer of the pancreas)	Low thoracic or lumbar pain	Palpation, blood tests.
Gynecological diseases	Low back pain	Gynecological examination
Drug-induced muscle pain	Neck/shoulder or proximal extremity	Case history: onset related to medication. It may be necessary to withdraw statins or ACE inhibitors

Table IV
Blood tests of relevance for muscle pain

Blood Test	Possible Diseases with Muscle Pain as a Symptom
Hemoglobin, leucocyte count	Anemia, leucemia
Erythrocyte sedimentation rate or C-reactive protein	Systemic inflammation
Thyroid-stimulating hormone	Hypo- or hyperthyroidism
Alkaline phosphatase	Malignancy, bone marrow disease
Calcium	Hypocalcemia

Note: More seldom seen: amylases (pancreatic diseases), creatine kinase (myositis), other transaminases (liver disease), and antibodies against various viruses.

Important red flags:
- Central distribution of muscle and joint pain close to the body in neck/shoulder/pelvic areas
- Diffuse spread of the muscle pain
- Lack of a precipitating factor

Table III gives examples of medical diseases that may be accompanied by muscle pain, sometimes as the primary symptom. *Generalized disease* or truncal muscle pain without reason should lead to a full clinical examination along with supplementary blood tests, which will uncover most relevant diseases (Tables IV–V).

Table V
Supplementary blood tests of relevance for joint pain

Blood Test	Possible Disease with Joint Pain as a Symptom
Erythrocyte sedimentation rate or C-reactive protein	Inflammatory joint disease
Uric acid	Gout
Rheumatoid factor	Rheumatoid arthritis
Anticyclic citrullinated peptide (anti CCP)	Rheumatoid arthritis
Antinuclear antibodies (ANA)	Collagenoses, e.g., lupus erythematosus

Therapy

This section presents some principles and examples of treatment. Space does not permit a more comprehensive overview of the treatment of muscle and joint pain.

If a precipitating factor can be discerned, it is of course relevant to try to avoid it. It must be admitted that this can be very difficult, even when a full explanation of the pain problem is possible. For example, it may prove very difficult to make radical changes so as to avoid the many problems in the arms and shoulders due to computer work. On the other hand, any therapy for such problems that does not take action against the precipitating factors is likely to meet with a negative result. A basic therapy aims at restoring malfunctioning joints, even while these may be difficult to diagnose precisely. In the case of tendon pathology, this underlying problem must be treated before the muscle pain can be relieved.

General information has definite merit and should be part of all patient instruction and therapy because well-informed patients fare better, with an especially remarkable difference during long-term follow-up (Indahl et al., 1998).

Table VI
Meta-analyses of various treatments in low back pain

Technique	Reference	Effect Size
Cognitive-behavioral therapy	van Tulder et al., 2000	0.62 (95% CI 0.25, 0.98)
Transcutaneous nerve stimulation	van Tulder et al., 2006a	No
Exercise	van Tulder et al., 2006a	Short-term effect; no long-term effect
Back school	Heymans et al., 2005	No
Bed rest	Hagen et al., 2005	0.22 (95% CI 0.02–0.41)
Injections	Nelemans et al., 2001	No
Epidural injections	van Tulder et al., 2006b	No

Note: Only cognitive-behavioral therapy and back school have reached some evidence of a little effect, although not in long-term follow up. Only activity has been proven to shorten sick leave.

Systematic reviews have found little, if any, evidence of effect of any one therapy against muscle pain. With respect to effect size, some recent reviews and meta-analyses of common therapies are summarized in Table VI. In most cases, some degree of chronicity will develop, along with periodic deterioration. While conditions as low back pain and lateral elbow pain may improve over time (Indahl et al., 1998; Smidt et al., 2005), recurrences will be frequent if the eliciting factors—including lifestyle—are not changed to prevent them.

Treatments for low back pain have been meticulously investigated for effects, and the results are meager. While investigators have failed to demonstrate an effect of controlled trials of rest therapy on muscle pain, neither has this very common intervention been proven disadvantageous.

The principles for treatment, however, are influenced by the wish to maintain—or obtain—as high a level of functioning as possible with any given muscle pain disorder. Therefore, a certain amount of exercise should be added to whatever treatment might be chosen for the individual. The threshold for activity with respect to muscle pain should not be the level of pain sensation, but rather, if possible, the level at which there is a risk of harm to the muscle.

More passive therapies, such as massage or acupuncture, are in general regarded as pain therapies and can be used for limited periods to facilitate other therapies with more functional prospects. Medication for localized muscle pain is supported by very little literature, whereas more recent studies of medications acting on the central nervous system seem to be promising in the field of FM and widespread pain. Thus, both anticonvulsants and similar drugs used originally for neuropathic pain have shown a definite effect on both pain and function in FM (Table VII).

In selected cases in which the causes cannot be cured and conservative treatments fail, invasive procedures may be considered. There are indications that radiofrequency denervation of the cervical and lumbar zygapophysial joints may improve the quality of life of patients with chronic cervical zygapophyseal joint pain (Lord et al., 1996; van Kleef et al., 1999).

Table VII
Suggested therapies in muscle pain syndromes

Treatment	Evidence
Local Muscle Pain	
Eccentric exercise	Some evidence in Achilles tendon disease (Norregaard et al., 2007)
Massage	May lead to addiction. One study points to a specific effect in myalgia (Danneskiold-Samsoe et al., 1983)
Articulation, manipulation	May lead to addiction. Some effect in acute back pain, has no place in chronic treatment (van Tulder et al., 2006a)
No evidence of effect of: electrotherapy, short-wave, ultrasound, laser, injections of steroid or NSAIDs (Gam et al., 1993; Gam and Johannsen, 1995). Contradictory evidence of acupuncture, which should not be used for long-term therapy (Furlan et al., 2005)	
Generalized Muscle Pain, Including Fibromyalgia	
Exercise	May have some effect in low-back pain and in fibromyalgia (van Tulder et al., 2000; Busch et al., 2007)
Multidisciplinary and cognitive-behavioral treatment	No effect has been shown, possible effect on subgroups (Carville et al., 2007)
Muscle relaxants	Possible effect in low back pain (van Tulder et al., 2003)
Antidepressants (nonspecific)	Evidence of effect on fibromyalgia (O'Malley et al., 2000)
Anticonvulsants	Evidence of effect on fibromyalgia (Mease et al., 2008)
No proven/little effect of: NSAIDs, serotonin-reuptake-inhibitors (Carville et al., 2007)	

Prevention

The question of how to prevent muscle pain is extensive and cannot be dealt with here in detail. Some general remarks, however, can be given. The modern working environment is characterized by specialization; many office jobs require repetitive uniform maneuvers, such as using a mouse for computer work, as do many blue collar jobs, including those in health care. These tasks cause a number of overuse injuries that are very difficult to treat. Campaigns are launched to encourage workers to change their body position during the work day and give their muscles and joints a more varied activation pattern. Preventive measures against another main cause of chronic muscle problems, whiplash injuries, have not been successful. Indications have been presented that working environment and lifestyle factors are just as important for chronification as the injury itself. Secondary prevention with exercise rather than passive therapies helps to increase the functional level of the patient, whatever the outcome of the muscle injury might be. This change to a more active attitude has obvious face validity, although long-term results are still needed to provide evidence of a relevant change in the level of pain and function in patients with chronic musculoskeletal pain.

References

Abramson SB, Attur M, Yazici Y. Prospects for disease modification in osteoarthritis. Nat Clin Pract Rheumatol 2006;2:304–312.

Andersen JH, Gaardboe O. Prevalence of persistent neck and upper limb pain in a historical cohort of sewing machine operators. Am J Ind Med 1993;24:677–687.

Ashina S, Jensen R, Bendtsen L. Pain sensitivity in pericranial and extracranial regions. Cephalalgia 2003;23:456–462.

Bagge E, Bjelle A, Eden S, Svanborg A. Osteoarthritis in the elderly: clinical and radiological findings in 79 and 85 year olds. Ann Rheum Dis 1991;50:535–539.

Barnsley L, Bogduk N. Medial branch blocks are specific for the diagnosis of cervical zygapophyseal joint pain. Reg Anesth 1993;18:343–350.

Barnsley L, Lord S, Bogduk N. Comparative local anaesthetic blocks in the diagnosis of cervical zygapophysial joint pain. Pain 1993;55:99–106.

Bliddal H, Danneskiold-Samsoe B. Chronic widespread pain in the spectrum of rheumatological diseases. Best Pract Res Clin Rheumatol 2007;21:391–402.

Breivik H, Collett B, Ventafridda V, Cohen R, Gallacher D. Survey of chronic pain in Europe: prevalence, impact on daily life, and treatment. Eur J Pain 2006;10:287–333.

Buckwalter JA. Sports, joint injury, and posttraumatic osteoarthritis. J Orthop Sports Phys Ther 2003;33:578–588.

Busch AJ, Barber KA, Overend TJ, Peloso PM, Schachter CL. Exercise for treating fibromyalgia syndrome. Cochrane Database Syst Rev 2007;CD003786.

Carli G, Suman AL, Biasi G, Marcolongo R. Reactivity to superficial and deep stimuli in patients with chronic musculoskeletal pain. Pain 2002;100:259–269.

Ceccato F, Roverano SG, Papasidero S, Barrionuevo A, Rillo OL, Paira SO. Peripheral musculoskeletal manifestations in polymyalgia rheumatica. J Clin Rheumatol 2006;12:167–171.

Clemmesen S, Kalbak K. Bevægelsessystemets rheumatiske sygdomme. Copenhagen: Store Nordiske Videnskabsboghandel; 1938.

Cooper G, Bailey B, Bogduk N. Cervical zygapophysial joint pain maps. Pain Med 2007;8:344–353.

Croft P, Schollum J, Silman A. Population study of tender point counts and pain as evidence of fibromyalgia. BMJ 1994;309:696–699.

Curatolo M, Arendt-Nielsen L, Petersen-Felix S. Evidence, mechanisms, and clinical implications of central hypersensitivity in chronic pain after whiplash injury. Clin J Pain 2004;20:469–476.

Danneskiold-Samsoe B, Christiansen E, Lund B, Andersen RB. Regional muscle tension and pain ("fibrositis"). Effect of massage on myoglobin in plasma. Scand J Rehabil Med 1983;15:17–20.

Dreyfuss P, Michaelsen M, Fletcher D. Atlanto-occipital and lateral atlanto-axial joint pain patterns. Spine 1994;19:1125–1131.

Dreyfuss P, Schwarzer AC, Lau P, Bogduk N. Specificity of lumbar medial branch and L5 dorsal ramus blocks. A computed tomography study. Spine 1997;22:895–902.

Dreyfuss P, Tibiletti C, Dreyer SJ. Thoracic zygapophyseal joint pain patterns. A study in normal volunteers. Spine 1994;19:807–811.

Dwyer A, Aprill C, Bogduk N. Cervical zygapophyseal joint pain patterns. I: A study in normal volunteers. Spine 1990;15:453–457.

Fukui S, Ohseto K, Shiotani M, Ohno K, Karasawa H, Naganuma Y. Distribution of referred pain from the lumbar zygapophyseal joints and dorsal rami. Clin J Pain 1997;13:303–307.

Furlan AD, van Tulder M, Cherkin D, Tsukayama H, Lao L, Koes B, Berman B. Acupuncture and dry-needling for low back pain: an updated systematic review within the framework of the Cochrane Collaboration. Spine 2005;30:944–963.

Gam AN, Johannsen F. Ultrasound therapy in musculoskeletal disorders: a meta-analysis. Pain 1995;63:85–91.

Gam AN, Thorsen H, Lonnberg F. The effect of low-level laser therapy on musculoskeletal pain: a meta-analysis. Pain 1993;52:63–66.

Graven-Nielsen T, Mense S. The peripheral apparatus of muscle pain: evidence from animal and human studies. Clin J Pain 2001;17:2–10.

Gupta A, McBeth J, Macfarlane GJ, Morriss R, Dickens C, Ray D, Chiu YH, Silman AJ. Pressure pain thresholds and tender point counts as predictors of new chronic widespread pain in somatising subjects. Ann Rheum Dis 2007;66:517–521.

Hagen KB, Jamtvedt G, Hilde G, Winnem MF. The updated Cochrane review of bed rest for low back pain and sciatica. Spine 2005;30:542–546.

Heymans MW, van Tulder MW, Esmail R, Bombardier C, Koes BW. Back schools for nonspecific low back pain: a systematic review within the framework of the Cochrane Collaboration Back Review Group. Spine 2005;30:2153–2163.

Indahl A, Haldorsen EH, Holm S, Reikeras O, Ursin H. Five-year follow-up study of a controlled clinical trial using light mobilization and an informative approach to low back pain. Spine 1998;23:2625–2630.

Janda V. The significance of muscular faulty posture as pathogenetic factor of vertebral disorders. Arch Phys Ther (Leipz) 1968;20:113–116.

Kidd BL. Osteoarthritis and joint pain. Pain 2006;123:6–9.

Lord SM, Barnsley L, Wallis BJ, McDonald GJ, Bogduk N. Percutaneous radio-frequency neurotomy for chronic cervical zygapophyseal-joint pain. N Engl J Med 1996;335:1721–1726.

Mease PJ, Russell IJ, Arnold LM, Florian H, Young JP Jr, Martin SA, Sharma U. A randomized, double-blind, placebo-controlled, phase III trial of pregabalin in the treatment of patients with fibromyalgia. J Rheumatol 2008;35:502–514.

Nelemans PJ, deBie RA, de Vet HC, Sturmans F. Injection therapy for subacute and chronic benign low back pain. Spine 2001;26:501–515.

Norregaard J, Larsen CC, Bieler T, Langberg H. Eccentric exercise in treatment of Achilles tendinopathy. Scand J Med Sci Sports 2007;17:133–138.

O'Malley PG, Balden E, Tomkins G, Santoro J, Kroenke K, Jackson JL. Treatment of fibromyalgia with antidepressants: a meta-analysis. J Gen Intern Med 2000;15:659–666.

O'Neill CW, Kurgansky ME, Derby R, Ryan DP. Disc stimulation and patterns of referred pain. Spine 2002;27:2776–2781.

Ostergaard M, Szkudlarek M. Magnetic resonance imaging of soft tissue changes in rheumatoid arthritis wrist joints. Semin Musculoskelet Radiol 2001;5:257–274.

Shah JP, Danoff JV, Desai MJ, Parikh S, Nakamura LY, Phillips TM, Gerber LH. Biochemicals associated with pain and inflammation are elevated in sites near to and remote from active myofascial trigger points. Arch Phys Med Rehabil 2008;89:16–23.

Shiri R, Viikari-Juntura E, Varonen H, Heliovaara M. Prevalence and determinants of lateral and medial epicondylitis: a population study. Am J Epidemiol 2006;164:1065–1074.

Simons DG, Travell JG, Simons LS. Myofascial pain and dysfunction, the trigger point manual. Baltimore: Williams & Wilkins; 1999.

Smidt N, Lewis M, Hay EM, van der Windt DA, Bouter LM, Croft P. A comparison of two primary care trials on tennis elbow: issues of external validity. Ann Rheum Dis 2005;64:1406–1409.

van Kleef M, Barendse GA, Kessels A, Voets HM, Weber WE, de Lange S. Randomized trial of radiofrequency lumbar facet denervation for chronic low back pain. Spine 1999;24:1937–1942.

van Tulder MW, Koes B, Malmivaara A. Outcome of non-invasive treatment modalities on back pain: an evidence-based review. Eur Spine J 2006a;15(Suppl 1):S64–S81.

van Tulder MW, Koes B, Seitsalo S, Malmivaara A. Outcome of invasive treatment modalities on back pain and sciatica: an evidence-based review. Eur Spine J 2006b;15(Suppl 1):S82–S92.

van Tulder MW, Ostelo R, Vlaeyen JW, Linton SJ, Morley SJ, Assendelft WJ. Behavioral treatment for chronic low back pain: a systematic review within the framework of the Cochrane Back Review Group. Spine 2000;25:2688–2699.

van Tulder M, Malmivaara A, Esmail R, Koes B. Exercise therapy for low back pain: a systematic review within the framework of the Cochrane Collaboration Back Review Group. Spine 2000;25:2784–2796.

van Tulder MW, Touray T, Furlan AD, Solway S, Bouter LM. Muscle relaxants for nonspecific low back pain: a systematic review within the framework of the Cochrane Collaboration. Spine 2003;28:1978–1992.

Wolfe F, Smythe HA, Yunus MB, Bennett RM, Bombardier C, Goldenberg DL, Tugwell P, Campbell SM, Abeles M, Clark P. The American College of Rheumatology 1990 criteria for the classification of fibromyalgia. Report of the Multicenter Criteria Committee. Arthritis Rheum 1990;33:160–172.

Correspondence to: Henning Bliddal, DMSc, The Parker Institute, Frederiksberg Hospital, Ndr Fasanvej 57, 2000 Frederiksberg, Denmark. Email: hb@frh. regionh.dk.

Translational Aspects of Musculoskeletal Pain: From Animals to Patients

Lars Arendt-Nielsen and Thomas Graven-Nielsen

Department of Health Sciences and Technology, Center for Sensory-Motor Interaction, Aalborg University, Aalborg, Denmark

Studies in animals or healthy volunteers cannot be translated directly into clinical applications or act as proxies for clinical conditions, but they can provide mechanistic knowledge to enhance our fundamental understanding of clinical signs and symptoms. Such translational steps can provide the theoretical basis for developing better diagnostic tools and targeted drugs to improve the treatment of disabling chronic musculoskeletal pain conditions.

Over the last 25 years, pain research has mainly focused on sensitization of nociceptors in the periphery, sensitization of dorsal horn neurons, changes in functionality of neurotransmitter regulatory processes, and phenotypic changes. The non-neuronal component of neuronal sensitization, including the involvement of glial cells, is currently a major target in drug discovery. Pain researchers first turned their attention to glia in the early 1990s when Garrison et al. (1991) reported that peripheral nerve damage activated spinal cord glia. Today, drug companies are competing to develop the first useful drug for this target. Research attention to this area in musculoskeletal pain is still limited, but work has begun in animals (Tenschert et al., 2004).

The obvious translation between animal models of nerve injury and the clinical manifestation of neuropathic pain has caused a prioritization of clinical pain research and drug development in this area. Neuropathic pain occurs in only 2–3% of the population, whereas musculoskeletal pain is far more prevalent. Translational work on musculoskeletal pain research thus has enormous potential to benefit a large section of the population.

This chapter will focus on some of the fundamental musculoskeletal pain mechanisms that can be translated from animals via experimental human studies to patients with musculoskeletal pain. These mechanisms are related to peripheral sensitization, central sensitization (expanded receptive fields), facilitated central integration, and disturbed descending modulation. Other chapters provide details of these mechanisms and their manifestations, so this chapter will focus on translational issues.

Translational Aspects of Peripheral Sensitization

Changes in the excitability of peripheral receptors have attracted the most research interest because signs of peripheral sensitization are clearly seen in patients.

Animal Studies

Muscle group III and IV nociceptors often respond to algesic chemical stimulation, for example to intramuscular (i.m.) or intra-arterial injections of bradykinin, serotonin, histamine, hypertonic saline (Fig. 1), or potassium ions (see Chapter 1, Mense and Hoheisel and Chapter 11, Graven-Nielsen and Arendt-Nielsen). Muscle nociception is normally evoked by overuse, trauma, or inflammation. Damaged muscle tissue releases substances including potassium ions, prostaglandin E_2, bradykinin, serotonin, and adenosine triphosphate (ATP), and nerve endings release neuropeptides such as substance P (SP), calcitonin gene-related peptide (CGRP), and somatostatin (Molander et al., 1987). Most of the sensitizing

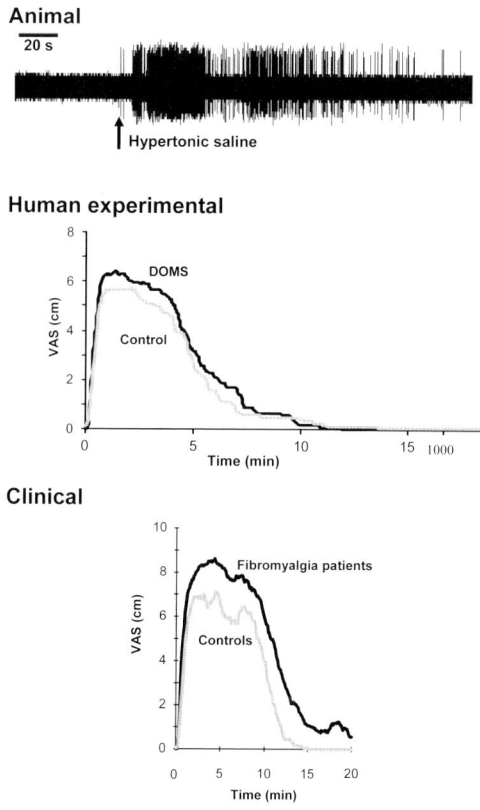

Fig. 1. Translational manifestations related to excitation of muscle nociceptors in animal studies, in experimental human studies, and in patients. *Animal:* Neuronal activity of muscle nociceptor after application of hypertonic saline (5%, 25 μL). Recording provided by courtesy of S. Mense. *Human experimental:* Mean visual analogue scale (VAS) scores ($N = 12$) after injections of hypertonic saline into the extensor carpi radialis brevis muscle of the exercised arm with delayed-onset muscle soreness (DOMS) and the control arm. The maximal VAS score was significantly higher for saline-induced pain in the DOMS arm compared with the control arm. Based on data from Slater et al. (2003). *Clinical:* Mean VAS scores ($N = 12$) following infusion of hypertonic saline (2.8 mL over 480 seconds) into the tibialis anterior muscle in controls and fibromyalgia patients. The area below the VAS-time curve is significantly larger for fibromyalgia patients compared with age- and sex-matched control subjects. Based on data from Sörensen el al. (1998).

substances released in muscles are similar to those released in other tissues, but ATP seems more specific for muscles as it reaches high concentrations in muscle cells. During muscle inflammation, the density of nerve endings containing SP and nerve growth factor increases (Reinert et al., 1998).

When the muscle is in a state of hyperalgesia or allodynia, the sensitized muscle nociceptors are more easily activated and may respond to weak,
normally innocuous stimuli such as light pressure and muscle movement (Fig. 2).

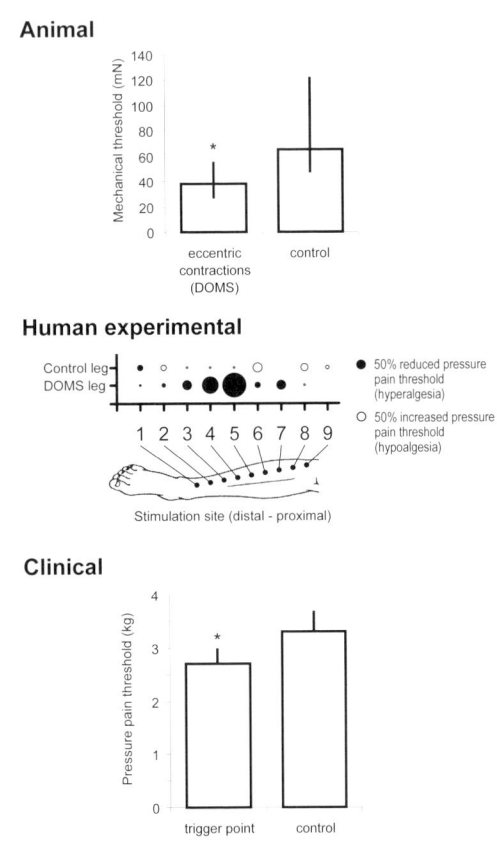

Fig. 2. Translational manifestations related to peripheral sensitization in animal studies, in
experimental human studies, and in patients. *Animal:* The mechanical threshold (median
and interquartile range, $N = 25–33$) for excitation of rat muscle nociceptors is significantly
decreased (* $P < 0.05$) 2 days after eccentric muscle contractions were performed to induce delayed-onset muscle soreness (DOMS). Based on data from Chapter 4, Mizumura.
Human experimental: Sites of hyperalgesia to pressure stimulation after DOMS was induced by eccentric exercise in one subject. Each circle represents the change of pressure
pain thresholds for the DOMS leg and the control leg. The width of the circles represents
the amount of either hyperalgesia (filled circles) or hypoalgesia (open circles) compared
with pre-exercise recordings taken 2 days previously. One site with extensive hyperalgesia
is located close to a site with no or very little change in the deep tissue sensitivity. Based on
data from Andersen et al. (2006). *Clinical:* Subjects with myofascial trigger points had significantly (* $P < 0.05$) decreased pressure pain threshold (mean + SEM, $N = 12$) compared
with neighboring sites without a trigger point (H. Andersen, unpublished observations).

Human Experimental Studies

Microneurographic recordings in volunteers have shown that the responses of human muscle nociceptors to injections of algesic substances were very similar to those of nociceptors in rats or cats (Marchettini et al., 1996). Experimental induction and assessment of pain and peripheral sensitization in humans can be performed by a variety of chemical (Fig. 1), mechanical, thermal, and electrical methods (Fig. 2, see Chapter 11, Graven-Nielsen and Arendt-Nielsen). Generally, the induced sensitization is brief, but it may still mimic some of the signs and symptom seen in patients. Assessment possibilities are limited, so in most cases it is difficult to differentiate between peripheral and central manifestations.

Brief muscle hyperalgesia (lasting only minutes) can be evoked by i.m. injections of capsaicin, glutamate, or a combination of serotonin (5-HT) and bradykinin. Ernberg et al., (2000) found that i.m. co-injection of 5-HT and the $5-HT_3$-receptor antagonist granisetron reduced the spontaneous pain evoked by injection of 5-HT and prevented hyperalgesia to mechanical pressure stimuli. Thus, peripheral serotonergic receptors could be involved in regulating musculoskeletal pain disorders. Glutamate receptors are known to be involved in muscle pain because glutamate-evoked pain can be reduced by coadministration of an NMDA antagonist (Cairns et al., 2006).

Brief muscle hyperalgesia that lasts for a few days can be induced if a muscle is eccentrically exercised; it will become sore after 1–2 days (Fig. 2). This model of delayed-onset muscle soreness (DOMS) causes hyperalgesia to pressure and has been used as a model of muscle hyperalgesia in patients (Slater et al., 2003). Interestingly, increased sensitivity to pressure was detected at different sites among subjects (Andersen et al., 2006); these localized spots of hyperalgesia might be linked to the initial mechanisms for hyperalgesic trigger points in myofascial pain patients.

Long-lasting muscle hyperalgesia that persists for about a week can be induced in healthy subjects by i.m. injection of nerve growth factor (Svensson et al., 2003). In this case, the hyperalgesia might be related to central sensitization (Hoheisel et al., 2007).

Clinical Studies

Muscle damage and inflammation of deep tissue are typical examples of conditions likely to involve peripheral sensitization. Peripheral sensitization may also contribute to the manifestation of trigger points in myofascial pain patients (Simons et al., 1999). Increased sensitivity of trigger points has often been assessed by pressure or electrical i.m. stimulation (Vecchiet et al., 1994). The continued presence of hyperalgesia (temporal summation) and the presence of multiple hyperalgesic points (spatial summation) might sensitize the spinal cord and supraspinal structures by the continued nociceptive afferent barrage to the central nervous system (CNS).

Translational Aspects of Central Sensitization

In animals it is possible to assess the expansion of the receptive fields of dorsal horn neurons. In humans, the spread of pain over time as well as referred pain are important proxies to assess (Fig. 3). Pain involving central sensitization and related mechanisms is a therapeutic challenge and unfortunately few patients with musculoskeletal pain gain complete relief after even the most advanced treatments. Better understanding of the underlying mechanisms is thus crucial for developing rational management protocols.

Animal Studies

Animal experiments suggest that expansion of receptive fields is brought about by the opening of "silent" (ineffective) synapses in the spinal cord by nociceptive input from muscle (Hoheisel et al., 1994). Neurokinin-1 (NK-1) and N-methyl-D-aspartate (NMDA) receptors are involved in this process (Hoheisel et al., 1997a). Within 2 hours after induction of experimental myositis, a local anesthetic block of the muscle afferents can prevent the development of central sensitization. If the block is given later (2 to 4 hours after induction of myositis), it has no influence on the development of central sensitization (Hoheisel et al., 1997b). This

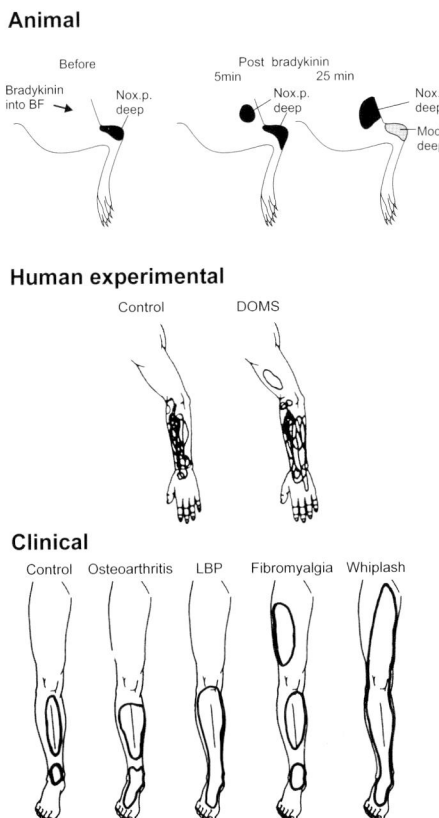

Fig. 3. Translational manifestations related to expansion of receptive fields (central sensitization) in animal studies, in experimental human studies, and in patients. *Animal:* Appearance of new receptive fields in rat dorsal horn neurons following noxious stimulation of skeletal muscle. Receptive field properties of a dorsal horn neuron following intramuscular injection of a painful dose of bradykinin into the biceps femoris (BF). Location and size of the original receptive field before bradykinin injection (left) and after a few minutes (right); note that one new receptive field has developed. Nox. p. deep = noxious deep pressure; mod. p. deep = moderate deep pressure. Modified from Hoheisel et al. (1993). *Human experimental:* Superimposed areas of experimental pain in 12 subjects after injections of hypertonic saline into the extensor carpi radialis brevis muscle of an exercised arm (DOMS) and the control arm. There was a trend ($P = 0.06$) for larger areas of saline-induced pain in the DOMS arm compared with the control arm. Based on data from Slater et al. (2003). *Clinical:* Examples of normal and abnormal referred pain patterns. The normal referred pattern following bolus injection of hypertonic saline in the anterior tibialis muscle is projected around the ankle joint. In patients with chronic musculoskeletal pain (osteoarthritis, low back pain [LBP], fibromyalgia, or whiplash), the same injection caused a highly abnormal referred pain pattern where the pain also spread in the proximal direction.

finding underlines the importance of delivering early and effective analgesic therapy so as to prevent central hyperexcitability.

As with other tissues, when a muscle is in a state of hyperalgesia or allodynia, its sensitized nociceptors are more easily activated and may respond to weak, normally innocuous stimuli such as light pressure or muscle movement. Animal studies have found that new receptive fields develop after noxious muscle stimuli are applied (Hoheisel et al., 1993). In the context of referred pain, the emergence of new receptive fields could be the mechanism behind referred pain due to central sensitization or hyperexcitability (Mense, 1994; Graven-Nielsen, 2006). The forming of new receptive fields is suggested to underlie the phenomenon of secondary hyperalgesia in deep tissue. Furthermore, an expansion of the receptive fields proximal to the normal receptive field was found in a study where experimental myositis was induced, and afterwards application of antagonists to three different neurokinin receptors was effective in preventing hyperexcitability (Sessle et al., 1986). An important factor, not yet substantiated in patients, is the contralateral spread of sensitization after localized muscle trauma (Sluka et al., 2003).

Human Experimental Studies

Referred pain is a pain sensation that is perceived at an area other than the site of nociceptive stimulation; it may arise from central spinal and other sensitization events. Referred pain patterns have been described using experimental stimuli applied to different structures, mostly muscles, joints, and viscera. It is still controversial whether hyperalgesia is present in referred muscle pain areas; Kellgren (1938) and Feinstein et al. (1954) found hyperalgesia, Steinbrocker et al. (1953) found no changes, and Graven-Nielsen et al. (1997b, 1998) found hypoalgesia to pressure. In the area of referred pain from osteoarthritis of the knee, trophic changes in the skin have been found (Galletti et al., 1990).

Referred muscle pain is probably a combination of central processing and peripheral input because it is possible to induce referred pain in limbs with complete sensory loss resulting from an anesthetic block (Laursen et al., 1999). The size of the area of referred pain is correlated with the intensity of the muscle pain. Referred pain begins 20–40 seconds later than local muscle pain (Graven-Nielsen et al., 1997b; Laursen et al., 1997). This delay indicates that a time-dependent process, perhaps the unmasking of new synaptic connections, is involved in the neural mediation of referred pain. Saline-induced referred pain occurs less frequently in healthy subjects treated with ketamine compared with a placebo treatment (Schulte et al., 2003), indicating the involvement of central sensitization.

Clinical Studies

The manifestations of expanded receptive fields (central sensitization) in chronic musculoskeletal pain conditions have been less studied, probably because those patient groups have not been recognized to the same degree as patients with neuropathic pain due to the difficulties in assessing chronic syndromes such as fibromyalgia. The assessment of musculoskeletal pain requires quantitative tests. Laursen et al. (2005) showed generalized sensitization to pressure stimulation (reduced pressure pain thresholds) in chronic musculoskeletal and visceral pain conditions. The more widespread a musculoskeletal pain problem becomes, the more numerous are the sensory abnormalities observed(Carli et al., 2002).

Besides standard clinical examinations, a simple clinical tool to assess pain in patients is the use of pain drawings to illustrate the localization and extent of myofascial pain areas. Pain intensity during rest and movement can be assessed on a visual analogue scale, pain quality using the McGill Pain Questionnaire, and quality of life using an assessment tool such as Short Form 36 of the Medical Outcomes Study Health Survey. Information on concomitant sites of pain has been largely neglected, even though their presence points to the involvement of widespread pathophysiological mechanisms. More advanced signs can be increased hyperalgesic reaction to cutaneous capsaicin in fibromyalgia (Morris et al., 1998) or rheumatoid arthritis (Morris et al., 1997), increased numbers of trigger points in osteoarthritis (Bajaj et al., 2001b), or spread of pain over time in lateral epicondylitis (Slater et al., 2005; Fernándcz-Carnero et al., 2007). Central sensitization in patients with fibromyalgia or whiplash patients is also suggested based on increased nociceptive withdrawal reflexes in those patients compared with controls (Banic et al., 2004).

Patients with fibromyalgia, compared with healthy subjects, experience stronger pain intensity (Fig. 1) and larger referred areas (Fig. 3) after i.m. injection of hypertonic saline in the leg (Sörensen et al., 1998); patients had no spontaneous leg pain. Results were similar in studies on other chronic musculoskeletal pain syndromes, such as whiplash (Johansen et al., 1999), knee osteoarthritis (Bajaj et al., 2001a), and low back pain (O'Neill et al., 2007). Expansion of the referred areas in fibromyalgia patients was prevented by ketamine (Graven-Nielsen et al., 2000). This finding may indicate generalized sensitization in those patient populations (Arendt-Nielsen and Graven-Nielsen, 2003).

Viscerosomatic hyperalgesia can be seen in patients with conditions such as urinary calculosis. In these patients, pain thresholds to electrical muscular stimulation in referred pain areas were significantly lower on the side with calculosis than on the control side (Vecchiet et al., 1989). In patients with urinary calculosis, those experiencing a larger number of colics showed more hyperalgesia than those having a limited number of episodes (Giamberardino et al., 2005). Similar somatic hyperalgesia is found in referred pain areas in acute appendicitis (Stawowy et al., 2002) and cholecystolithiasis (Stawowy et al., 2005). Patients who had previously suffered from renal colics but had spontaneously eliminated the stone a long time (3–10 years) ago still showed marked muscle hyperalgesia (Vecchiet et al., 1992). This finding suggests that once the central sensitization is established it may persist, becoming relatively independent of the primary triggering event (see Giamberardino et al., 1999). This view is still controversial, although a subsequent study also showed that a certain amount of hyperalgesia remains for quite some time after cessation of the spontaneous pain (Coderre et al., 1993). More than 100 years ago, Sturge (1883) noted that attacks of angina are associated with a persistent tenderness after the attack.

Mechanisms of referred somatic hyperalgesia can be explained on the basis of the convergence-projection theory where visceral and somatic afferent fibers converge upon the same neurons in the CNS. There is a great deal of experimental support for the existence of viscerosomatic convergence at various levels of the CNS (see Cervero, 1995). The pathophysiological basis of referred visceral pain with hyperalgesia is incompletely understood. Similar to the changes found in areas of referred muscle pain, trophic changes of the skin occur in areas of referred visceral pain (Giamberardino et al., 2005).

Translational Aspects of Temporal Integration

Repeated neural firing will lead to temporal integration in dorsal horn neurons and enhanced nociceptive responses. As a result, more pain is perceived (see Fig. 4).

Animal Studies

Repeated strong C-fiber stimulation of somatic nociceptive fibers causes a frequency-dependent increase in neuronal excitability that outlasts the stimuli. The response of spinal cord neurons to successive stimuli of this type is a progressive increase in the magnitude of the Aδ- and C-fiber input (Schouenborg and Sjolund, 1983), often followed by the development of afterdischarge. Wind-up has been used as a model of neural plasticity and central sensitization in the spinal cord. Postsynaptic actions of the neurotransmitters released by repeated noxious stimuli, such as SP and glutamate, can contribute to the enhanced excitability.

Wind-up and central sensitization are not identical phenomena. Wind-up does not persist for a long time after stimulation, whereas sensitization can be long-lasting. Nonetheless, there are apparent similarities in transmitters and pathways underlying wind-up and sensitization, and wind-up initiates and maintains central sensitization (Woolf, 1996). Wind-up increases the receptive field area of dorsal horn neurons (Cervero et al., 1984); this expansion of receptive field area is a feature of central sensitization.

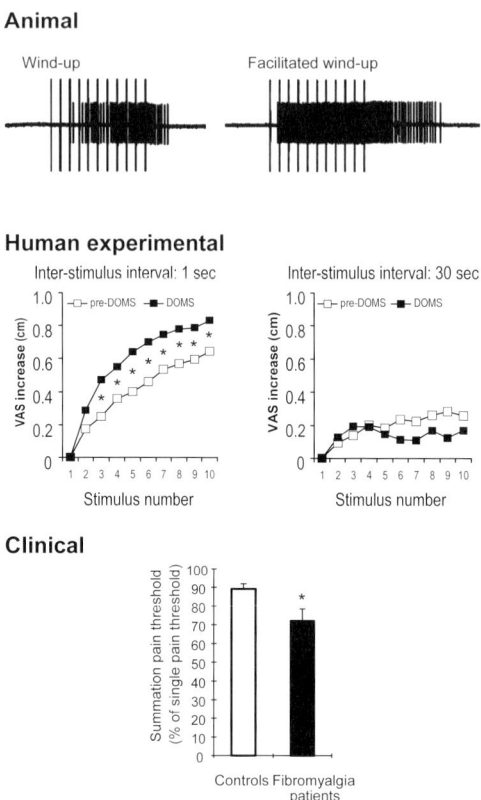

Fig. 4. Translational manifestations related to temporal integration in animal, experimental human and patients. *Animal:* Activity of dorsal horn neurons (wide-dynamic range, recorded in spinalized, anesthetized rats) related to peripheral nociceptive electrical stimulation (1 Hz). The wind-up phenomenon is facilitated after peripheral nociceptors are activated by bee venom and the central neurons are sensitized. Modified from You et al. (2003). *Human experimental:* Mean visual analogue scale (VAS) scores (N = 16) after pressure stimuli applied to the trapezius muscle with 1-second and 30-seconds interstimulus intervals at an intensity equal to the pressure pain threshold for each stimulation. The subject scored the pain intensity on a VAS after each stimulus. Temporal summation was clearly seen for the 1-second interstimulus interval by the increase in VAS scores during sequential stimulation. Temporal summation was significantly (* P < 0.05) facilitated in the condition of delayed-onset muscle soreness (DOMS) 1 day after eccentric muscle contractions. Based on data from Nie el al. (2006). *Clinical:* Mean (+ SEM, N = 12) summation pain thresholds determined by intramuscular electrical stimulations in the tibialis anterior muscle. Temporal summation was significantly more expressed in fibromyalgia patients compared with age- and sex-matched control subjects. Based on data from Sörensen el al. (1998).

Human Experimental Studies

In human studies, the initial phase of the wind-up process can be measured by increased pain response to consecutive stimuli. Various modalities have been used to induce temporal summation in muscles (electrical stimulation, pressure, or algesic substances; see Chapter 11, Graven-Nielsen and Arendt-Nielsen). Temporal summation of pain stimuli applied to skin, joint, and muscle showed the highest reproducibility for muscle tissue (Wright et al., 2002). If i.m. chemical stimulations are repeated, the pain will increase and at the same time the referred pain area will expand (Graven-Nielsen et al., 1997a). Increased temporal summation to pressure is found under experimental conditions with experimentally induced muscle hyperalgesia (Nie et al., 2006).

Clinical Studies

Muscular temporal stimulation is significantly facilitated in patients with fibromyalgia (Sörensen et al., 1998) and chronic whiplash pain (Curatolo et al., 2001) compared with controls. Facilitated temporal summation suggests the involvement of central sensitization in patients with chronic musculoskeletal pain (Arendt-Nielsen and Graven-Nielsen, 2003). Recently, the increased efficacy of temporal summation in fibromyalgia patients has been reproduced with cutaneous heat stimulation (Staud et al., 2001). This finding indicates that the sensitization in fibromyalgia is not tissue specific. In a study in fibromyalgia patients, the exaggerated temporal summation was partly inhibited by ketamine (Graven-Nielsen et al., 2000).

Translational Aspects of Descending Modulation

In previous studies on descending modulation, the main focus has been on the descending inhibitory modulation of spinal nociceptive processes. However, emerging evidence indicates that descending facilitation, and hence the balance between inhibition and facilitation, is just as important.

Animal Studies

Inhibitory control of nociceptive neuronal excitability in animals is sub-served by inhibitory circuits operating principally at the segmental lev-el and by pathways that originate at higher (central) levels, such as the cerebral cortex, thalamus, and brainstem. These pathways include the periaqueductal gray (PAG), the raphe nuclei, and the rostroventral me-dial medulla (RVM). One manifestation of inhibitory influences, known as diffuse noxious inhibitory control (DNIC), has been explored mostly in the spinal system and is reported to be selectively expressed on "con-vergent" or wide-dynamic-range (WDR) nociceptive neurons (Millan, 2002). The inhibitory bulbospinal pathways are serotoninergic and inhib-it the activity of WDR neurons of the spinal dorsal horn, but additional nonserotoninergic mechanisms are also involved, including endogenous opioid pathways.

Descending facilitatory influences on nociceptive neuronal ex-citability are manifested via pathways that originate in the midbrain and brainstem structures. The PAG, raphe nuclei, and RVM are key struc-tures in the descending modulatory repertoire. Together, the descending facilitatory and inhibitory networks allow for the bidirectional control of spinal cord activity in processing nociceptive information (Millan, 2002; Vanegas and Schaible, 2004).

Human Experimental Studies

In human experimental and clinical studies it is not possible to dissociate the two competing systems—inhibition and facilitation. It is only pos-sible to assess the net effect. Most human studies have addressed DNIC, although the results may reflect influences other than DNIC alone. Pain-ful heterotopic conditioning by means of tonic thermal, mechanical, electrical, or chemical stimuli decreases pain perception induced by pha-sic noxious stimulation given elsewhere in the body (Arendt-Nielsen and Gotliebsen, 1992; Graven-Nielsen et al., 1998; Bouhassira et al., 2003). One study found that μ-opioid receptors were activated in multiple cor-tical and subcortical brain regions during saline-induced muscle pain; for example, μ-opioid receptor availability in the amygdala was reduced by muscle pain and was negatively correlated with pain intensity (Zubieta et al., 2001). The amygdala is known to be involved in antinociception via descending inhibition (Millan, 2002).

Many of the conditions associated with impaired DNIC have a female predominance. Experimental studies have shown that females show less efficient inhibition as compared with males (Ge et al., 2004), indicating that gender may be an important parameter. Moreover, μ-opioid receptor availability in the amygdala during saline-induced muscle pain is higher in females compared to males (Zubieta et al., 2002), illustrating a more pronounced hypoalgesic effect in men compared to women (Ge et al., 2004). In a later study, Zubieta et al. (2003) reported that the level of μ-opioid receptor activation during saline-induced muscle pain was related to genetic variations. This possibility might add to the variability of somatosensory changes in experimental muscle pain studies.

Clinical Studies

DNIC-like mechanisms are less efficient in musculoskeletal pain conditions such with myofascial temporomandibular disorder (Bragdon et al., 2002), chronic low back pain (Peters et al., 1992), fibromyalgia (Kosek and Hansson, 1997), painful osteoarthritis (Kosek and Ordeberg, 2000), and chronic tension-type headaches (Sandrini et al., 2006). Interestingly, the patients in the osteoarthritis study initially had deficient DNIC-like pain inhibition but showed normal inhibition when pain-free after having surgery relieve their pain (Kosek and Ordeberg, 2000). This finding suggests that chronic pain was maintaining the DNIC dysfunction and that ongoing pain from one site may interact with DNIC evoked by pain from another area. Stimuli applied to patients with neuropathic pain to evoke DNIC decreased the area of brush-evoked pain, but did not change the intensity of brush-evoked pain or spontaneous pain intensity (Witting et al., 2003), suggesting differential effects of DNIC on different aspects of nociceptive processing. The mechanism of descending control seems intact in patients with short- or long-term rheumatoid arthritis compared with controls (Leffler et al., 2002).

Discussion

The relationship between the origin of pain, actual tissue damage, pain intensity, and the manifestations of sensitization is not always causal. The severity of a nerve injury, for example, does not predict the severity of pain. The same simple standard surgical procedures (e.g., to repair inguinal hernia) may cause postsurgical chronic neuropathic pain in up to 37% of patients, but not in the remaining patients (Perkins and Kehlet, 2000). It is well known that degree of radiologically verified cartilage damage in osteoarthroses is not correlated with the severity of pain and that the amount of abnormal endometrium in endometriosis or the size of a peptic ulcer are not related to the pain complaints. In patients with disorders such as temporomandibular pain, chronic low back pain, fibromyalgia, whiplash pain, interstitial cystitis, or irritable bowel syndrome, clear pathologies are rarely found, despite severe pain intensity and widespread pain, and/or sensitization. One reason for lack of the expected relationship between muscle or joint damage and pain can be sensitization along the neuroaxis.

Management approaches for chronic musculoskeletal pain are less systematic compared with treatments for neuropathic pain. The reasons include the greater diversity in conditions and the fact that patients are referred to many different specialists—rheumatologists, orthopedic surgeons, neurologists, neurosurgeons, gastroenterologists, urologists, and gynecologists. It is now generally accepted that some of the pain manifestations in chronic musculoskeletal pain conditions are consequences of sensitization (Arendt-Nielsen and Graven-Nielsen, 2003). Therefore, some of the management strategies used to manage neuropathic pain also apply to chronic musculoskeletal pain conditions. This concept is slowly being clinically accepted, and the drugs used in neuropathic pain are being used in conjunction with traditional musculoskeletal pain management regimes.

Translational research in the field of musculoskeletal pain still lags behind efforts in the area of neuropathic pain. Mechanisms such as sensitization, descending control, central integration, and expansion of receptive fields (referred pain) have been identified in animal studies on musculoskeletal nociception, and emerging evidence indicates that similar manifestations can be assessed in volunteers and pain patients. These promising advances are sure to lead to better diagnosis and management of musculoskeletal pain disorders.

References

Andersen H, Arendt-Nielsen L, Danneskiold-Samsoe B, Graven-Nielsen T. Pressure pain sensitivity and hardness along human normal and sensitized muscle. Somatosens Mot Res 2006;23:97–109.

Arendt-Nielsen L, Graven-Nielsen T. Central sensitization in fibromyalgia and other musculoskeletal disorders. Curr Pain Headache Rep 2003;7:355–361.

Arendt-Nielsen L, Gotliebsen K. Segmental inhibition of laser-evoked brain potentials by ipsi- and contralaterally applied cold pressor pain. Eur J Appl Physiol Occup Physiol 1992;64:56–61.

Bajaj P, Bajaj P, Graven-Nielsen T, Arendt-Nielsen L. Osteoarthritis and its association with muscle hyperalgesia: an experimental controlled study. Pain 2001a; 93:107–114.

Bajaj P, Graven-Nielsen T, Arendt-Nielsen L. Trigger points in patients with lower limb osteoarthritis. J Musculoskel Pain 2001b;9:17–33.

Banic B, Petersen-Felix S, Andersen OK, Radanov BP, Villiger PM, Arendt-Nielsen L, Curatolo M. Evidence for spinal cord hypersensitivity in chronic pain after whiplash injury and in fibromyalgia. Pain 2004;107:7–15.

Bouhassira D, Danziger N, Attal N, Guirimand F. Comparison of the pain suppressive effects of clinical and experimental painful conditioning stimuli. Brain 2003;126:1068–1078.

Bragdon EE, Light KC, Costello NL, Sigurdsson A, Bunting S, Bhalang K, Maixner W. Group differences in pain modulation: pain-free women compared to pain-free men and to women with TMD. Pain 2002;96:227–237.

Cairns BE, Svensson P, Wang K, Castrillon E, Hupfeld S, Sessle BJ, Arendt-Nielsen L. Ketamine attenuates glutamate-induced mechanical sensitization of the masseter muscle in human males. Exp Brain Res 2006;169:467–472.

Carli G, Suman AL, Biasi G, Marcolongo R. Reactivity to superficial and deep stimuli in patients with chronic musculoskeletal pain. Pain 2002;100:259–269.

Cervero F. Mechanisms of visceral pain: past and present. In: Gebhart GF, editor. Visceral pain. Seattle: IASP Press; 1995. p 25–40.

Cervero F, Shouenborg J, Sjolund BH, Waddell PJ. Cutaneous inputs to dorsal horn neurones in adult rats treated at birth with capsaicin. Brain Res 1984;301:47–57.

Coderre TJ, Katz J, Vaccarino AL, Melzack R. Contribution of central neuroplasticity to pathological pain: review of clinical and experimental evidence. Pain 1993;52:259–285.

Curatolo M, Petersen-Felix S, Arendt-Nielsen L, Giani C, Zbinden AM, Radanov BP. Central hypersensitivity in chronic pain after whiplash injury. Clin J Pain 2001;17:306–315.

Ernberg M, Lundeberg T, Kopp S. Effect of propranolol and granisetron on experimentally induced pain and allodynia/hyperalgesia by intramuscular injection of serotonin into the human masseter muscle. Pain 2000;84:339–346.

Feinstein B, Langton JNK, Jameson RM, Schiller F. Experiments on pain referred from deep somatic tissues. J Bone Joint Surg Am 1954;36-A:981–997.

Fernández-Carnero J, Fernandez-de-Las-Penas C, de la Llave-Rincon AI, Ge HY, Arendt-Nielsen L. Prevalence of and referred pain from myofascial trigger points in the forearm muscles in patients with lateral epicondylalgia. Clin J Pain 2007;23:353–360.

Galletti R, Obletter G, Giamberardino MA, Formica LG, Cicchitti G, Vecchiet L. Pain from osteoarthritis of the knee. Adv Pain Res Ther 1990;13:183–191.

Garrison CJ, Dougherty PM, Kajander KC, Carlton SM. Staining of glial fibrillary acidic protein (GFAP) in lumbar spinal cord increases following a sciatic nerve constriction injury. Brain Res 1991;565:1–7.

Ge HY, Madeleine P, Arendt-Nielsen L. Sex differences in temporal characteristics of descending inhibitory control: an evaluation using repeated bilateral experimental induction of muscle pain. Pain 2004;110:72–78.

Giamberardino MA. Recent and forgotten aspects of visceral pain. Eur J Pain 1999;3:77–92.

Giamberardino MA, Affaitati G, Lerza R, Lapenna D, Costantini R, Vecchiet L. Relationship between pain symptoms and referred sensory and trophic changes in patients with gallbladder pathology. Pain 2005;114:239–249.

Graven-Nielsen T. Fundamentals of muscle pain, referred pain, and deep tissue hyperalgesia. Scand J Rheumatol 2006;35(Suppl 122):1–43.

Graven-Nielsen T, Arendt-Nielsen L, Svensson P, Jensen TS. Quantification of local and referred muscle pain in humans after sequential i.m. injections of hypertonic saline. Pain 1997a;69:111–117.

Graven-Nielsen T, Arendt-Nielsen L, Svensson P, Jensen TS. Stimulus-response functions in areas with experimentally induced referred muscle pain—a psychophysical study. Brain Res 1997b;744:121–128.

Graven-Nielsen T, Babenko V, Svensson P, Arendt-Nielsen L. Experimentally induced muscle pain induces hypoalgesia in heterotopic deep tissues, but not in homotopic deep tissues. Brain Res 1998;787:203–210.

Graven-Nielsen T, Kendall SA, Henriksson KG, Bengtsson M, Sörensen J, Johnson A, Gerdle B, Arendt-Nielsen L. Ketamine reduces muscle pain, temporal summation, and referred pain in fibromyalgia patients. Pain 2000;85:483–491.

Hoheisel U, Mense S, Simons DG, Yu X-M. Appearance of new receptive fields in rat dorsal horn neurons following noxious stimulation of skeletal muscle: a model for referral of muscle pain? Neurosci Lett 1993;153:9–12.

Hoheisel U, Koch K, Mense S. Functional reorganization in the rat dorsal horn during an experimental myositis. Pain 1994;59:111–118.

Hoheisel U, Sander B, Mense S. Myositis-induced functional reorganisation of the rat dorsal horn: Effects of spinal superfusion with antagonists to neurokinin and glutamate receptors. Pain 1997a;69:219–230.

Hoheisel U, Sardy M, Mense S. Experiments on the nature of the signal that induces spinal neuroplastic changes following a peripheral lesion. Eur J Pain 1997b;1:243–259.

Hoheisel U, Unger T, Mense S. Sensitization of rat dorsal horn neurons by NGF-induced subthreshold potentials and low-frequency activation. A study employing intracellular recordings in vivo. Brain Res 2007;1169:34–43.

Johansen MK, Graven-Nielsen T, Olesen AS, Arendt-Nielsen L. Generalised muscular hyperalgesia in chronic whiplash syndrome. Pain 1999;83:229–234.

Kellgren JH. Observations on referred pain arising from muscle. Clin Sci 1938;3:175–190.

Kosek E, Hansson P. Modulatory influence on somatosensory perception from vibration and heterotopic noxious conditioning stimulation (HNCS) in fibromyalgia patients and healthy subjects. Pain 1997;70:41–51.

Kosek E, Ordeberg G. Lack of pressure pain modulation by heterotopic noxious conditioning stimulation in patients with painful osteoarthritis before, but not following, surgical pain relief. Pain 2000;88:69–78.

Laursen BS, Bajaj P, Olesen AS, Delmar C, Arendt-Nielsen L. Health related quality of life and quantitative pain measurement in females with chronic non-malignant pain. Eur J Pain 2005;9:267–275.

Laursen RJ, Graven-Nielsen T, Jensen TS, Arendt-Nielsen L. Quantification of local and referred pain in humans induced by intramuscular electrical stimulation. Eur J Pain 1997;1:105–113.

Laursen RJ, Graven-Nielsen T, Jensen TS, Arendt-Nielsen L. The effect of compression and regional anaesthetic block on referred pain intensity in humans. Pain 1999;80:257–263.

Leffler AS, Kosek E, Lerndal T, Nordmark B, Hansson P. Somatosensory perception and function of diffuse noxious inhibitory controls (DNIC) in patients suffering from rheumatoid arthritis. Eur J Pain 2002;6:161–176.

Marchettini P, Simone DA, Caputi G, Ochoa JL. Pain from excitation of identified muscle nociceptors in humans. Brain Res 1996;740:109–116.

Mense S. Referral of muscle pain. New aspects. Am Pain Soc J 1994;3:1–9.

Millan MJ. Descending control of pain. Prog Neurobiol 2002;66:355–474.

Molander C, Ygge J, Dalsgaard C-J. Substance P-, somatostatin- and calcitonin gene-related peptide-like immunoreactivity and fluoride resistant acid phosphatase-activity in relation to retrogradely labeled cutaneous, muscular and visceral primary sensory neurons in the rat. Neurosci Lett 1987;74:37–42.

Morris VH, Cruwys SC, Kidd BL. Characterisation of capsaicin-induced mechanical hyperalgesia as a marker for altered nociceptive processing in patients with rheumatoid arthritis. Pain 1997;71:179–186.

Morris V, Cruwys S, Kidd B. Increased capsaicin-induced secondary hyperalgesia as a marker of abnormal sensory activity in patients with fibromyalgia. Neurosci Lett 1998;250:205–207.

Nie H, Arendt-Nielsen L, Madeleine P, Graven-Nielsen T. Enhanced temporal summation of pressure pain in the trapezius muscle after delayed onset muscle soreness. Exp Brain Res 2006;170:182–190.

O'Neill S, Manniche C, Graven-Nielsen T, Arendt-Nielsen L. Generalized deep-tissue hyperalgesia in patients with chronic low-back pain. Eur J Pain 2007;11:415–420.

Perkins FM, Kehlet H. Chronic pain as an outcome of surgery. A review of predictive factors. Anesthesiology 2000;93:1123–1133.

Peters ML, Schmidt AJ, Van den Hout MA, Koopmans R, Sluijter ME. Chronic back pain, acute postoperative pain and the activation of diffuse noxious inhibitory controls (DNIC). Pain 1992;50:177–187.

Reinert A, Kaske A, Mense S. Inflammation-induced increase in the density of neuropeptide-immunoreactive nerve endings in rat skeletal muscle. Exp Brain Res 1998;121:174–180.

Sandrini G, Rossi P, Milanov I, Serrao M, Cecchini AP, Nappi G. Abnormal modulatory influence of diffuse noxious inhibitory controls in migraine and chronic tension-type headache patients. Cephalalgia 2006;26:782–789.

Schouenborg J, Sjolund BH. Activity evoked by A- and C-afferent fibers in rat dorsal horn neurons and its relation to a flexion reflex. J Neurophysiol 1983;50:1108–1121.

Schulte H, Graven-Nielsen T, Sollevi A, Jansson Y, Arendt-Nielsen L, Segerdahl M. Pharmacological modulation of experimental phasic and tonic muscle pain by morphine, alfentanil and ketamine in healthy volunteers. Acta Anaesthesiol Scand 2003;47:1020–1030.

Sessle BJ, Hu JW, Amano N, Zhong G. Convergence of cutaneous, tooth pulp, visceral, neck and muscle afferents onto nociceptive and non-nociceptive neurones in trigeminal subnucleus caudalis (medullary dorsal horn) and its implications for referred pain. Pain 1986;27:219–235.

Simons, DG, Travell, JG, Simons L. Myofascial pain and dysfunction. The trigger point manual. Philadelphia: Lippincott Williams & Wilkins, USA, 1999.

Slater H, Arendt-Nielsen L, Wright A, Graven-Nielsen T. Experimental deep tissue pain in wrist extensors—a model of lateral epicondylalgia. Eur J Pain 2003;7:277–288.

Slater H, Arendt-Nielsen L, Wright A, Graven-Nielsen T. Sensory and motor effects of experimental muscle pain in patients with lateral epicondylalgia and controls with delayed onset muscle soreness. Pain 2005;114:118–130.

Sluka KA, Price MP, Breese NM, Stucky CL, Wemmie JA, Welsh MJ. Chronic hyperalgesia induced by repeated acid injections in muscle is abolished by the loss of ASIC3, but not ASIC1. Pain 2003;106:229–239.

Staud R, Vierck CJ, Cannon RL, Mauderli AP, Price DD. Abnormal sensitization and temporal summation of second pain (wind-up) in patients with fibromyalgia syndrome. Pain 2001;91:165–175.

Stawowy M, Funch-Jensen P, Arendt-Nielsen L, Drewes AM. Somatosensory changes in the referred pain area in patients with cholecystolithiasis. Eur J Gastroenterol Hepatol 2005;17:865–870.

Stawowy M, Rössel P, Bluhme C, Funch-Jensen P, Arendt-Nielsen L, Drewes AM. Somatosensory changes in the referred pain area following acute inflammation of the appendix. Eur J Gastroenterol Hepatol 2002;14:1079–1084.

Steinbrocker O, Isenberg SA, Silver M, Neustadt D, Kuhn P, Schittone M. Observations on pain produced by injections of hypertonic saline into muscles and other supportive tissues. J Clin Invest 1953;32:1045–1051.

Sturge WA. The phenomena of angina pectoris and their bearing upon the theory of counter-irritation. Brain 1883;5:492–510.

Svensson P, Cairns BE, Wang K, Arendt-Nielsen L. Injection of nerve growth factor into human masseter muscle evokes long-lasting mechanical allodynia and hyperalgesia. Pain 2003;104:241–247.

Sörensen J, Graven-Nielsen T, Henriksson KG, Bengtsson M, Arendt-Nielsen L. Hyperexcitability in fibromyalgia. J Rheumatol 1998;25:152–155.

Tenschert S, Reinert A, Hoheisel U, Mense S. Effects of a chronic myositis on structural and functional features of spinal astrocytes in the rat. Neurosci Lett 2004;361:196–199.

Vanegas H, Schaible HG. Descending control of persistent pain: inhibitory or facilitatory? Brain Res Brain Res Rev 2004;46:295–309.

Vecchiet L, Giamberardino MA, de Bigontina P. When the symptom persist despite the extinction of the visceral focus. In: Sicuteri F, Terenius L, Vecchiet L, Maggi CA, editors. Pain versus man, Vol. 20. New York: Raven Press; 1992. p 101–110.

Vecchiet L, Giamberardino MA, de Bigontina P, Dragani L. Comparative sensory evaluation of parietal tissues in painful and nonpainful areas in fibromyalgia and myofascial pain syndrome. In: Gebhart GF, Hammond DL, Jensen TS, editors. Proceedings of the 7th World Congress on Pain. Seattle: IASP Press; 1994. p 177–185.

Vecchiet L, Giamberardino MA, Dragani L, Albe-Fessard D. Pain from renal/ureteral calculosis: evaluation of sensory thresholds in the lumbar area. Pain 1989;36:289–295.

Witting N, Svensson P, Jensen TS. Differential recruitment of endogenous pain inhibitory systems in neuropathic pain patients. Pain 2003;103:75–81.

Woolf CJ. Windup and central sensitization are not equivalent. Pain 1996;66:105–108.

Wright A, Graven-Nielsen T, Davies II, Arendt-Nielsen L. Temporal summation of pain from skin, muscle and joint following nociceptive ultrasonic stimulation in humans. Exp Brain Res 2002;144:475–482.

You HJ, Morch CD, Chen J, Arendt-Nielsen L. Differential antinociceptive effects induced by a selective cyclooxygenase-2 inhibitor (SC-236) on dorsal horn neurons and spinal withdrawal reflexes in anesthetized spinal rats. Neuroscience 2003;121:459–472.

Zubieta J-K, Heitzeg MM, Smith YR, Bueller JA, Xu K, Xu Y, Koeppe RA, Stohler CS, Goldman D. COMT val[158]met genotype affects mu-opioid neurotransmitter responses to a pain stressor. Science 2003;299:1240–1243.

Zubieta J-K, Smith YR, Bueller JA, Xu Y, Kilbourn MR, Jewett DM, Meyer CR, Koeppe RA, Stohler CS. Regional mu opioid receptor regulation of sensory and affective dimensions of pain. Science 2001;293:311–315.

Zubieta J-K, Smith YR, Bueller JA, Xu Y, Kilbourn MR, Jewett DM, Meyer CR, Koeppe RA, Stohler CS. Mu-opioid receptor-mediated antinociceptive responses differ in men and women. J Neurosci 2002;22:5100–5107.

Correspondence to: Prof. Lars Arendt-Nielsen, Dr Med Sci, PhD, Department of Health Sciences and Technology, Center for Sensory-Motor Interaction (SMI), Aalborg University, Fredrik Bajers Vej 7, D3, DK-9220 Aalborg, Denmark. Email: lan@hst.aau.dk.

Part III

Effects of Muscle Pain on Motor Function

Effects of Experimental Muscle Pain on Muscle Spindle Sensitivity

Jin Y. Ro,[a,c] Norman F. Capra,[a,c] and Radi Masri[b,c]

[a]Department of Biomedical Sciences, [b]Department of Endodontics, Prosthodontics and Operative Dentistry, [c]Program in Neuroscience, University of Maryland Baltimore School of Dentistry, Baltimore, Maryland, USA

Sensory signals arising from muscle spindle receptors are essential for optimal performance of motor behaviors, and motor performance is compromised when such sensory feedback is abolished or disturbed (Gandevia and Burke, 1992; McCloskey and Prochazka, 1994). It is now well established that conditions such as acute and chronic muscle pain or muscle fatigue alter motor performance (Lund et al., 1994; Arendt-Nielsen et al., 1996; Pedersen et al., 1999). Mechanisms that contribute to motor disturbances under painful conditions have been the subject of investigation for many decades (Travell and Rinzler, 1952; Johansson and Sojka, 1991; Lund et al., 1991). Jaw muscle pain is associated with a reduced range of motion and decreased maximum voluntary contractions in patients with temporomandibular disorder (TMD) (Stohler et al., 1988). These patients also show significant impairment in performing interdental discrimination and mandibular positioning tasks, which suggests defective processing of proprioceptive signals (Ransjö and Thilander, 1963; Morimoto, 1983). Jaw muscle spindles have been particularly implicated in providing feedback necessary for interdental discrimination and mandibular positioning and may be involved in matching the spa-tiotemporal pattern of the moving jaw by modulating the output of the central pattern generator (Hidaka et al., 1999). More recent studies have reported that the stretch reflex is facilitated by modulation of the muscle spindle-fusimotor system under various experimental muscle pain condi-tions (Wang et al., 2002, 2004). Thus, painful stimulation of muscle tissue produces profound changes in simple as well as in complex motor func-tions, along with changes in sensory sensitivities (Graven-Nielsen, 2006). This chapter summarizes experimental data on how painful conditions in the jaw muscle alter proprioceptive signals arising from muscle spindle afferents and describes how these nociceptive–proprioceptive interac-tions occur in the trigeminal system.

Experimental Muscle Pain and Central Modulation of Jaw Muscle Spindle Afferent Signals

The influence of experimentally induced jaw muscle pain on propriocep-tive processing was first demonstrated in central neurons that receive jaw muscle spindle afferent (JMSA) inputs (Capra and Ro, 2000). JMSAs are innervated by the trigeminal mesencephalic nucleus (Vmes), a unique collection of primary afferent cell bodies located in the central nervous system. In addition to making monosynaptic connections onto trigemi-nal motoneurons (Vmot), Vmes provides primary afferent input to the principal sensory nucleus, the supratrigeminal region, the dorsomedial spinal trigeminal nucleus, and the reticular formation subjacent to the spinal trigeminal nucleus (PcRF) as far caudally as the upper cervical spi-nal cord (Luschei, 1987; Luo et al., 2006). Transganglionic transport and autoradiographic studies show that this caudal projection specifically includes muscle spindle input, which travels via Probst's tract (Nomura and Mizuno, 1985).

Ro and Capra (1999b) have physiologically identified neurons located on the medial edge of the subnucleus interpolaris (Vi) and the adjacent PcRF as recipients for the caudal projections from JMSAs. Two groups of cells were delineated based on their responses to passive jaw movements. One group of neurons exhibited a clear and consistent dynamic response consisting of an initial burst of activity during the onset of muscle stretch followed by significantly lower but relatively constant activity during the hold phase. These neurons were classified as dynamic-static units because their mean firing rates during jaw opening varied as a function of opening speed, responses that are characteristic of muscle spindle primary afferents. The other group of cells showed a linear increase in firing rate with the onset of jaw opening that persisted as long as the jaw was held open. These units lacked a clear dynamic response, and they were classified as static units because their firing rates varied as a function of jaw opening amplitude, resembling responses from muscle spindle secondary afferents.

Capra and Ro (2000) subsequently studied the effect of experimental muscle pain on discharge properties from these neurons. Masseter nociceptors were activated with a bolus injection of 5% hypertonic saline (HS), which is known to cause intense muscle pain when injected into human muscles (Stohler et al., 1996; Graven-Nielsen et al., 1997). Single-unit responses to passively imposed ramp-and-hold jaw stretches were compared before and after the injection. Seventy-six percent of the cells tested showed a significant modulation of mean firing rate during opening and/or holding phases. The most remarkable HS-induced change was a significant reduction of mean firing rate during the hold phase in all static units. Sixty-nine percent of the dynamic-static units were also modulated by HS during the hold phase. HS injections made into the contralateral masseter muscle also altered jaw movement-related responses with a pattern and time course similar to those following ipsilateral injections.

It is unlikely that the injection procedure or volume of HS in the muscle altered the movement-related responses because injections of an equal volume of isotonic saline rarely produced a significant effect. It is also unlikely that HS directly activated muscle spindle receptors and altered jaw-movement-related responses. Intramuscular injections with algesic substances, including HS, preferentially activate group III and IV muscle afferents, but rarely activate muscle spindle receptors (Paintal,

1960; Mense, 1977; Mense and Meyer, 1985). The data from HS injection in the contralateral muscle provide convincing evidence that the effect of HS on central proprioceptive neurons requires a centrally mediated mechanism. This mechanism may involve small-diameter muscle afferent input onto interneurons that provide bilateral connections. These results unequivocally demonstrate that intramuscular injection with an algesic substance, sufficient to evoke pain, significantly modulates proprioceptive signals arising from JMSAs.

A Model for Nociceptive-Proprioceptive Interactions in the Trigeminal System

Intramuscular injections with algesic chemicals cause dramatic changes in muscle spindle discharge in neck and limb muscles (Johansson et al., 1993; Djupsjöbacka et al., 1995; Pedersen et al., 1997; Wenngren et al., 1998). In the spinal system, the interaction between nociceptive and proprioceptive neurons is thought to be mediated by gamma motoneurons. Johansson and Sojka (1991) proposed that the changes in muscle spindle discharge are mediated by gamma motoneurons that are stimulated by muscle nociceptors. Algesic chemical stimulation of small-diameter muscle afferents increases fusimotor activity (Jovanovic et al., 1990). Electrical stimulation of group III muscle afferents causes strong reflex activation, as well as inhibition, of static gamma motoneurons (Appelberg et al., 1982, 1983). These studies have led to the hypothesis that stimulation of muscle nociceptors initiates a chain of events that activate gamma motoneurons, which ultimately influence muscle spindle discharges by providing the "final integrated input" to muscle spindle afferents.

The neural linkage between nociceptor activation and alterations in proprioceptive signals from orofacial muscles needs to be demonstrated independently because the reflex control of muscle spindle afferents by gamma motoneurons in the trigeminal and spinal systems may be quite different. Unlike jaw-closing muscles, jaw-opening muscles and the muscles of facial expression have very few muscle spindles (Kubota et al., 1980, 1983). Therefore, the agonist-antagonist pairing of spindle elements in spinal circuits is not a feature of the craniofacial system. In addition, by virtue of the mandibular symphysis, the jaw joints function in concert bilaterally, whereas limb joints typically act independently to maintain balance (e.g., crossed extensor reflex; Lund et al., 1983). Relatively few, if any, jaw muscle motoneurons have recurrent collaterals, and type Ia inhibitory interneurons are lacking (Luschei and Goldberg, 1981). These fundamental differences in neuronal circuitry require a systematic evaluation of how the kinematic properties of JMSAs change in the presence of craniofacial muscle pain and subsequently affect motor function. To this end, we proposed the underlying circuitry that mediates nociceptive-proprioceptive interactions that are unique to the trigeminal system (Fig. 1). We hypothesized that (1) noxious chemical stimulation of the muscle differentially modulates responses from muscle spindle primaries

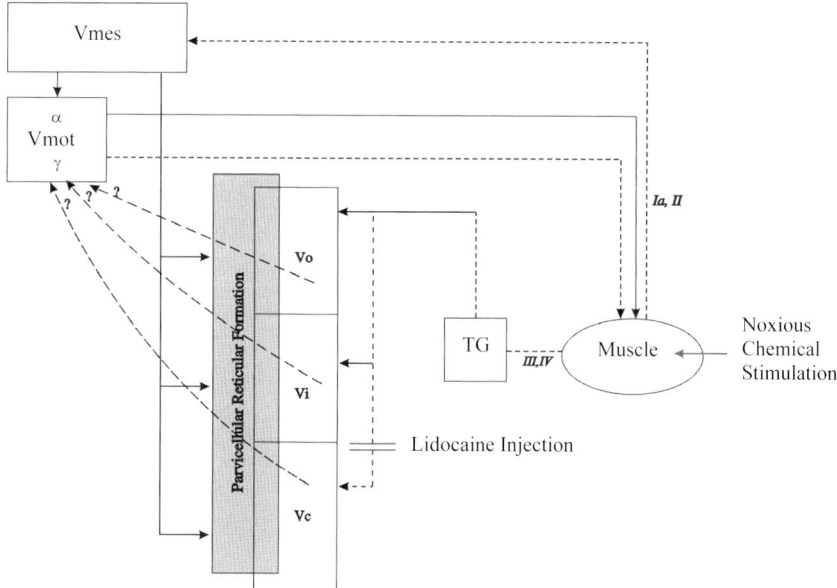

Fig. 1. A model diagram for nociceptive modulation of proprioceptive signals in the trigeminal system. Noxious chemical stimulation of the jaw muscle will activate trigeminal neurons in the caudal brainstem, which in turn will modulate trigeminal gamma motoneurons. The gamma motoneurons will ultimately influence discharge properties of muscle spindle afferents in jaw-closing muscles. TG = trigeminal ganglion, Vc = subnucleus caudalis, Vi = subnucleus interpolaris, Vmes = trigeminal mesencephalic nucleus, Vmot = trigeminal motor nucleus, Vo = subnucleus oralis.

and secondaries to proprioceptive stimuli, (2) the caudal brainstem neurons that process muscle nociceptive input are an integral link in the circuit for proprioceptive modulation, and (3) the modulation of spindle afferents following noxious chemical stimulation of the muscle is mediated through the gamma-fusimotor system.

Muscle Spindle Afferent Responses to Intramuscular Algesic Injection

We first determined whether the modulation of proprioceptive responses that we observed in dorsomedial Vi and PcRF reflected nociceptor-induced changes in spindle afferents by recording directly from JMSAs in the Vmes (Ro and Capra, 2001). Twenty-nine JMSAs were tested with 5% HS, of which 79% (23/29) showed significant modulation of mean firing rates during one or more phases of ramp-and-hold movements. Among the 12 muscle spindle primary-like units, mean firing rates were facilitated in four units, were reduced in five, showed mixed responses in two, and were unchanged in one. In 17 muscle spindle secondary-like units, mean firing rates were facilitated in nine units, reduced in three, and unchanged in five. Further analysis revealed that HS not only affected the overall output of muscle spindle afferents, but also increased the variability of firing and altered the relationship between afferent signal and muscle length. These experiments show that activation of muscle nociceptors either facilitated or reduced mean firing rates during various phases of ramp-and-hold jaw movements. Hypertonic saline produced more heterogeneous responses in primary-like units than in secondary-like units. The heterogeneity in response recorded from muscle spindle afferents reflects a similar heterogeneity in the response of gamma motoneuron activity reported in spinal circuits (Hellstrom et al., 2000) and suggests the involvement of gamma-mediated circuits in the brainstem.

A greater proportion of muscle spindle secondary-like units from the Vmes showed facilitation than inhibition of movement-related responses following HS injection. This observation is not entirely compatible with HS-induced responses recorded from the caudal brainstem neurons (i.e., Vi and PcRF), which showed predominantly inhibitory responses. Muscle spindle primary-like and secondary-like afferents project preferentially to different regions in and around the Vmot (Dessem et al., 1997). Thus, it is possible that caudal brainstem neurons receive selective inputs from muscle spindle secondary-like units that are inhibited upon noxious stimulation of the muscle. Another possibility is that the caudal brainstem neurons with muscle spindle input may receive additional modulation from other central and peripheral sources. Most experimental studies show that muscle nociceptive information is processed primarily in more caudal regions of the spinal trigeminal nucleus (Capra and Dessem, 1992). Thus, central processing of proprioceptive signals following noxious stimulation of the muscle may be different at various levels of the rostrocaudal extent of muscle spindle afferent distribution in the brainstem.

We then investigated whether masseteric HS significantly compromises amplitude and velocity sensitivities of JMSAs (Masri et al., 2005). Velocity sensitivity was assessed in spindle primary-like afferents by calculating the mean dynamic index of each unit in response to three different velocities of jaw opening before and after intramuscular injection with HS. Amplitude sensitivity of jaw muscle spindle afferents was assessed by calculating the mean firing rate of each unit in response to three different amplitudes of jaw openings before and after HS injection. Best-fit lines for velocity and amplitude changes before and after HS injection were obtained using linear regression analysis. The variance of the two regression lines obtained was compared using the coincidence test, and changes in intercept and slope were determined. Seventy-five percent of the primary-like units and 80% of the secondary-like units showed changes in amplitude-related responses after HS injection. Only about 30% of the primary-like units showed HS-induced changes in velocity-related responses. Typically, the changes were characterized by either an increase or a decrease in the intercept but not in the slope, suggesting alterations in gain of response rather than sensitivity, per se. However, in some cases, HS caused amplitude-related responses to become "nonlinear," completely disrupting the amplitude sensitivity. Our results demonstrated that the predominant effect of HS was a shift in amplitude sensitivity of both primary-like and secondary-like afferents and, to a lesser extent, velocity sensitivity of the primary-like unit.

Dynamic and static fusimotor activity on intrafusal fibers of muscle spindle afferents is independently controlled (Murthy, 1978). In the spinal system, the predominant effect of noxious muscle stimulation is facilitation of the fusimotor drive (Jovanovic et al., 1990; Hellstrom et al., 2002), but an inhibitory effect on the gamma fusimotor system has also been observed (Mense and Skeppar, 1991). In our studies, HS-induced responses have consistently been mixed responses (Capra and Ro, 2000; Ro and Capra, 2001; Masri et al., 2005). Electrical stimulation of group III muscle afferents causes activation as well as inhibition of static gamma motoneurons, with a weaker effect on dynamic gamma moto-neurons (Appelberg et al., 1982, 1983). The observation that HS effects on spindle afferents were more evident during changing amplitudes than during changing velocities also suggests a preferential activation of the static gamma fusimotor system as opposed to the dynamic fusimotor system. Spindles of jaw-closing muscles have a different pattern of inner-vation from spindles of the hindlimb muscles and other muscles of the body. Like the neck muscles, a high proportion of jaw muscle spindle af-ferents are influenced by intrafusal static nuclear bag fibers (bag 2) and chain fibers (Richmond and Abraham, 1979; Taylor et al., 1992; Masri et al., 2006). Reduced influence on dynamic bag 1 intrafusal fibers pre-disposes a principal effect on static fusimotor neurons. Taken together, these data suggest that muscle pain independently modulates static and dynamic gamma motoneurons and that the effect is more pronounced in static gamma motoneurons.

Subnucleus Caudalis and Caudal Subnucleus Interpolaris Form an Integral Link in the Circuit for Proprioceptive Modulation

Although our data strongly suggest that noxious chemical stimulation of the masseter muscle modulates muscle spindle afferent responses, it is not likely that the effect is mediated by direct projections of muscle nociceptors to the Vmes. Therefore, the neural circuitry between muscle nociceptors and JMSAs needs to be demonstrated. Anatomical studies have shown that most of the input from small-diameter trigeminal ganglion muscle afferents terminates in Vc and Vi (Nishimori et al., 1986; Capra and Wax, 1989). The importance of Vc in orofacial muscle pain is well established (Sessle, 2000). The role of muscle nociceptive inputs into Vi has received little attention, despite observations that Vi also contains neurons that process nociceptive signals from deep structures, including the muscles of mastication (Hayashi et al., 1984; Ro and Capra, 1999b). We hypothesized that these Vc and caudal Vi neurons are interneurons that form a necessary link in the modulation of muscle spindle responses (Fig. 1).

To test this hypothesis, we documented jaw muscle spindle responses before and after intramuscular injection of 5% HS as described in previous sections (Capra and Ro, 2000; Ro and Capra, 2001). Following a complete documentation of the HS effects, unilateral injection of lidocaine (4%, 0.5-0.7 µL/2 min) was made in the vicinity of the obex to reversibly inactivate the region of Vc/Vi. An hour was allowed between the HS injection and the lidocaine block. Five minutes after the lidocaine injection, HS was reinjected into the same muscle, and responses were documented. As a group, 81% of the Vmes muscle spindle afferents studied (29/36) were modulated by HS. Following lidocaine blockade, 65% of the HS-modulated units were no longer responsive to reinjection with HS.

Fig. 2A illustrates examples of HS-induced changes in jaw-movement-related responses from a spindle primary-like neuron before and after the lidocaine injection. This unit exhibited a significant HS-induced modulation of mean firing rates during both open and hold phases of the jaw movements. The same volume of HS injected into the masseter 5 minutes after the microinjection of lidocaine resulted in a negligible increase in the mean firing rate during the opening phase. The partial blockade of HS effect was due to temporary inactivation of the Vc/Vi region, as inferred from the histological evaluation of the brainstem sections. Another unit shown in Fig 2B responded to the initial HS injection with a 35% increase in firing rate during the open phase and a 15%

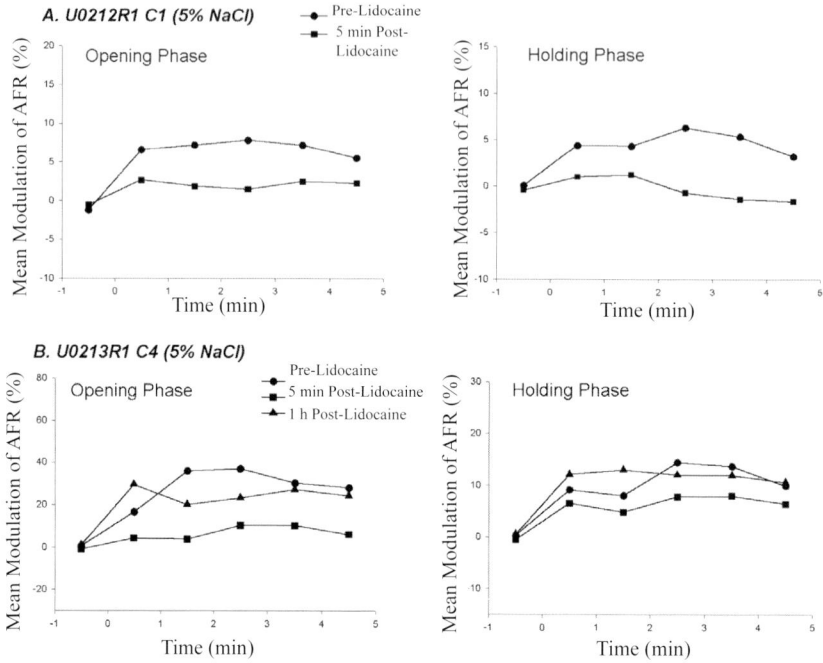

Fig. 2. Mean percentage modulation of average firing rates of muscle spindle afferents following hypertonic saline (HS) injections before and after lidocaine was microinjected into the caudal spinal trigeminal nucleus. Changes in firing rates during both opening and holding phases of passive jaw stretches are shown. Time 0 is when HS was injected into the masseter muscle.

increase during the hold phase. The microinjection of lidocaine 1 mm caudal to the obex almost completely blocked the HS-induced increase during the open phase and produced a partial block (a reduction in firing) during the hold phase. Interestingly, another HS injection given 1 hour after the lidocaine treatment produced responses that were similar in magnitude to those following the initial HS injection. These results support the idea that HS-induced changes in spindle afferent responses depend, in part, upon input from either Vc or caudal Vi. Our failure to observe a more profound reduction of HS modulation may be due to technical issues or to the likelihood that some masseter nociceptive afferents provide axon collaterals to rostral trigeminal subnuclei (Capra and Dessem, 1992).

Intramuscular Hypertonic Saline Alters Spontaneous Discharge of Gamma Motoneurons

In addition to their role in the initial relay of information from muscle nociceptors in the spinal trigeminal nuclei (Vc and caudal Vi), we proposed that gamma motoneurons are part of the essential neural circuitry that ultimately influences afferent discharge from jaw-closing muscle spindles. Physiological evidence for modulation of the fusimotor system following intramuscular injections with algesic substances is provided by directly recording from single gamma motoneurons (Capra et al., 2007). Using several criteria including background activity, response to stretch, and conduction velocity (Sessle, 1977; Appenteng et al., 1980), we identified a group of putative gamma motoneurons from the Vmot (Capra et al., 2007). The effect of algesic stimulation on these neurons was studied by injecting a small volume of 5% HS into the masseter muscle. Responses of one gamma motoneuron to passive jaw stretches are shown in Fig. 3A. For this particular unit, average firing rates were elevated during all phases of ramp and hold jaw movements for 2 minutes after the HS injection and returned to preinjection levels within 3 minutes. The extent of modulation of resting discharge of seven putative gamma motoneurons was normalized and plotted as percentage modulation of average firing rates over time (Fig. 3B). This type of analysis allows comparisons of the magnitude and temporal characteristics of gamma motoneurons with those documented for muscle spindle afferents (Capra et al., 2007). Consistent with muscle spindle afferent responses, HS produced both facilitation and reduction of resting discharge in gamma motoneurons that lasted for several minutes. These response patterns were strikingly similar to those obtained from muscle spindle afferents. Therefore, algesic substances can either enhance or inhibit discharge of gamma motoneurons, which may explain the bidirectional responses observed in muscle spindle afferents. Further studies are needed for more complete documentation of modulation of responses of static and dynamic gamma motoneurons to algesic stimulation of muscle nociceptors.

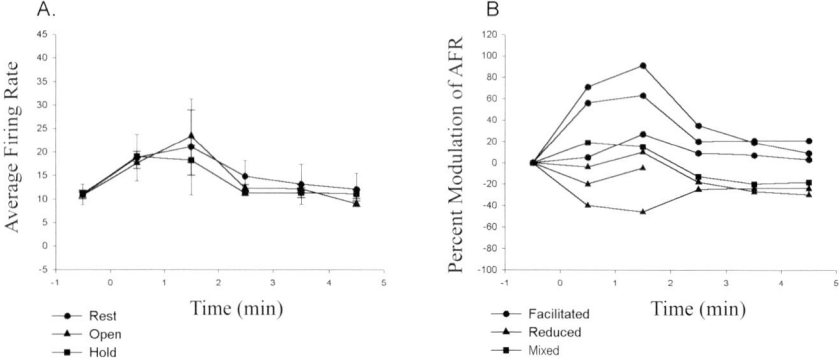

Fig. 3. Changes in average firing rate (AFR) during passive jaw movements in a gamma motoneuron. (B). Mean percentage modulation of resting discharge of a group of gamma motoneurons following intramuscular injections with 5% hypertonic saline (HS). Time 0 is when HS was injected into the masseter muscle.

Summary and Functional Significance

Experimental induction of masseter pain modulates proprioceptive signal processing at multiple levels in the trigeminal circuitry. Intramuscular injection of algesic substances does not appear to directly change muscle spindle sensitivity at the receptor ending because activation of muscle nociceptors in the contralateral or synergistic muscle produces similar alterations in muscle spindle responses. Instead, nociceptive signals arising from craniofacial muscle tissue are relayed by small-diameter muscle afferents in trigeminal ganglia onto the neurons in the trigeminal sensory nuclear complex, especially those located in Vc or caudal Vi. These neurons subsequently provide muscle nociceptive input sufficient to modulate gamma motoneurons, which in turn alter the overall output of spindle afferents in jaw-closing muscles. Algesic chemical injections of masseter muscle preferentially influence the amplitude-related responses of JMSAs, consistent with actions on static gamma motoneurons. Functional implications of pain-induced modulation of muscle spindle afferent responses are numerous because JMSAs are known to project diffusely throughout the rostrocaudal extent of the brainstem.

Observations that algesic chemical stimulation produced both enhanced and reduced responses in fusimotor neurons and jaw muscle spindle afferents complicate predictions by the pathophysiological model (Johansson and Sojka, 1991) that accumulation of metabolites invariably leads to increased spindle sensitivity via gamma motoneurons. The bidirectional responses to noxious stimulation we have seen may be more compatible with the predictions of the pain adaptation model (Lund et al., 1991), in such a way that appropriate patterns of excitation and inhibition protect the injured muscle by subtle, yet coordinated, peripheral modulation of motor activity during mastication by influencing specific elements of the pattern generator (Capra et al., 2007). Craniofacial pain is associated with acute malocclusion, altered sensation of jaw position, and altered swallowing patterns. The disturbance of proprioceptive signals in primary afferents and in subsequent levels of processing observed after experimental induction of masseter muscle pain may well contribute to impaired oral motor function.

Acknowledgments

We would like to thank Ms. Youping Zhang and Mr. Gregory Haynes for their contribution in this project. Research was supported by National Institute of Dental and Craniofacial Research Grant DE06027.

References

Appelberg B, Hulliger M, Johansson H, Sojka P. Fusimotor reflexes in triceps surae elicited by natural stimulation of muscle afferents from the cat ipsilateral hind limb. J Physiol (Lond) 1982;329:211–229.

Appelberg B, Hulliger M, Johansson H, Sojka P. Actions on gamma-motoneurons elicited by electrical stimulation of group I muscle afferent fibres in the hind limb of the cat. J Physiol (Lond) 1983: 335:237–253.

Appenteng K, Morimoto T, Taylor A. Fusimotor activity in masseter nerve of the cat during reflex jaw movements. J Physiol (Lond) 1980;305:415–431.

Arendt-Nielsen L, Graven-Nielsen T, Svarrer H, Svensson P. The influence of low back pain on muscle activity and coordination during gait: a clinical and experimental study. Pain 1996;64:231–240.

Capra NF, Dessem D. Central connections of trigeminal primary afferent neurons: topographical and functional considerations. Crit Rev Oral Biol Med 1992;4:1–52.

Capra NF, Hisley CK, Masri R. The influence of pain on masseter spindle afferent discharge. Arch Oral Biol 2007;52:387–390.

Capra NF, Ro JY. Experimental muscle pain produces central modulation of proprioceptive signals arising from jaw muscle spindles. Pain 2000;86:151–162.

Capra NF, Wax TD. Distribution and central projection of primary afferent neurons that innervate the masseter muscle and mandibular periodontium: a double-label study. J Comp Neurol
1989;279:341–352.

Dessem D, Donga R, Luo P. Primary- and secondary-like jaw-muscle spindle afferents have characteristic topographic distributions. J Neurophysiol 1997;77:2925–2944.

Djupsjöbacka M, Johansson H, Bergenheim M, Wenngren BI. Influences on the gamma-muscle
spindle system from muscle afferents stimulated by increased intramuscular concentrations of
bradykinin and 5-HT. Neurosci Res 1995;22:325–333.

Gandevia SC, Burke D. Does the nervous system depend on kinesthetic information to contralateral
limb movements? Behav Brain Sci 1992;15:614–632.

Graven-Nielsen T. Fundamentals of muscle pain, referred pain, and deep tissue hyperalgesia. Scand J
Rheumatol Suppl 2006;122:1–43.

Graven-Nielsen T, McArdle A, Phoenix J, Arendt-Nielsen L, Jensen TS, Jackson MJ, Edwards RH.
In vivo model of muscle pain: quantification of intramuscular chemical, electrical, and pressure
changes associated with saline-induced muscle pain in humans. Pain 1997;69:137–143.

Hayashi H, Sumino R, Sessle BJ. Functional organization of trigeminal subnucleus interpolaris: nociceptive and innocuous afferent inputs, projections to thalamus, cerebellum and spinal cord, and
descending modulation from periaqueductal gray. J Neurophysiol 1984;51:890–905.

Hellstrom F, Thunberg J, Bergenheim M, Sjolander P, Pedersen J, Johansson H. Elevated intramuscular concentration of bradykinin in jaw muscle increases the fusimotor drive to neck muscles in
the cat. J Dent Res 2000;79:1815–1822.

Hidaka O, Morimoto T, Kato T, Masuda Y, Inoue T, Takada K. Behavior of jaw muscle spindle afferents during cortically induced rhythmic jaw movements in the anesthetized rabbit. J Neurophysiol 1999;82:2633–2640.

Johansson H, Sojka P. Pathophysiological mechanisms involved in genesis and spread of muscular
tension in occupational muscle pain and in chronic musculoskeletal pain syndromes: a hypothesis. Med Hypotheses 1991;35:196–203.

Johansson H, Djupsjöbacka M, Sjölander P. Influences on the gamma-muscle spindle system from
muscle afferents stimulated by KCl and lactic acid. Neurosci Res 1993;16:49–57.

Jovanovic K, Anastasijevic R, Vuco J. Reflex effects on gamma fusimotor neurons of chemically induced discharges in small-diameter muscle afferents in decerebrate cats. Brain Res 1990;521:89–94.

Kubota K, Komatsu S, Nakamura M. Muscle spindle supply in the pig masticatory muscles. Anat
Anz 1983;153:415–428.

Kubota K, Komatsu S, Nakamura M, Masegi T. Muscle spindle supply to the bovine jaw muscles.
Anat Rec 1980;197:413–422.

Lund JP, Donga R, Widmer CG, Stohler C.S. The pain-adaptation model: a discussion of the relationship between chronic musculoskeletal pain and motor activity. Can J Physiol Pharmacol
1991;69:683–694.

Lund JP, Lamarre Y, Lavigne G, Duquet G. Human jaw reflexes. Adv Neurol 1983;39:739–755.

Lund JP, Stohler CS, Widmer CG. The relationship between pain and muscle activity in fibromyalgia
and similar conditions. In: Vaeroy H, Merskey H, editors. Progress in fibromyalgia and myofascial pain. Amsterdam: Elsevier; 1994.

Luo P, Wong R, Dessem D. Projection of jaw-muscle spindle afferents to the caudal brainstem in rats
demonstrated using intracellular biotinamide. J Comp Neurol 1995;358:63–78.

Luo P, Zhang J, Yang R, Pendlebury W. Neuronal circuitry and synaptic organization of trigeminal
proprioceptive afferents mediating tongue movement and jaw-tongue coordination via hypo-
glossal premotor neurons. Eur J Neurosci 2006;23:3269–3283.

Luschei ES. Central projections of the mesencephalic nucleus of the fifth nerve: autoradiographic
study. J Comp Neurol 1987;263:137–145.

Luschei ES, Goldberg LG. Neural mechanisms of mandibular control: mastication and voluntary bit-
ing. In: Brooks VB, editor. Handbook of physiology, Section 1, Motor control, Vol. II. Bethesda,
MD: American Physiological Society; 1981. p. 1237– 1274 (Part 1).

Masri R, Ro JY, Capra N. The effect of experimental muscle pain on the amplitude and velocity sensitivity of jaw closing muscle spindle afferents. Brain Res 2005;1050:138–147.

Masri R, Ro JY, Dessem D, Capra N. Classification of muscle spindle afferents innervating the masseter muscle in rats. Arch Oral Biol 2006;51:740–747.

McCloskey DI, Prochazka A. The role of sensory information in the guidance of voluntary movement: reflections on a symposium held at the 22nd Annual Meeting of the Society of Neuroscience. Somatosens Mot Res 1994;11:69–76.

Mense S. Muscular nociceptors. J Physiol (Paris) 1977;73:233–240.

Mense S, Meyer H. Different types of slowly conducting afferent units in cat skeletal muscle and tendon. J Physiol 1985;363:403–417.

Mense S, Skeppar P. Discharge behaviour of feline gamma-motoneurones following induction of an artificial myositis. Pain 1991;46:201–210.

Morimoto T. Mandibular position sense in man. In: Kawamura Y, editor. Frontiers of oral physiology: Oral sensory mechanisms, Vol. 4. Basel: Karger; 1983. p. 80–101.

Murthy KSK. Vertebrate fusimotor neurones and their influences on motor behavior. Prog Neurobiol 1978;11:249–307.

Nishimori T, Sera M, Suemune S, Yoshida A, Tsura K, Tsuiki Y, Akisaka T, Okamoto T, Dateoka Y, Shigenaga Y. The distribution of muscle primary afferents from the masseter nerve to the trigeminal sensory nuclei. Brain Res 1986;372:375–381.

Nomura S, Mizuno N. Differential distribution of cell bodies and central axons of mesencephalic trigeminal nucleus neurons supplying the jaw-closing muscles and periodontal tissue: a transganglionic tracer study in the cat. Brain Res 1985;359:311–319.

Paintal AS. Functional analysis of group III afferent fibers of mammalian muscles. J Physiol 1960;52:250–270.

Pedersen J, Sjölander P, Wenngren BI, Johansson H. Increased intramuscular concentration of bradykinin increases the static fusimotor drive to muscle spindles in neck muscles of the cat. Pain 1997;70:83–91.

Ransjö K, Thilander B. Perception of mandibular position in cases of temporomandibular joint disorders. Odont Tijdschr 1963;71:134–144.

Richmond FJ, Abrahams VC. Physiological properties of muscle spindles in dorsal neck muscles of the cat. J Neurophysiol 1979;42:604–617.

Ro JY, Capra NF. Physiological evidence for caudal brainstem projections of jaw muscle spindle afferents. Exp Brain Res 1999a;128:425–434.

Ro JY, Capra NF. Evidence for subnucleus interpolaris in craniofacial muscle pain mechanisms demonstrated by intramuscular injections with hypertonic saline. Brain Res 1999b;842:166–183.

Ro JY, Capra NF. Modulation of jaw muscle spindle afferent activity following intramuscular injections with hypertonic saline. Pain 2001;92:117–127.

Sessle BJ. Identification of alpha and gamma trigeminal motoneurons and effects of stimulation of amygdala, cerebellum, and cerebral cortex. Exp Neurol 1977;54:303–322.

Sessle BJ. Acute and chronic craniofacial pain: brainstem mechanisms of nociceptive transmission and neuroplasticity, and their clinical correlates. Crit Rev Oral Biol Med 2000;11:57–91.

Stohler CS, Ashton-Miller JA, Carlson DS. The effects of pain from the mandibular joint and muscles on masticatory motor behaviour in man. Arch Oral Biol 1988;33:175–182.

Stohler CS, Zhang X, Lund JP. The effect of experimental jaw muscle pain on postural muscle activity. Pain 1996;66:215–221.

Taylor A, Durbaba R, Rodgers JF. The classification of afferents from muscle spindles of the jaw-closing muscles of the cat. J Physiol 1992;456:609–628.

Travell JG, Rinzler S. The myofascial genesis of pain. Postgrad Med 1952;11:425–434.

Wang K, Arendt-Nielsen L, Svensson P. Capsaicin-induced muscle pain alters the excitability of the human jaw-stretch reflex. J Dent Res 2002;81:650–654.

Wang K, Sessle BJ, Svensson P, Arendt-Nielsen L. Glutamate evoked neck and jaw muscle pain facilitate the human jaw stretch reflex. Clin Neurophysiol 2004;115:1288–1295.

Wenngren BI, Pedersen J, Sjölander P, Bergenheim M, Johansson H. Bradykinin and muscle stretch alter contralateral neck muscle spindle output. Neurosci Res 1998;32:119–129.

Correspondence to: Jin Y. Ro, PhD, Department of Biomedical Sciences, University of Maryland Baltimore School of Dentistry, 650 W. Baltimore Street, Baltimore, MD 21201, USA. Tel: 1-410-706-6027; fax: 1-410-706-0865; email: jro@umaryland.edu.

Proprioception and Neck/Shoulder Pain

Mats Djupsjöbacka

Center for Musculoskeletal Research, University of Gävle, Umeå, Sweden

Chronic neck and shoulder pain constitutes an extensive health problem. The point prevalence has been estimated to be as high as 18% in the general population, according to a Swedish study (Guez et al., 2003). The symptoms usually involve pain and stiffness in the neck and shoulder area as well as impaired neck mobility. A history of neck or head trauma is common. Guez and colleagues found that more than a quarter of cases of neck and shoulder pain were associated with a history of trauma. Nevertheless, due to limited knowledge on the underlying pathological mechanisms, the source of the symptoms can only rarely be established. This problem clearly hampers efficient treatment and rehabilitation of patients. It is thus important to develop sensitive and specific tools for characterization of patients with chronic neck and shoulder pain.

Assessment should take into account many different patient characteristics. One aspect that has received increasing attention is assessment of sensorimotor functions such as muscle coordination and proprioception. The growing interest in this area is based on an increasing number of studies reporting atypical, or impaired, sensorimotor function in persons with chronic neck and shoulder pain, along with the fact that several models of the pathophysiology behind musculoskeletal disorders involve various aspects of sensorimotor functioning.

This chapter will focus on one of these sensorimotor functions: proprioception. It provides a background to the topic and a review of the research on proprioception in relation to chronic neck and shoulder pain, along with a discussion on methodology. Research and clinical implications are also discussed.

Proprioception

The sense of proprioception is commonly defined as the perception of the positions and movements of the body segments in relation to each other, without the aid of vision or the sense of touch (Djupsjöbacka and Domkin, 2005). Afferent information from mechanoreceptors in the muscles, joints, and skin provides the basis for proprioception. This information is processed by the central nervous system (CNS) to form internal models of body configuration (Wolpert et al., 1995), which at a conscious level represent proprioception.

For voluntary movements, the information that gives rise to proprioception originates not only from mechanoreceptors, but also from an internal copy of the motor command that activates the muscles producing the movement. This internal copy is known as the efference copy. That is, for voluntary movements, the brain uses the efference copy to predict the new body configuration while using afferent feedback (proprioceptive information) to improve this prediction (Wolpert et al., 1995). In general, when the CNS fuses different sources of information to estimate body configuration, the relative weight for each source seems to be adapted according to the precision of the information. In this way, the available information can be used optimally in the estimation (Wolpert et al., 1995; van Beers et al., 1999). Hence, in conditions that may affect the quality of an information source, such as illness or muscle fatigue, the relative weight of each source of information could be different than under normal conditions.

The internal models of body configuration formed in the CNS from the efference copy and from proprioceptive information are of great importance for both planning and correcting motor commands (see, e.g., Wolpert et al., 1995). Proprioceptive information is used to correct relatively fast movements with a time delay of only 100–250 milliseconds. Thus, this information is crucial for optimal motor control in general. Proprioceptive information from the neck region is especially important for oculomotor function and control of posture (for references see Karlberg et al., 1991).

Consequently, any disturbance of the proprioceptive information from the neck and shoulder region could have a negative impact on motor control, such as impaired control of posture and increased muscle coactivation. Impaired, or inefficient, motor control is a predictor of musculoskeletal pain conditions (see, e.g., Kilbom and Persson 1987; Veiersted et al., 1993). Thus, impaired proprioceptive information may increase the risk for developing a pain condition, or it may contribute to the persistence of an existing condition.

Possible Mechanisms behind Proprioceptive Impairments

Most of the present models for the mechanisms behind chronic musculoskeletal pain conditions (e.g., Johansson et al., 2003; O'Leary et al., 2003) involve some aspect of sensorimotor control. In one of these models, impaired proprioception constitutes an important aspect of the mechanisms of musculoskeletal pain (Johansson et al., 2003). This part of the model largely relies on data from acute experiments in animal models, which have shown that activation of chemoreceptive and nociceptive muscle and joint afferents can affect the sensitivity of muscle spindles, which are considered to be the type of mechanoreceptor most important for proprioception. Specifically, intramuscular injections of inflammatory or algesic substances to hindlimb and neck muscles in anesthetized cats elicited strong effects on both primary and secondary muscle spindle afferents from the injected muscle as well as adjacent muscles (for references, see Djupsjöbacka, 2003). These effects were mediated by reflex effects from chemosensitive muscle afferents onto gamma-motoneurons. In general, the effects on the spindles consisted of an increase in the mean rate of discharge along with a decrease in stretch sensitivity. Also, injection of bradykinin into cervical facet joints (Thunberg et al., 2001) affected the sensitivity of neck muscle spindles in a similar manner. However, these results, obtained by recording individual afferents separately, permit no firm conclusions on how activation of chemosensitive and nociceptive afferents affects the quality of proprioceptive information.

To address this issue, the information content in ensembles of simultaneously recorded spindle afferents should be evaluated (Johansson et al., 1995). Using a method for objective measurement of the ability of ensembles of spindle afferents to distinguish muscle stretches of different amplitudes (Johansson et al., 1995), Pedersen and coworkers (1998) showed that muscle fatigue considerably reduced the quality of the proprioceptive information from the spindle afferents. The authors determined that this effect was due to reflex effects onto gamma-motoneurons from $A\delta$ and/or C fibers from the fatigued muscle. Thus, the model by Johansson et al. (2003) suggests that the quality of proprioceptive information from muscle spindle afferents can be impaired by muscle pain or muscle fatigue as well as by inflammation. In line with these results, Ro and Capra (2001) were able to show that noxious chemical stimulation of jaw muscles modulates the proprioceptive responses of caudal brainstem neurons. For further details on this work, see Chapter 23 by Ro et al.

In the context of neck and shoulder disorders, it is relevant to note that the density of muscle spindles is not uniform. The number of muscle spindles serving a joint increases the more proximal the joint is (Scott and Loeb, 1994). Thus, the deep muscles of the cervical spine have a very high density of spindles (Bakker and Richmond, 1982).

Another tentative mechanism that may affect proprioception in pain conditions was suggested by Matre and coworkers (2002). They proposed that modulation of the sensitivity of dorsal horn neurons by nociceptive input, as well as the mechanisms behind reduced cutaneous sensitivity in response to experimental muscle pain, could also affect the processing and transmission of proprioceptive inflow (for references see Matre et al., 2002).

It is also possible that the level of physical activity may have an impact on proprioception. Thus, an inactive lifestyle is associated with impaired sensorimotor control compared to a physically active one (Lord et al., 1993). Experimental support for the role of physical inactivity comes from a study by Karlberg et al. (1991), where healthy subjects wore a rigid neck-collar for 5 days. After this period of restrained neck mobility, subjects showed reduced peak velocity of voluntary saccades and smooth pursuit eye movements, along with a slight impairment of postural control. Since all these functions depend, at least partly, on proprioceptive input from the neck (for references see Karlberg et al., 1991), one possible interpretation of the results is that the deconditioning period impaired the ability of the CNS to utilize cervical proprioceptive input. Along these lines, it has also been proposed that the reduced activation of deep cervical flexor muscles that has been documented in chronic neck pain conditions (O'Leary et al., 2003) might reduce the important proprioceptive function of these muscles (Jull et al., 2007). Thus, if a chronic neck pain condition leads to reduced neck movements, it seems plausible that this could be reflected in tests of cervical proprioception as well as other tests of sensorimotor functions that depend on proprioceptive information from the cervical region. The mechanisms behind reduced proprioception proposed above are summarized schematically in Fig. 1.

Clinical Studies on Proprioception in Neck/Shoulder Pain

Assessment of Proprioception by Repositioning Tests

A substantial number of investigations have used cervical repositioning tests to study cervical proprioceptive function in chronic neck pain. This type of test involves a procedure in which a blindfolded subject attempts to relocate the head, usually to the natural head position. An average repositioning error is calculated from a series of such trials (a discussion on this methodology is provided below). Greater repositioning errors are

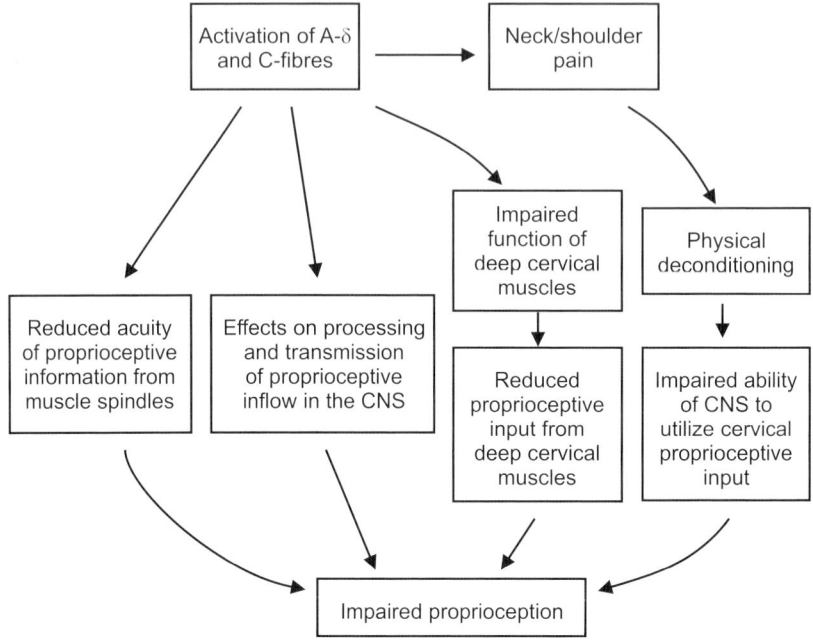

Fig. 1. Schematic illustration of putative mechanisms behind impaired proprioception in neck/shoulder pain.

more common in people with neck pain due to trauma (Heikkila and As-trom, 1996; Loudon et al., 1997; Kristjansson et al., 2003; Treleaven et al., 2003; Sjölander et al., 2008) as well as those with neck pain with nontrau-matic etiology (Revel et al., 1991; Heikkila et al., 2000; Kristjansson et al., 2003). However, several studies have also presented negative results (Rix and Bagust, 2001; Armstrong et al., 2005; Teng et al., 2007). The reason for this discrepancy between studies could be differences in the severity of the pain condition between the study samples. However, it is difficult to compare this aspect across studies due to the large variation in how the samples were characterized. Among studies with negative findings, it is relevant to note that in the study by Teng et al. (2007), the participants with neck pain had only mild disability, rated at 15 points or less on the 0–50-point Neck Disability Index (NDI), and in the study by Armstrong et al. (2005) the neck pain group presented a mean NDI of 12. Only one of the positive studies (those reporting greater repositioning errors in the neck pain group) used the NDI instrument, and it reported a much higher mean score of 22 for a group of patients with whiplash-associated disorder (Sjölander et al., 2008). It is also worth noting that two of the studies reporting greater repositioning errors in groups with neck pain included subjects with symptoms of dizziness (Heikkila et al., 2000; Treleaven et al., 2003).

Repositioning tests have also been used to assess proprioception of the upper extremities in chronic neck pain. A recent study showed reduced acuity of shoulder repositioning in persons with chronic neck pain of traumatic origin (Sandlund et al., 2006). Results were similar for subjects with nonspecific neck and shoulder pain (Djupsjöbacka et al., unpublished data). Additionally, Knox et al. (2006) showed that repositioning errors of the elbow joint were more affected by changes in head position in subjects with chronic neck pain of traumatic origin than in healthy controls.

Considering the common use of repositioning tests to evaluate proprioception in neck and shoulder pain, some methodological aspects are relevant for the interpretation of data. A repositioning test is a psychophysical measurement technique. In general, psychophysical tests involve presentation of a stimulus to a subject and monitoring of the subject's response (Gescheider, 1997). In a repositioning test, a blindfolded subject attempts to reposition a limb or joint to a memorized target position or joint angle. The information underlying the subject's response will be based on different factors depending on whether movements are performed voluntarily (subject-generated) or passively (externally generated). In tests involving active movements, both the efference copy and proprioceptive information will influence the outcome, whereas tests using passive movements will rely on proprioceptive information alone.

The outcome variables of repositioning tests are the variance and the mean of the repositioning errors over a series of trials. These outcome variables are denoted the variable error (VE) and constant error (CE), respectively. VE represents the differential sensory threshold, that is, the threshold for discriminating between two stimuli of different magnitudes, whereas CE represents systematic errors from factors such as a change in the subject's memory of the target position (Craske and Crawshaw, 1975; Gescheider, 1997). In the clinical studies cited above, the discrimination threshold (VE) is rarely reported. Instead, the absolute error (AE), which is the average of the absolute values of the errors for each trial, and thus a composite of VE and CE, is commonly used as the outcome measure. However, AE is hard to interpret (Schutz and Roy, 1973) because it is a nonlinear combination of VE and CE. To measure the quality of sensory information, the VE is preferred (e.g., Clark et al., 1995; van Beers et al., 1998; Djupsjöbacka and Domkin, 2005). In line with this reasoning, Lee et al. (2006) recently emphasized the importance of reporting both CE and VE in studies of cervical repositioning to allow for clearer interpretation of test results.

Another relevant aspect with respect to repositioning tests is that the outcome will not only represent the quality of the efference copy and proprioceptive information, as well as the basic processing of this information in the CNS, but will also involve factors such as cognitive strategies, attention, and memory. While some confounding variables may be kept under reasonable control by careful standardization of the testing procedure, other may pose a greater problem. One such factor is the effect of memory. Given that repositioning tests involve matching a short-term memory representation of a previously presented target position, the time delay will affect performance (Adams and Dijkstra, 1966). The fact that individuals with chronic pain can have reduced memory functions (e.g., Söderfjell et al., 2006) highlights the importance of taking this factor into consideration when evaluating differences in repositioning acuity in chronic pain patients compared to healthy subjects. Surprisingly, no studies to date have taken this potential confounding factor into consideration.

Indirect Assessment of Proprioceptive Function

Clearly, measuring proprioception is a difficult endeavor. However, measurement of proprioception is seldom the final goal. Rather, the research questions in studies attempting to measure proprioception are almost always related to the quality of proprioceptive information. This question can also be addressed by testing motor functions that depend on proprioceptive information.

Measurement of postural sway is often used to evaluate cervical proprioceptive function. This approach is based on evidence for an important role of cervical proprioceptive information for postural control. For example, activation of muscle spindles by muscle vibration has revealed that proprioceptive input from the neck contributes to balance and helps regulate body position (Kavounoudias et al., 1999). A number of studies have reported increased postural sway in various conditions of quiet standing in persons with chronic neck pain either due to trauma (Kogler et al., 2000; Michaelson et al., 2003; Madeleine et al., 2004; Field et al., 2008) or of nontraumatic etiology (Ålund et al., 1993; Karlberg et al., 1995, 1996; Koskimies et al., 1997; McPartland et al., 1997; Field et al., 2008). Due to the complexity of the postural control system, these findings do not necessarily reflect impaired cervical proprioceptive function. However, the link between cervical proprioceptive information and balance in neck pain conditions is supported by the finding that vibration of neck muscles in individuals with neck pain causes greater perturbations of postural control than in controls (Koskimies et al., 1997).

Similar to postural control, oculomotor control depends on cervical proprioceptive information (for references see Karlberg et al., 1991) and has therefore been used for indirect evaluation of cervical proprioceptive function in neck pain conditions. Several studies have shown that smooth pursuit eye movements are affected to a greater extent by neck torsion in persons with chronic neck pain than in healthy controls (e.g., Treleaven et al., 2005a; 2006).

Associations between Sensorimotor Functions and Symptoms and Self-Rated Functioning

One way to address the clinical relevance of the different sensorimotor dysfunctions described above, and to gain better understanding of the mechanisms behind these dysfunctions, is to study associations between sensorimotor variables and symptoms and self-rated functioning. Several investigations have addressed this issue and have found that more pronounced symptoms of dizziness or vertigo are related to greater errors in head repositioning (Treleaven et al., 2003) or greater postural sway

(Ålund et al., 1993; Michaelson et al., 2003; Treleaven et al., 2005b) in persons with neck pain. An association between self-rated physical functioning and acuity of shoulder repositioning has also been reported for subjects with neck and shoulder pain with traumatic etiology (Sandlund et al., 2006). Furthermore, our unpublished results (Djupsjöbacka et al.) indicate an association between shoulder repositioning acuity and the cognitive-behavioral aspect of kinesiophobia in subjects with nonspecific neck and shoulder pain.

Summary

Taken together, the results from the clinical studies reviewed above provide substantial evidence that chronic neck pain with either traumatic or nontraumatic etiology is associated with impaired cervical proprioceptive function. Evidence also suggests that chronic neck pain may be associated with deficits in shoulder proprioception. The reported association between sensorimotor functions and symptoms and self-rated functioning supports the clinical validity of these findings (Ålund et al., 1993; Michaelson et al., 2003; Treleaven et al., 2003, 2005b; Sandlund et al., 2006). Nevertheless, given the complexity of chronic musculoskeletal pain conditions, it is not possible to solely attribute reduced repositioning performance or altered postural activity to proprioceptive deficits. Hence, other factors related to information processing as well as cognitive aspects may play a role.

Implications for Future Research

Studies using repositioning tests should report the differential sensory thresholds (variable errors), and preferably also constant errors, to allow for clearer interpretation of test results (Lee et al., 2006). Repositioning tests involve matching a short-term memory representation of a previously presented target position (Adams and Dijkstra, 1966), and chronic pain can be associated with reduced memory functions (e.g., Söderfjell et al., 2006), so investigators must consider the potentially confounding effect of memory function.

The mechanisms behind the impaired ability in repositioning the upper extremities in persons with neck and shoulder pain could be explored further by incorporating knowledge from basic motor control research. Studies of goal-directed reaching without blindfolding subjects show that precision depends on a weighting of sensory information so that the horizontal (left-right) direction depends more on vision, while the depth (near-far) direction relies more on proprioceptive information from the arm (van Beers et al., 1998). These data provide an opportunity to design tests to evaluate whether the impaired acuity of shoulder (Sandlund et al., 2006) and elbow repositioning (Knox et al., 2006) found in individuals with chronic neck pain is reflected in the quality of proprioceptive information used for everyday functional movements such as reaching.

Cross-sectional studies investigating proprioceptive functioning in pain conditions should collect data on physical activity levels to control for the potential confounding variable of physical fitness.

Another important aspect for future research is to study associations between the outcomes of different tests that may reflect proprioceptive functioning. Recently, Treleaven et al. (2006) studied associations between cervical repositioning errors, standing balance in different conditions, and eye movement control. The authors found only weak to moderate correlations between the outcomes, which suggests that several underlying factors were affecting the outcome of the different tests. Such results can provide valuable insights into the mechanisms reflected by different tests as well as important information for the design of protocols for evaluating patients in rehabilitation.

Lastly, human experimental pain models (e.g., Capra and Ro, 2004) are an attractive way to study the influence of muscle nociceptive input on sensorimotor control. However, such models have yet not been applied extensively in studies on neck/shoulder proprioceptive functioning (but see Madeleine et al., 2004). The acute pain that these models generate may elicit effects on sensorimotor functioning that differ substantially from those in effect in chronic pain conditions (e.g., Moseley et al., 2005). Nevertheless, studies on the effect of experimental muscle pain on neck/shoulder proprioceptive functioning could still add to our understanding of the relationship between neck and shoulder pain and proprioception.

Clinical Implications

Are there interventions that can improve proprioceptive function? Unfortunately, research on this issue is scarce. More than a century ago, Slinger and Horsley (1906) reported that blind subjects could perform a finger-matching task with superior precision compared to subjects with intact vision. On this basis the authors concluded that "if the information gained by sight is permanently blotted out, the muscular sense under necessity can, by education, be brought to a point at least one-fourth better than that learnt by a normal seeing individual." More recently, Tsang and coworkers (2003) presented evidence that long-term Tai Chi practitioners had improved knee joint proprioception and superior stability when shifting their weight in standing positions, compared to matched controls. Also, Jull and coworkers (2007) found that craniocervical flexion exercises as well as exercises directly targeting cervical relocation ability both reduced errors in cervical repositioning.

In support of the role of proprioception in the mechanisms behind chronic neck and shoulder pain, several studies have found that different interventions have beneficial effects on symptoms in people with chronic neck pain. These interventions feature components that may enhance proprioceptive acuity, such as body awareness training (Kadi et al., 2000); exercises involving coordinated rapid eye, head, neck, and arm movements (Fitz-Ritson, 1995); Feldenkrais therapy (Lundblad et al., 1999); multimodal treatment involving exercises to improve balance, neck coordination, and oculomotor control (Taimela et al., 2000); a proprioceptive training program to improve coordination of eye and head movement (Revel et al., 1994; Jull et al., 2007); and craniocervical flexion exercises (Jull et al., 2007).

Together, this information suggests that proprioception can be improved by training and that specially designed exercises can improve symptoms in people with neck pain. When implementing these exercises in clinical practice, it is probably also beneficial to incorporate knowledge from the field of motor learning. Thus, to promote retention of training effects and to help patients to transfer the effects of the exercises to more general functions, it is important to design the exercises so that they are cognitively challenging for the patient, include a progression of difficulty, and contain unpredictable task variations as well as changes in the context in which the task is performed (Jarus, 1994; Guadagnoli and Lee, 2004).

References

Adams JA, Dijkstra S. Short-term memory for motor responses. J Exp Psychol 1966;71:314–318.

Ålund M, Ledin T, Ödkvist L, Larsson SE. Dynamic posturography among patients with common neck disorders. A study of 15 cases with suspected cervical vertigo. J Vestib Res 1993;3:383–389.

Armstrong BS, McNair PJ, Williams M. Head and neck position sense in whiplash patients and healthy individuals and the effect of the cranio-cervical flexion action. Clin Biomech 2005;20:675–684.

Bakker DA, Richmond FJR. Muscle spindle complexes in muscles around upper cervical vertebrae in the cat. J Neurophysiol 1982;48:62–74.

Capra NF, Ro JY. Human and animal experimental models of acute and chronic muscle pain: intramuscular algesic injection. Pain 2004;110:3–7.

Clark FJ, Larwood KJ, Davis ME, Deffenbacher KA. A Metric for Assessing Acuity in Positioning Joints and Limbs. Exp Brain Res 1995;107:73–79.

Craske B, Crawshaw M. Shifts in kinesthesis through time and after active and passive movement. Percept Mot Skills 1975;40:755–761.

Djupsjöbacka M. Effects of physical work exposure on proprioception. In: Johansson JH, Windhorst U, Djupsjöbacka M, Passatore M, editors. Chronic work-related myalgia: neuromuscular mechanisms behind work-related chronic muscle pain syndromes. Gävle University Press; 2003. p 175–183.

Djupsjöbacka M, Domkin D. Correlation analysis of proprioceptive acuity in ipsilateral position-matching and velocity-discrimination. Somatosens Mot Res 2005;22:85–93.

Field S, Treleaven J, Jull G. Standing balance: a comparison between idiopathic and whiplash-induced neck pain. Man Ther 2008;13:183–191.

Fitz-Ritson D. Phasic exercises for cervical rehabilitation after "whiplash" trauma. J Manipulative Physiol Ther 1995;18:21–24.

Gescheider GA. Psychophysics: the fundamentals. Mahwah, NJ: Lawrence Erlbaum Associates, 1997.

Guadagnoli MA, Lee TD. Challenge point: a framework for conceptualizing the effects of various practice conditions in motor learning. J Mot Behav 2004;36:212–224.

Guez M, Hildingsson C, Stegmayr B, Toolanen G. Chronic neck pain of traumatic and non-traumatic origin: a population-based study. Acta Orthop Scand 2003;74:576–579.

Heikkila H, Åstrom PG. Cervicocephalic kinesthetic sensibility in patients with whiplash injury. Scand J Rehabil Med 1996;28:133–138.

Heikkila H, Johansson M, Wenngren BI. Effects of acupuncture, cervical manipulation and NSAID therapy on dizziness and impaired head repositioning of suspected cervical origin: a pilot study. Man Ther 2000;5:151–157.

Jarus T. Motor learning and occupational therapy: the organization of practice. Am J Occup Ther 1994;48:810–816.

Johansson H, Arendt-Nilsson L, Bergenheim M, et al. Epilogue: an integrated model for chronic work-related myalgia "Brussels Model." In: Johansson H, Windhorst U, Djupsjöbacka M, Passatore M, editors. Chronic work-related myalgia: neuromuscular mechanisms behind work-related chronic muscle pain syndromes. Gävle University Press; 2003. p 291–300.

Johansson H, Bergenheim M, Djupsjöbacka M, Sjölander P. A method for analysis of encoding of stimulus separation in ensembles of afferents. J Neurosci Methods 1995;63:67–74.

Jull G, Falla D, Treleaven J, Hodges P, Vicenzino B. Retraining cervical joint position sense: the effect of two exercise regimes. J Orthop Res 2007;25:404–412.

Kadi F, Ahlgren C, Waling K, Sundelin G, Thornell LE. The effects of different training programs on the trapezius muscle of women with work-related neck and shoulder myalgia. Acta Neuropathol (Berl) 2000;100:253–258.

Karlberg M, Magnusson M, Johansson R. Effects of restrained cervical mobility on voluntary eye movements and postural control. Acta Otolaryngol 1991;111:664–670.

Karlberg M, Persson L, Magnusson M. Impaired postural control in patients with cervico-brachial pain. Acta Otolaryngol Suppl 1995;520:440–442.

Karlberg M, Johansson R, Magnusson M, Fransson PA. Dizziness of suspected cervical origin distinguished by posturographic assessment of human postural dynamics. J Vestib Res 1996;6:37–47.

Kavounoudias A, Gilhodes JC, Roll R, Roll JP. From balance regulation to body orientation: two goals for muscle proprioceptive information processing? Exp Brain Res 1999;124:80–88.

Kilbom Å, Persson J. Work technique and its consequences for musculoskeletal disorders. Ergonomics 1987;30:273–279.

Knox JJ, Beilstein DJ, Charles SD, Aarseth GA, Rayar S, Treleaven J, Hodges PW. Changes in head and neck position have a greater effect on elbow joint position sense in people with whiplash-associated disorders. Clin J Pain 2006;22:512–518.

Kogler A, Lindfors J, Ödkvist LM, Ledin T. Postural stability using different neck positions in normal subjects and patients with neck trauma. Acta Otolaryngol 2000;120:151–155.

Koskimies K, Sutinen P, Aalto H, Starck J, Toppila E, Hirvonen T, Kaksonen R, Ishizaki H, Alaranta H, Pyykko I. Postural stability, neck proprioception and tension neck. Acta Otolaryngol 1997;95–97.

Kristjansson E, Dall'Alba P, Jull G. A study of five cervicocephalic relocation tests in three different subject groups. Clin Rehabil 2003;17:768–774.

Lee HY, Teng CC, Chai HM, Wang SF. Test-retest reliability of cervicocephalic kinesthetic sensibility in three cardinal planes. Man Ther 2006;11:61–68.

Lord SR, Caplan GA, Ward JA. Balance, reaction-time, and muscle strength in exercising and non-exercising older women—a pilot-study. Arch Phys Med Rehabil 1993;74:837–839.

Loudon JK, Ruhl M, Field E. Ability to reproduce head position after whiplash injury. Spine 1997;22:865–868.

Lundblad I, Elert J, Gerdle B. Randomized controlled trial of physiotherapy and Feldenkrais interventions in female workers with neck-shoulder complaints. J Occup Rehabil 1999;9:179–194.

Madeleine P, Prietzel H, Svarrer H, Arendt-Nielsen L. Quantitative posturography in altered sensory conditions: a way to assess balance instability in patients with chronic whiplash injury. Arch Phys Med Rehabil 2004;85:432–438.

Matre D, Arendt-Nielsen L, Knardahl S. Effects of localization and intensity of experimental muscle pain on ankle joint proprioception. Eur J Pain 2002;6:245–260.

McPartland JM, Brodeur RR, Hallgren RC. Chronic neck pain, standing balance, and suboccipital muscle atrophy—a pilot study. J Manipulative Physiol Ther 1997;20:24–29.

Michaelson P, Michaelson M, Jaric S, Latash ML, Sjölander P, Djupsjöbacka M. Vertical posture and head stability in patients with chronic neck pain. J Rehabil Med 2003;35:229–235.

Moseley GL, Sim DF, Henry ML, Souvlis T. Experimental hand pain delays recognition of the contralateral hand - evidence that acute and chronic pain have opposite effects on information processing? Brain Res Cogn Brain Res 2005;25(1):188–194.

O'Leary S, Falla D, Jull G. Recent advances in therapeutic exercise for the neck: implications for patients with head and neck pain. Aust Endod J 2003;29:138–142.

Pedersen J, Ljubisavljevic M, Bergenheim M, Johansson H. Alterations in information transmission in ensembles of primary muscle spindle afferents after muscle fatigue in heteronymous muscle. Neuroscience 1998;84:953–959.

Revel M, Andre-Deshays C, Minguet M. Cervicocephalic kinesthetic sensibility in patients with cervical pain. Arch Phys Med Rehabil 1991;72:288–291.

Revel M, Minguet M, Gregoy P, Vaillant J, Manuel JL. Changes in cervicocephalic kinesthesia after a proprioceptive rehabilitation program in patients with neck pain: a randomized controlled study. Arch Phys Med Rehabil 1994;75:895–899.

Rix GD, Bagust J. Cervicocephalic kinesthetic sensibility in patients with chronic, nontraumatic cervical spine pain. Arch Phys Med Rehabil 2001;82:911–919.

Ro JY, Capra NF. Modulation of jaw muscle spindle afferent activity following intramuscular injections with hypertonic saline. Pain 2001;92:117–127.

Sandlund J, Djupsjöbacka M, Ryhed B, Hamberg J, Björklund M. Predictive and discriminative value of shoulder proprioception tests for patients with whiplash-associated disorders. J Rehabil Med 2006;38:44–49.

Schutz RW, Roy EA. Absolute error: the devil in disguise. J Mot Behav 1973;5:141–153.

Scott SH, Loeb GE. The computation of position sense from spindles in mono- and multiarticular muscles. J Neurosci 1994;14:7529–7540.

Sjölander P, Michaelson P, Jaric S, Djupsjöbacka M. Sensorimotor disturbances in chronic neck pain: range of motion, peak velocity, smoothness of movement, and repositioning acuity. Man Ther 2008;13:122–131.

Slinger RT, Horsley V. Upon the orientation of points in space by the muscular, arthrodial, and tactile senses of the upper limbs in normal individuals and blind persons. Brain 1906;April:1–27.

Söderfjell S, Molander B, Johansson H, Barnekow-Bergkvist M, Nilsson LG. Musculoskeletal pain complaints and performance on cognitive tasks over the adult life span. Scand J Psychol 2006;47:349–359.

Taimela S, Takala EP, Asklof T, Seppala K, Parviainen S. Active treatment of chronic neck pain: a prospective randomized intervention. Spine 2000;25:1021–1027.

Teng CC, Chai H, Lai DM, Wang SF. Cervicocephalic kinesthetic sensibility in young and middle-aged adults with or without a history of mild neck pain. Man Ther 2007;12:22–28.

Thunberg J, Hellstrom F, Sjölander P, Bergenheim M, Wenngren B, Johansson H. Influences on the fusimotor-muscle spindle system from chemosensitive nerve endings in cervical facet joints in the cat: possible implications for whiplash induced disorders. Pain 2001;91:15–22.

Treleaven J, Jull G, LowChoy N. Smooth pursuit neck torsion test in whiplash-associated disorders: Relationship to self-reports of neck pain and disability, dizziness and anxiety. J Rehabil Med 2005a;37:219–223.

Treleaven J, Jull G, LowChoy N. Standing balance in persistent whiplash: a comparison between subjects with and without dizziness. J Rehabil Med 2005b;37:224–229.

Treleaven J, Jull G, LowChoy N. The relationship of cervical joint position error to balance and eye movement disturbances in persistent whiplash. Man Ther 2006;11:99–106.

Treleaven J, Jull G, Sterling M. Dizziness and unsteadiness following whiplash injury: characteristic features and relationship with cervical joint position error. J Rehabil Med 2003;35:36–43.

Tsang WW, Hui-Chan CW. Effects of tai chi on joint proprioception and stability limits in elderly subjects. Med Sci Sports Exerc 2003;35:1962–1971.

van Beers RJ, Sittig AC, Denier van der Gon JJ. The precision of proprioceptive position sense. Exp Brain Res 1998;122:367–377.

van Beers RJ, Sittig AC, van der Gon JJD. Integration of proprioceptive and visual position-information: an experimentally supported model. J Neurophysiol 1999;81:1355–1364.

Veiersted KB, Westgaard RH, Andersen P. Electromyographic evaluation of muscular work pattern as a predictor of trapezius myalgia. Scand J Work Environ Health 1993;19:284–290.

Wolpert DM, Ghahramani Z, Jordan MI. An internal model for sensorimotor integration. Science 1995;269:1880–1882.

Correspondence to: Mats Djupsjöbacka, PhD, Center for Musculoskeletal Research, University of Gävle, Box 7629, SE-907 12 Umeå, Sweden. Tel: +46 90 106076; Fax: +46 90 106099; email: mda@hig.se.

Functional Adaptations in Work-Related Pain Conditions

Pascal Madeleine

Laboratory for Work-Related Pain and Biomechanics, Center for Sensory-Motor Interaction, Department of Health Science and Technology, Aalborg University, Aalborg, Denmark

This chapter reviews the risk factors leading to work-related musculoskeletal disorders and describes pain and structural muscle changes associated with these disorders. Details follow on the functional adaptations that take place in both static and dynamic work-related musculoskeletal pain conditions. The chapter describes the existing neurophysiological models for muscle pain and motor control interactions and discusses the clinical implications of current research knowledge for the prevention of chronic disorders. This brief chapter focuses on disorders of the low back and shoulder regions.

Work-Related Pain

Risk Factors Leading to Work-Related Musculoskeletal Disorders

Despite a decline in the proportion of workers employed in physically demanding sectors such as manufacturing and agriculture, many physical

risk factors are still prevalent in the workplace. In a recent European survey, 62% of the working population reported exposure to repetitive hand
or arm movements, and 45% mentioned spending at least 25% of their
working hours in painful, tiring positions (European Foundation for the
Improvement of the Living and Working Conditions, 2007). These recent
results are corroborated by a number of epidemiological studies identifying risk factors for the development of work-related musculoskeletal
disorders (WMSDs) in the low back and upper extremities (Punnett and
Wegman, 2004). These risk factors are divided into internal and external
risk factors (Sjøgaard et al., 1995). Among the internal risk factors are
age, gender, muscle strength, endurance, fitness, personality, and muscle
tension. The external risk factors can be expressed in terms of physical
and psychosocial factors. A relatively fixed erect posture, repetitive arm
movements, heavy work, insufficient rest, vibrations, cold temperature,
and static posture are the known physical risk factors (Winkel and Westgaard, 1992; Sommerich et al., 1993). Stress and pain behavior are two
of the most important psychological risk factors (Sjøgaard et al., 1995;
Vlaeyen and Linton, 2000).

Exposure-response-effect models (Winkel and Westgaard, 1992;
Sjøgaard et al., 1995) have been designed to evaluate the importance of
external and internal risk factors for the development of WMSDs. The
responses reflect acute physiological changes such as adenosine triphosphate breakdown and actin-myosin coupling related to physical
and mental loads (Sjøgaard et al., 1995). Repeated acute responses over
a long period will result either in adaptation mechanisms or in the development of WMSDs, depending on the capacity or ability of the individual and the risk factors to which he or she is exposed. However, the
complex interrelations among internal and external risk factors make it
impossible to rank them in terms of their importance for risk of further
development of disorders in the low back or shoulder region (Visser and
van Dieën, 2006). The large number of risk factors and their complex relationships explain why WMSDs are characterized by both diffuse symptoms (constant fatigue, stiffness, and referred pain) and specific symptoms (increased muscle tone, pain in different parts of the body, and
trigger points).

Pain in Work-Related Musculoskeletal Disorders

Pain in deep structures including cartilage, tendons, ligaments, and muscles is one of the most consistent symptoms associated with WMSDs in the low back and upper extremity. In musculoskeletal pain, the pain sensation is mediated by nociceptive free nerve endings in the wall of arterioles and related structures such as the connective tissue between muscle fibers (Mense, 1993; see Chapter 1 by Mense and Hoheisel). Free nerve endings are connected to primary afferent neurons that are group III and IV sensory fibers. Fast, thin, myelinated muscle afferents (group III/Aδ) terminate in free nerve endings and other receptor types, whereas thick, unmyelinated muscle afferents (group IV/C) terminate only in free nerve endings. Muscle nociceptors are usually polymodal and respond to high-intensity stimuli or to algogenic agents. The activation of muscle nociceptors arises with the release of mediators such as bradykinin, potassium, prostaglandin, and serotonin (Cairns, 2007). Increased muscle load or sustained repetitive muscle activity could result in a higher accumulation of Ca^{2+} and metabolites in the muscles (Edwards, 1988; Gissel, 2000; Rosendal et al., 2004), which might be sufficient to activate nociceptors. Muscle nociceptive afferents terminate in laminae I, II, and V of the dorsal horn or of the subnucleus caudalis in the brain (Mense, 1993). In consequence, noxious sensory input influences both alpha- and gamma-motoneurons. Nociceptive input interacts with the motor system through connections between interneurons and alpha-motoneurons. For gamma-motoneurons, a general central inhibitory effect on agonist and antagonist muscles and on proprioception has been demonstrated (Mense and Skeppar, 1991; see Chapter 23 by Ro et al.). Recurrent acute pain episodes may induce sensitization and can in turn lead to chronic work-related pain. Due to lack of knowledge on the etiology of WMSDs in general, there is to date no effective treatment. Indeed, the prevention of WMSDs is still the best treatment.

One way to gain insight into the transduction, transmission, and projection of nociceptive input is to use experimental pain models. Experimental muscle pain models are of great interest because they cause transitory well-controlled muscle pain that mimics clinical conditions (see Chapter 11 by Graven-Nielsen and Arendt-Nielsen). Experimental muscle pain can be induced endogenously or exogenously (Svensson and Arendt-Nielsen, 1995). Repetitive eccentric loadings at a supramaximal level causing delayed-onset muscle soreness and intramuscular injection of hypertonic saline (Fig. 1a) are the two modalities most often used to induce experimental pain in the shoulder region (Madeleine et al., 1998; Nie et al., 2005). Such models enable researchers to quantify the outcome of a treatment or an intervention and delineate the transition from acute to chronic stages.

Muscle Structural Changes in Work-Related Musculoskeletal Disorders

In addition to pain, morphological changes have also been reported in relation to low back and upper extremity disorders. Clear evidence shows the effects of occupational workload on type I muscle fibers

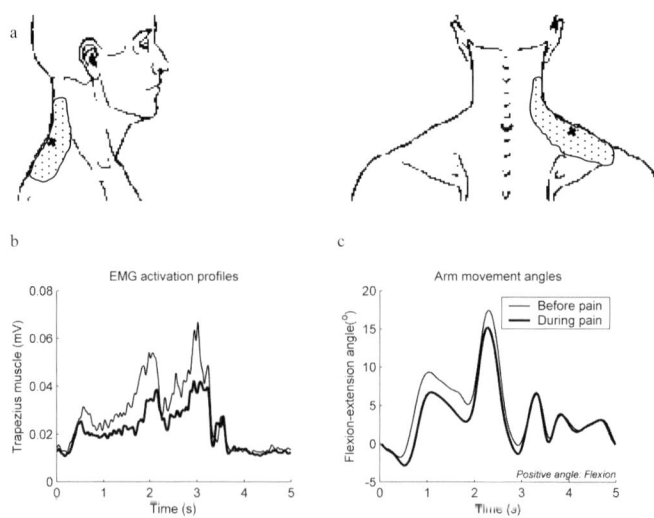

Fig. 1. Example of (a) local and referred endogenous muscle pain pattern following injection of 0.75 mL hypertonic saline (6%) into the right trapezius muscle (x: injection site), (b) averaged surface electromyogram profiles (mV) of the right trapezius muscle, and (c) offset corrected mean arm movement angles (°) in the flexion-extension direction during repetitive work before pain (36 cycles) and after hypertonic saline injection (during pain, 50 cycles). For more details, see Madeleine et al. (1999).

(Hägg, 2000). In the paraspinal muscles, a predominance of type II fibers has been found in low back patients compared with controls (Mannion, 1999). The percentage of type I fibers, in contrast, was increased or unchanged in patients with trapezius myalgia (Hägg, 2000). Reduced microcirculation has also been reported, most likely due to an inability to relax the muscles. Long-time static work is suggested to lead to "moth-eaten" or "ragged red" type I fibers. "Ragged red" fibers are closely related to repetitive assembly work (Hägg, 2000). Moreover, the cross-sectional area of fibers is also increased in painful muscles. The appearance of such morphological changes could indicate mitochondrial disturbances, with a loss of oxidative capacity; a reduced concentration of adenosine diphosphate, adenosine triphosphate, and creatinine; and increased enzyme cytochrome-c oxydase activity in the painful muscle (Hägg, 2000). Although questions remain concerning the relationship between muscle fiber abnormalities and pain intensity, and about the extent of structural changes in low back and trapezius muscles, we know that these structural changes have important implications in terms of general physical capacity. Moreover, we know that muscle fiber abnormalities are likely to be related to degenerative processes due to metabolic overuse or overload. These findings give credit to the "Cinderella hypothesis," which posits the overloading of type I muscle fibers during long-term repetitive work (Hägg, 1991).

Functional Adaptations in Work-Related Conditions

Physical exposure is usually described in terms of four different modes of activity: static sustained, static repetitive, dynamic concentric, and dynamic eccentric activity (Sjøgaard et al., 1995). This section will be limited to two modes of action: static and dynamic work. Static work is associated with postural load, and dynamic work is correlated with repetitive work. This section will emphasize low back and shoulder functional adaptations, focusing mainly on the trapezius muscle, which is considered the most important muscle of the shoulder region due to its functional implications: the upper part of the muscle is responsible for elevation of shoulders and rotation of the glenoid fossa, the lower part of the muscle assists with this rotation, and the middle part of the muscle performs adduction of the scapula.

Static Conditions

Static contractions are performed extensively in the workplace. There are three distinct types of static conditions: resting conditions, submaximal (brief or sustained) static contractions, and maximal static contractions. Resting conditions and submaximal contraction levels are most commonly found in today's workplace, and they are of great interest due to their relationship to work-related pain.

In clinical conditions, either unchanged or increased amplitude in the surface electromyographic (EMG) activity of muscles at rest may be reported in patients with low back pain (for review, see van Dieën et al., 2003b). Similarly, in patients with shoulder pain or other shoulder complaints, the upper trapezius muscle may show either unchanged EMG activity (Takala and Viikari-Juntura, 1991) or increased activity (Veiersted et al., 1990; Madeleine et al., 1999, 2003b). Interestingly, the variability in resting surface EMG activity is less pronounced in chronic shoulder pain patients and in subchronic pain conditions (pain that develops after 6 months of work) (Madeleine et al., 2008a,b). For the trapezius muscle, the resting period in the surface EMG signal is often analyzed by computing the number and frequency of gaps or resting events. A gap has been defined as a period of muscle surface EMG activity below 0.5% of the maximum voluntary contraction for at least 200 milliseconds (Veiersted et al., 1990). Cross-sectional and longitudinal studies (Veiersted et al., 1993; Hägg and Astrom, 1997) have revealed that workers who either have or are at risk for developing work-related shoulder disorders have fewer EMG gaps or resting events compared with controls. On the other hand, other studies have reported no differences between patients and control groups (Takala and Viikari-Juntura, 1991; Jensen et al., 1993).

Experimental muscle pain induced either endogenously or exogenously does not produce a sustained increase in surface EMG activity.

Either a transient increase occurs, or no change is reported in resting surface EMG activity (Svensson et al., 1998; Kawczynski et al., 2007).

At submaximal contraction levels, increased static EMG activity is found among patients with trapezius myalgia (Sandsjö et al., 2000; Szeto et al., 2005). Moreover, this increase in surface EMG activity has been reported as a risk factor for developing pain or other complaints in the shoulder region (Veiersted et al., 1993). The increased surface EMG activity observed in patients is not considered a favorable trait because it contributes to overloading the painful muscle. Moreover, relatively high surface EMG activity has been proposed as a predictor of the development of work-related disorders by the few longitudinal studies that have investigated the effects of pain on trapezius surface EMG activity (Veiersted et al., 1993; Madeleine et al., 2003b).

Experimentally induced muscle pain causes a functional reorganization of muscle activity that depends on the motor task and the ability of the motor system to recruit synergistic muscles. However, these changes are not always detected, mostly due to the specificity of the motor task investigated and the limited sensitivity of single-channel surface EMG in assessing changes in muscle activation (Birch et al., 2000; Madeleine and Arendt-Nielsen, 2005). In order to overcome such limitations, other quantitative methods can be used based on multichannel surface EMG and mechanomyographic (MMG) recordings. MMG is used to assess intrinsic mechanical properties of muscles (Orizio, 1993). Increased MMG is reported during experimental pain induced either endogenously or exogenously (Madeleine and Arendt-Nielsen, 2005; Kawczynski et al., 2007). The increase could reflect an increase in twitch force and a decreased number of active motor units (Sohn et al., 2004).

However, in the paraspinal or shoulder muscles, a reorganization of muscle synergies is observed in static conditions due to the redundancy of the motor system and the vast number of possibilities for stabilizing structures such as the shoulder girdle (Madeleine et al., 1999). For the upper trapezius muscle, most studies have shown reduced surface EMG activity in the painful muscle, which is interpreted as an inhibitory mechanism reflecting adaptation to pain (Ge et al., 2005; Madeleine et al., 2006). Moreover, the short-term reorganization observed in acute experimental conditions demonstrates spatial changes in surface EMG activity caused by inhibitory reflex mechanisms (Fig. 2). In the long run, such adaptive mechanisms among subdivisions of the upper trapezius muscle can explain the spreading of pain observed in clinical conditions to other parts of the same muscle and to synergistic muscles (Madeleine et al., 2006; Falla et al., 2007).

During sustained contraction, time to task failure is shorter among patients with trapezius myalgia performing a submaximal contraction compared with controls (Elert et al., 1993). Moreover, competing fatigue and pain mechanisms are reported with respect to the surface EMG changes (Madeleine et al., 2006). In clinical conditions, the explanation of the shorter time to task failure is likely to depend on physiological factors such as microcirculation and morphological changes.

At maximal contraction level, a general decrease of the maximum force is found in both experimental and clinical painful conditions (Thorstensson and Arvidson, 1982; Elert et al., 1991). These changes have been attributed to central effects and not to changes in the contractile properties of muscle fibers (Graven-Nielsen et al., 2002). Despite the fact that a large percentage of the workforce usually performs tasks at low contraction levels (less than 30% of MVC), the changes reported

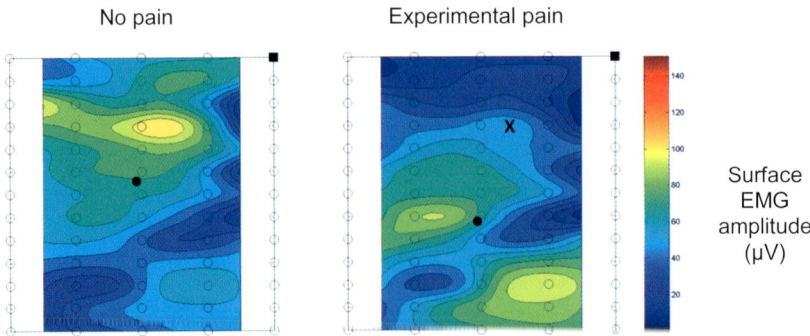

Fig. 2. Example of reorganization of surface electromyographic activity (5 × 13 electrodes) maps of the right trapezius muscle prior to and following injection of 0.5 mL hypertonic saline (6%) into the right trapezius muscle (X: injection site). Note the changes in trapezius activation on the topographical maps in response to acute experimental pain induced exogenously, underlined by the shift in the center of gravity (filled circles). For more details, see Madeleine et al. (2006).

at maximum level are important because they contribute to narrow the range of activity of painful muscles, leading to increased absolute load.

In conclusion, complex changes accompany pain in either the low back or shoulder region (Table I). Moreover, there are discrepancies between the effects of experimental and chronic pain on muscle activity as depicted by surface EMG and MMG. The changes in surface EMG amplitude and the amount of variability indicate a dynamic reorganization of muscle activity during painful conditions, indicating that new synergies develop as pain changes from acute to chronic stages. Furthermore, the reorganization occurring within and among synergistic muscles during experimental pain can explain the spreading of pain to remote areas. At subchronic and chronic stages, the relatively static surface EMG activity shows that patients are unable to relax the muscle, suggesting that the muscle has entered a "Cinderella" mode (Hägg, 1991).

Table I
Overall motor functional adaptations in the low back and the shoulder region in the presence of experimental and chronic pain during static and dynamic contractions

	Experimental Pain	Chronic Pain
Static Contractions		
Resting level	Transient increase/ unchanged EMG	Unchanged/increased EMG, lower EMG variability, fewer/ unchanged gaps
Submaximal contraction	Unchanged/decreased EMG, increased MMG, EMG spatial reorganization	Increased EMG
Sub-maximal sustained contraction	EMG spatial reorganization	Shorter endurance time
Maximal contraction level	Decreased force	Decreased force
Dynamic Contractions		
Timing	Slower movement, increased timing variability	Slower movement, increased timing variability
Force	Decreased force	Decreased force
Surface EMG	Decreased EMG	Increased EMG, muscle activation imbalance, increased co-contraction, lower EMG variability
Movement	Decreased posture and movement amplitude; increased variability	Decreased/increased movement amplitude, increased/decreased variability

Dynamic Conditions

Repetitive movements are a frequent component of many occupations and are associated with WMSDs. The effects of WMSDs on motor activity can be quantified by measuring the timing of tasks, the force exerted, muscle activity, and movement amplitude during tasks such as cyclic arm movements.

During sudden loading or cyclic arm movement, a time delay or a decrease in working rhythm is observed in the presence of either low back or shoulder pain (Madeleine et al., 1999; Radebold et al., 2000). The amount of variability of the duration of the work cycle increased in subjects with unilateral acute experimental shoulder pain and in patients with bilateral chronic shoulder pain. Moreover, unilateral experimental pain in the shoulder region induced bilateral changes in the performance of a motor task (Madeleine et al., 2008a). These results indicate that supraspinal and/or spinal mechanisms can mediate the spreading of motor effects to the contralateral pain-free side (Madeleine et al., 1999; Thunberg et al., 2002).

A decrease in the strength of lower trunk flexors and extensors has been found in low back patients (Takemasa et al., 1995) and in subjects with experimental or subchronic shoulder pain (Madeleine et al., 1999, 2003b). These results during cyclic movements corroborate findings in static conditions and underline a general protective response in the presence of experimental or clinical pain.

In patients with low back pain, the surface EMG activity of the paraspinal muscles during a dynamic exercise is higher in full extension compared with that of controls (Ahern et al., 1988). Imbalanced and variable surface EMG activation and increased co-contraction of trunk muscles are also reported in low back pain patients (Radebold et al., 2000; Oddsson and De Luca, 2003; Lamoth et al., 2006). During walking, increased surface EMG is only reported during the swing phase, both in low back pain patients and in subjects with experimental muscle pain (Arendt-Nielsen et al., 1996). This finding indicates that muscle activity is dependently modulated with specific changes in muscle function during agonist and antagonist phases. Co-contraction mechanisms aiming at stabilizing the lumbar spine can be added to this compensatory effect (Radebold et al., 2000).

Similar to findings in static conditions, experimental pain decreased the surface EMG activity of the trapezius muscle (Fig. 1b). In chronic shoulder pain conditions, the level of surface EMG activity was greater for patients than for controls during a nonactive part of a dynamic task (Madeleine et al., 1999). Moreover, a general lack of variation in surface EMG amplitude leading to increased static muscle activation is also found among workers with subchronic pain (Madeleine et al., 2003b). These results are in line with previous findings showing a higher level of static surface EMG for workers with previous shoulder pain episodes compared to workers with no shoulder complaints (Veiersted et al., 1990, 1993). All in all, the dynamic reorganization of surface EMG activity under painful conditions, or more precisely, the development of new synergies along with the spreading of pain, is likely to indicate a *learning effect* of motor strategies in response to nociceptive influx. The activation of group III and IV afferents and the lack of harmonious recruitment and derecruitment of muscles most likely play important roles in the development of WMSD.

A general reduction in movement amplitude is reported among low back pain patients (Ahern et al., 1988; Arendt-Nielsen et al., 1996). Fear avoidance, referring to the avoidance of movement or activities due to fear of pain, has been suggested as a precursor of long-term back disability (Vlaeyen and Linton, 2000). Both lower and higher amounts of variability in movement amplitude have been reported among patients with chronic low back pain, expressed for example as a counterrotation at higher walking speeds (Lamoth et al., 2006).

During experimental shoulder pain, both posture and movement change. In our study, the starting position changed, and the movement of the arm (Fig. 1c) decreased compared with before pain (Madeleine et al., 1999). It is more difficult to draw conclusions based on kinematic results for workers with subchronic and chronic pain (Madeleine et al., 1999, 2003b). In the arm, chronic pain leads to increased movement amplitude, while the opposite has been observed at the subchronic stage. Variability in the amplitude of arm movement is reported to increase in experimental pain, whereas a decrease is found in subchronic and chronic shoulder pain, underlining a decrease in the available degree of freedom and reduced flexibility of the motor system (Madeleine et al., 2008a,b). The reported changes in low back and especially shoulder pain conditions suggest that motor behavior also differs with pain at different stages and of different origins.

These findings show an interaction between work-related pain and motor strategies during dynamic tasks (Table I). The reported adaptive mechanisms confirm the importance of the known physical risk factors associated with repetitive work, namely repetitiveness, force level, surface EMG activity amplitude, arm and trunk posture, and movement amplitude. Relatively high surface EMG activity in symptom-free workers is reported to be a prognostic factor for WMSD development in the shoulder region. Quantification of sensory-motor interactions and their variability at various pain stages (acute, subchronic, and chronic) furnishes important data toward a better understanding of pain status transition.

Pathophysiological Models in Relation to Work-Related Musculoskeletal Disorders

Functional motor adaptive mechanisms are found in work-related pain and highlight both inhibitory and excitatory mechanisms and modulation in repetitive work tasks. A vicious cycle due to ischemia and leading to muscle hyperactivity has been proposed to explain the cause of muscle pain (Travell et al., 1942). However, limitations in the "vicious cycle" theory have been put forward based on a relative lack of evidence. This has led to the "pain adaptation model" to explain the interactions between muscle pain and motor strategies. The model predicts decreased surface EMG activity of the agonist muscle, increased surface EMG activity of the antagonist muscle, and less powerful and slower movements during muscle pain (Lund et al., 1991). Another physiological model based on animal data recently challenged existing models (see Chapter 23 by Ro et al.). This model suggests that group III and IV afferents activate the gamma-motoneuron system and lead to a vicious cycle including muscle hyperactivity (Schmidt et al., 1981; Johansson and Sojka, 1991). This facilitation could in turn cause increased muscle stiffness and explain the propagation of pain from one muscle to others via positive feedback.

A number of studies have given credit to the pain adaptation model. The motor reorganization observed in the low back and shoulder regions mainly follows the model's predictions (Arendt-Nielsen et al., 1996; Madeleine et al., 1999). However, the hardwired pain adaptation model provides no solutions regarding the behavior of the motor-neuron pool during isometric contraction, whereas the vicious cycle theory predicts an increase in muscle activation that is not always supported in the literature (van Dieën et al., 2003a). Moreover, the concept of agonist/antagonist muscles is not always consistent due to the co-contraction mechanisms reported in experimental and chronic pain (Radebold et al., 2000).

In conclusion, none of the existing models furnishes consistent proof that the muscle enters a vicious cycle or that the reported adaptive mechanisms solely reflect protective mechanisms aiming at minimizing the effects of work-related pain on the motor system. The pain adaptation model partly predicts changes in experimental pain conditions, whereas hyperactivity theories are better supported in chronic pain stages. The lack of consistency emphasizes the need for further generic neurophysiological models.

Clinical Impact of Work-Related Musculoskeletal Disorders

The main challenge for a clinician treating WMSDs is to serve heterogeneous patient groups with a number of nonspecific symptoms without an adequate clinical tool to quantify these symptoms. This explains the difficulty in treating WMSDs in an effective manner. Quantitative assessment of the functional motor adaptations in work-related conditions can be a way to benchmark pain status and can help to identify early signs of WMSDs. However, the identification of such signs is still a matter of debate and is difficult to integrate into clinical daily practice. Moreover, the lack of longitudinal studies does not enable the distinction between pain leading to less variable motor strategies or vice versa. For this reason, the prognostic value of the reported changes in motor strategies is a matter of debate. However, motor variability is an important characteristic in motor control, and fearful patients may benefit from graded exposure to movements and activities they were used to avoiding (Vlaeyen and Linton, 2000). Moreover, there are signs indicating a prognostic value of motor variability in relation to avoiding shoulder disorders (Madeleine et al., 2003a, 2008a) or recovering from acute low back pain (Moseley and Hodges, 2006). Finally, introducing variability to a defined work task may be a valuable way to reduce the development of acute or chronic musculoskeletal disorders.

References

Ahern DK, Follick MJ, Council JR, Laser-Wolston N, Litchman H. Comparison of lumbar paravertebral EMG patterns in chronic low back pain patients and non-patient controls. Pain 1988;34:153–160.

Arendt-Nielsen L, Graven-Nielsen T, Svarrer H, Svensson P. The influence of low back pain on muscle activity and coordination during gait: a clinical and experimental study. Pain 1996;64:231–240.

Birch L, Christensen H, Arendt-Nielsen L, Graven-Nielsen T, Sogaard K. The influence of experimental muscle pain on motor unit activity during low-level contraction. Eur J Appl Physiol 2000;83:200–206.

Cairns BE. Physiologic properties of thin-fiber muscle afferents: excitation and modulatory effects. In: Graven-Nielsen T, Arendt-Nielsen L, Mense S, editors. Fundamentals of musculoskeletal pain. Seattle: IASP Press; 2007.

Edwards RHT. Hypothesis of peripheral and central mechanisms underlying occupational muscle pain and injury. Eur J Appl Physiol 1988;57:275–281.

Elert JE, Dahlqvist SR, Almay B, Eisemann M. Muscle endurance, muscle tension and personality traits in patients with muscle or joint pain: a pilot study. J Rheumatol 1993;20:1550–1556.

Elert JE, Rantapää-Dahlqvist SB, Henriksson-Larsén K, Lorentzon R, Gerdle BUC. Muscle performance, electromyography and fibre type composition in fibromyalgia and work-related myalgia. Scand J Rheumatol 1991;21:28–34.

European Foundation for the Improvement of the Living and Working Conditions. Fourth European Working Conditions Survey 2005. Luxembourg: Office for Official Publications of the European Communities; 2007.

Falla D, Farina D, Graven-Nielsen T. Experimental muscle pain results in reorganization of coordination among trapezius muscle subdivisions during repetitive shoulder flexion. Exp Brain Res 2007;178:385–393.

Ge HY, Arendt-Nielsen L, Farina D, Madeleine P. Gender-specific differences in electromyographic changes and perceived pain induced by experimental muscle pain during sustained contractions of the upper trapezius muscle. Muscle Nerve 2005;32:726–733.

Gissel H. Ca²⁺ accumulation and cell damage in skeletal muscle during low frequency stimulation. Eur J Appl Physiol 2000;83:175–180.

Graven-Nielsen T, Lund H, Arendt-Nielsen L, Danneskiold-Samsoe B, Bliddal H. Inhibition of maximal voluntary contraction force by experimental muscle pain: a centrally mediated mechanism. Muscle Nerve 2002;26:708–712.

Hägg GM. Static work loads and occupational myalgia—a new explanation. In: Anderson PA, Hobart DJ, Danoff JV, editors. Electromyographical kinesiology. Amsterdam: Elsevier; 1991. p. 141–144.

Hägg GM. Human muscle fibre abnormalities related to occupational load. Eur J Appl Physiol 2000;83:159–165.

Hägg GM, Astrom A. Load pattern and pressure pain threshold in the upper trapezius muscle and psychosocial factors in medical secretaries with and without shoulder/neck disorders. Int Arch Occup Environ Health 1997;69:423–432.

Jensen C, Nilsen K, Hansen K, Westgaard RH. Trapezius muscle load as a risk indicator for occupational shoulder-neck complaints. Int Arch Occup Environ Health 1993;64:415–423.

Johansson H, Sojka P. Pathophysiological mechanisms involved in genesis and spread of muscular tension in occupational muscle pain and in chronic musculoskeletal pain syndromes: a hypothesis. Med Hypotheses 1991;35:196–203.

Kawczynski A, Nie H, Jaskolska A, Jaskolski A, Arendt-Nielsen L, Madeleine P. Mechanomyography and electromyography during and after fatiguing shoulder eccentric contractions in males and females. Scand J Med Sci Sports 2007;17:172–179.

Lamoth CJC, Meijer OG, Daffertshofer A, Wuisman PIJM, Beek PJ. Effects of chronic low back pain on trunk coordination and back muscle activity during walking: changes in motor control. Eur Spine J 2006;15:23–40.

Lund JP, Donga R, Widmer CG, Stohler CS. The pain-adaptation model: a discussion of the relationship between chronic musculoskeletal pain and motor activity. Can J Physiol Pharmacol 1991;69:683–694.

Madeleine P, Arendt-Nielsen L. Experimental muscle pain increases mechanomyographic signal activity during sub-maximal isometric contractions. J Electromyogr Kinesiol 2005;15:27–36.

Madeleine P, Leclerc F, Arendt-Nielsen L, Ravier P, Farina D. Experimental muscle pain changes the spatial distribution of upper trapezius muscle activity during sustained contraction. Clin Neurophysiol 2006;117:2436–2445.

Madeleine P, Lundager B, Voigt M, Arendt-Nielsen L. Sensory manifestations in experimental and work-related chronic neck-shoulder pain. Eur J Pain 1998;2:251–260.

Madeleine P, Lundager B, Voigt M, Arendt-Nielsen L. Shoulder muscle co-ordination during chronic and acute experimental neck-shoulder pain. An occupational study. Eur J Appl Physiol 1999;79:127–140.

Madeleine P, Lundager B, Voigt M, Arendt-Nielsen L. Standardized low-load repetitive work: evidence of different motor control strategies between experienced workers and a reference group. Appl Ergon 2003a;34:533–542.

Madeleine P, Lundager B, Voigt M, Arendt-Nielsen L. The effects of neck-shoulder pain development on sensory-motor interaction among female workers in poultry and fish industries. A prospective study. Int Arch Occup Environ Health 2003b;39–49.

Madeleine P, Mathiassen SE, Arendt-Nielsen L. Changes in the degree of motor variability associated with experimental and chronic neck-shoulder pain during a standardised repetitive arm movement. Exp Brain Res 2008a;185:689–698.

Madeleine P, Voigt M, Mathiassen SE. Cycle-to-cycle variability in biomechanical exposure among butchers performing a standardised cutting task. Ergonomics 2008b; in press.

Mannion AF. Fibre type characteristics and function of the human paraspinal muscles: normal values and changes in association with low back pain. J Electromyogr Kinesiol 1999;9:363–377.

Mense S. Nociception from skeletal muscle in relation to clinical muscle pain. Pain 1993;54:241–289.

Mense S, Skeppar P. Discharge behaviour of feline gamma-motoneurons following induction of an artificial myositis. Pain 1991;46:201–210.

Moseley GL, Hodges PW. Reduced variability of postural strategy prevents normalization of motor changes induced by back pain: a risk factor for chronic trouble? Behav Neurosci 2006;120:474–476.

Nie HL, Kawczynski A, Madeleine P, Arendt-Nielsen L. Delayed onset muscle soreness in neck/shoulder muscles. Eur J Pain 2005;9:653–660.

Oddsson LI, De Luca CJ. Activation imbalances in lumbar spine muscles in the presence of chronic low back pain. J Appl Physiol 2003;94:1410–1420.

Orizio C. Muscle sound: bases for the introduction of a mechanomyographic signal in muscle studies. Crit Rev Biomed Eng 1993;21:201–243.

Punnett L, Wegman DH. Work-related musculoskeletal disorders: the epidemiologic evidence and the debate. J Electromyogr Kinesiol 2004;14:13–23.

Radebold A, Cholewicki J, Panjabi MM, Patel TC. Muscle response pattern to sudden trunk loading in healthy individuals and in patients with chronic low back pain. Spine 2000;25:947–954.

Rosendal L, Larsson B, Kristiansen J, Peolsson M, Søgaard K, Kjaer M, Sorensen J, Gerdle B. Increase in muscle nociceptive substances and anaerobic metabolism in patients with trapezius myalgia: microdialysis in rest and during exercise. Pain 2004;112:324–334.

Sandsjö L, Melin B, Rissen D, Dohns I, Lundberg U. Trapezius muscle activity, neck and shoulder pain, and subjective experiences during monotonous work in women. Eur J Appl Physiol 2000;83:235–238.

Schmidt RF, Kniffki K-D, Schomburg ED. Der Einfluss kleinkalibriger Muskelafferenzen auf den Muskeltonus. In: Bauer H, Koella WP, Struppler H, editors. Therapie der Spastic. Munich: Verlag for angewandte Wissenschaft; 1981. p 71–86.

Sjøgaard G, Sejersted OM, Winkel J, Smolander J, Jørgensen K, Westgaard RH. Exposure assessment and mechanisms of pathogenesis in work-related musculoskeletal disorders: significant aspects in the documentation of risk factors. Luxembourg: European Commission; 1995. p 75–87.

Sohn MK, Graven-Nielsen T, Arendt-Nielsen L, Svensson P. Effects of experimental muscle pain on mechanical properties of single motor unit in human masseter. Clin Neurophysiol 2004;115:76–84.

Sommerich CM, McGlothin J, Marras WS. Occupational risk factors associated with soft tissue disorders of the shoulder: a review of recent investigations in the literature. Ergonomics 1993;36:697–717.

Svensson P, Arendt-Nielsen L. Induction and assessment of experimental muscle pain. J Electromyogr Kinesiol 1995;5:131–140.

Svensson P, Graven-Nielsen T, Matre D, Arendt-Nielsen L. Experimental muscle pain does not cause long-lasting increases in resting electromyographic activity. Muscle Nerve 1998;21:1382–1389.

Szeto GPY, Straker LM, O'Sullivan PB. A comparison of symptomatic and asymptomatic office workers performing monotonous keyboard work. 1: Neck and shoulder muscle recruitment patterns. Man Ther 2005;10:270–280.

Takala E-P, Viikari-Juntura E. Muscular activity in simulated light work among subjects with frequent neck-shoulder pain. Int J Ind Ergon 1991;8:157–164.

Takemasa R, Yamamoto H, Tani T. Trunk muscle strength in and effect of trunk muscle exercises for patients with chronic low-back-pain—the differences in patients with and without organic lumbar lesions. Spine 1995;20:2522–2530.

Thorstensson A, Arvidson Å. Trunk muscle strength and low back pain. Scand J Rehab Med 1982;14:69–75.

Thunberg J, Ljubisavljevic M, Djupsjobacka M, Johansson H. Effects on the fusimotor-muscle spindle system induced by intramuscular injections of hypertonic saline. Exp Brain Res 2002;142:319–326.

Travell JG, Rinzler S, Herman M. Pain and disability of the shoulder and arm. JAMA 1942;120:417–422.

van Dieën JH, Selen LPJ, Cholewicki J. Trunk muscle activation in low-back pain patients, an analysis of the literature. J Electromyogr Kinesiol 2003a;13:333–351.

van Dieën JH, Selen LPJ, Cholewicki J. Trunk muscle activation in low-back pain patients, an analysis of the literature. J Electromyogr Kinesiol 2003b;13:333–351.

Veiersted KB, Westgaard RH, Andersen P. Pattern of muscle activity during stereotyped work and its relation to muscle pain. Int Arch Occup Environ Health 1990;62:31–41.

Veiersted KB, Westgaard RH, Andersen P. Electromyographic evaluation of muscular work pattern as a predictor of trapezius myalgia. Scand J Environ Health 1993;19:284–290.

Visser B, van Dieën JH. Pathophysiology of upper extremity muscle disorders. J Electromyogr Kinesiol 2006;16:1–16.

Vlaeyen JWS, Linton SJ. Fear-avoidance and its consequences in chronic musculoskeletal pain: a state of the art. Pain 2000;85:317–332.

Winkel J, Westgaard RH. Occupational and individual risk factors for neck-shoulder complaints: Part II. The scientific basis (literature review) for the guide. Int J Ind Ergon 1992;10:85–104.

Correspondence to: Pascal Madeleine, PhD, Laboratory for Work-Related pain and Biomechanics, Center for Sensory-Motor Interaction (SMI), Dept. of Health Science and Technology, Aalborg University, Fredrik Bajers Vej 7, Bldg. D-3, DK-9220 Aalborg, Denmark. Tel: +45 99 40 88 20; fax: +45 98 15 40 08; email: pm@hst.aau.dk.

Neuromuscular Control of the Cervical Spine in Neck Pain Disorders

Deborah Falla

Center for Sensory-Motor Interaction, Aalborg University, Aalborg, Denmark

The cervical spine is a complex structure responsible for stabilizing head posture and controlling head movement. The abundance of muscle spindles in the cervical region (Boyd Clark et al., 2002) is an indicator of the involvement of this spinal region in proprioception and in reflexes controlling postural orientation and stability (Roberts, 1978; Wilson, 1984; Taylor and McCloskey, 1988; Dutia, 1991). Neural control of the cervical spine includes demands for stabilization of the head in three-dimensional space, in addition to the execution of voluntary movements, such as following a visual stimulus through coordinated control of eye and head movements (Schor et al., 1988; Dutia, 1991). The cervical spine has elaborate musculature to achieve these goals, and the coordinated activity of all muscles influences the orientation of the cervical spine and head position (Dutia, 1991).

Neck pain is a common complaint that affects up to 70% of individuals at some point in their lives (Fejer et al., 2006). Moreover, reports suggest that the incidence of neck pain is increasing (Borghouts et al., 1998). Neck pain may present in many forms, including whiplash-associated disorders, cervicogenic headache, and cervicobrachial pain. In many cases, the pain is persistent or recurrent, with up to 60% of those affected experiencing some degree of ongoing pain for many years after their first episode (Gore et al., 1987). Given the complexity of the head-neck system, it is likely that pain affects muscle function. It is well documented that individuals with neck pain display limitations in strength (Vernon et al., 1992; Barton and Hayes, 1996), endurance (Watson and Trott, 1993; Placzek et al., 1999), steadiness of contraction (O'Leary et al., 2007), and range of active cervical motion (Dall'Alba et al., 2001; Zwart, 2007). In addition, the intricacy of the cervical spine dictates that nociception will have a profound influence on motor control of head movement and stability as well as postural orientation. This chapter reviews evidence for specific alterations of cervical motor control associated with neck pain; highlights the histological, morphological, and biochemical changes that occur in the cervical muscles in neck pain patients; and discusses the implications of these findings for the rehabilitation of patients with cervical spine disorders.

Biochemical and Morphological Changes

Biochemical alterations in the upper trapezius muscle of persons with neck pain include increased interstitial levels of glutamate that are positively correlated to pain intensity in those with trapezius myalgia (Rosendal et al., 2004) and higher interstitial interleukin and serotonin in those with chronic whiplash-associated disorders (Gerdle et al., 2008). Other changes include disturbed oxidative metabolism of muscle fibers ("moth-eaten" fibers) (Larsson et al., 1998b, 2004) and impaired intramuscular microcirculation (Larsson et al., 1998a) (Fig. 1A).

Biopsies of the cervical flexor and extensor muscles in individuals with neck pain showed a significant increase in the proportion of type IIC fibers, which suggests preferential atrophy of slow-twitch oxidative type I fibers and is consistent with reduced endurance of the cervical muscles in patients with neck pain (Watson and Trott, 1993; Placzek et al., 1999; O'Leary et al., 2007). In addition, findings of greater myoelectric

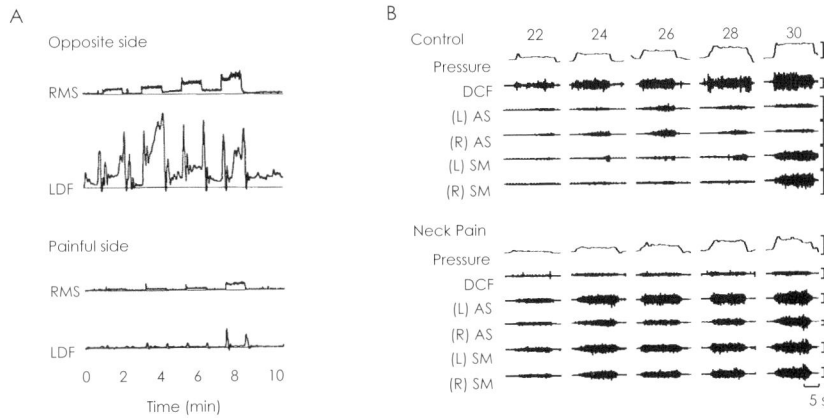

Fig. 1. (A) Continuous recordings of muscle microcirculation using laser Doppler flow-metry (LDF) and electromyographic root mean square (RMS) values recorded from the upper trapezius muscle on the painful and opposite side of a patient with cervico-brachial pain during alternating 1-minute periods of rest and stepwise increased static contraction of shoulder elevation at increments of 30°, 60°, 90°, and 135°. Note that both LDF and RMS values are lower on the painful left side compared with the opposite side. Reprinted with permission from Larsson et al. (1998a). (B) Representative raw EMG data are shown for a control subject and a person with neck pain during a task of staged craniocervical flexion. Data are shown for the deep cervical flexors (DCF) and left (L) and right (R) anterior scalene (AS) and sternocleidomastoid (SM) muscles. Note the in-cremental increase in EMG activity for all muscles with increasing craniocervical flex-ion (recorded as an increase in pressure in a pressure sensor under the cervical spine). The lesser activity in the deep cervical flexors and greater activity in the superficial mus-cles for the neck pain patient suggest a reorganization of muscle activity to perform the task. EMG calibration: 0.5 mV. Reprinted with permission from Falla et al. (2004d).

manifestations of cervical muscle fatigue during sustained contractions (Falla et al., 2003) as well as a greater decrease in muscle fiber conduction velocity of the upper trapezius during repetitive shoulder elevation (Falla and Farina, 2005) in persons with cervical spine disorders indirectly support the histological and biochemical observations.

An additional observation in patients with chronic neck pain of both traumatic and idiopathic onset is atrophy and connective tissue in-filtration of the extensor muscles, especially for the deeper muscles in-cluding the rectus capitis minor and major and the multifidi (Hallgren et al., 1994; McPartland et al., 1997; Elliott et al., 2006; Jull et al., 2007a).

Motor Strategies

Electromyographic studies have demonstrated a reorganization of cervical flexor, extensor, and axioscapular muscle activity in persons with neck pain. In particular, neck pain is consistently associated with inhibition of the deep cervical flexor muscles, longus colli and longus capitis (Jull et al., 1999; Sterling et al., 2003; Falla et al., 2004d; Chiu et al., 2005), together with increased activation of the superficial muscles, the sternomastoid and anterior scalenes (Jull, 2000; Falla et al., 2004d) (Fig. 1B). People with neck pain show augmented activity of the superficial cervical flexor muscles during isometric cervical contractions (Falla et al., 2004b) and during tasks involving dynamic movement of the upper limb (Falla et al., 2004a). There may be changes in the activation of the cervical extensor muscles and upper trapezius during functional upper limb activities (Nederhand et al., 2000; Falla et al., 2004a; Szeto et al., 2005). Heightened muscle activity may induce motion in and mechanically load the cervical spine (Behrsin and Maguire, 1986; Moore and Dalley, 1999), which may reflect a compensatory strategy for impairment of the deeper intersegmental muscles of the cervical spine (Falla, 2004).

In addition to experiencing changes in the magnitude of muscle activation under various conditions, when individuals with neck pain perform a rapid arm movement they experience delayed activation of both the deep and superficial cervical muscles (Falla et al., 2004c). This delay indicates a significant deficit in the automatic feed-forward control of the cervical spine. Moreover, persons with neck pain demonstrate reduced ability to relax the anterior scalene, sternocleidomastoid, and upper trapezius muscles following activation (Barton and Hayes, 1996; Nederhand et al., 2002; Falla et al., 2004a). The upper trapezius also shows decreased ability to relax between repetitive arm movements (Fredin et al., 1997) and has shorter periods of rest during repetitive tasks (Veiersted et al., 1990; Hagg and Anstrom, 1997).

Although persons with neck pain consistently have impaired activation of the deep cervical muscles, together with augmented superficial muscle activity, the change in muscle activity is highly variable among individuals. This variability is reflected in EMG data reported for persons with neck pain (e.g., Falla et al., 2004a). Although there is some evidence that the variability may be related to the magnitude of pain and disability (Falla et al., 2004a), it is also in accordance with the notion of redundancy in the cervical muscle system.

Proprioception

In addition to changes in muscle activation, persons with neck pain show other alterations in sensorimotor interaction, including reduced proprioceptive acuity. Alterations in proprioception may reflect abnormal spindle afferent discharge that may result from activation of chemo- and nociceptive sensory afferents (Pedersen et al., 1997; Wenngren et al., 1998; Thunberg et al., 2001; Hellstrom et al., 2002), from direct trauma to cervical structures, or from increased sympathetic drive (Roatta et al., 2002). The abnormal discharge results in a conflict of inputs from visual, vestibular, and somatosensory sources and may underlie the sensation of unsteadiness and dizziness frequently reported in those with neck pain (Treleaven et al., 2003).

Although errors in positioning the head following voluntary movement are greater in persons with neck pain of both insidious (Revel et al., 1991) and traumatic onset (Heikkila and Astrom, 1996; Kristjansson et al., 2003; Treleaven et al., 2006), proprioceptive acuity appears to be more affected in persons with chronic whiplash pain (Kristjansson et al., 2003), especially in those reporting higher pain and disability (Sterling et al., 2003; Feipel et al., 2006) and dizziness (Treleaven et al., 2003). In addition to greater repositioning errors with head movement, persons with whiplash-induced neck pain show reduced proprioception in both the shoulder and elbow (Knox et al., 2006; Sandlund et al., 2006).

Postural Control

Disturbed postural stability has been found in patients with neck pain, whether of insidious onset or caused by whiplash (Karlberg et al., 1995; McPartland et al., 1997; Michaelson et al., 2003). Changes include greater postural trunk sway, both in standing tasks and in tasks such as walking up and down stairs (Michaelson et al., 2003; Sjostrom et al., 2003; Madeleine et al., 2004). They also include reduced head stability in response to predictable and unpredictable postural perturbations (Michaelson et al., 2003). Although balance disturbances have been reported in both traumatic and nontraumatic neck pain disorders, consistent with observations for head relocation, in persons with whiplash-induced pain the disturbances are generally greater (Field et al., 2007), and postural instability is positively associated with dizziness (Treleaven et al., 2005b).

Disturbances of postural control are also thought to reflect disruption of cervical somatosensory input and a mismatch among somatosensory, visual, and vestibular inputs. Consistent with this hypothesis, changes in oculomotor control occur in persons with neck pain, suggesting disturbances in the cervicocollic and cervico-ocular reflexes (Tjell and Rosenhall, 1998; Heikkila and Wenngren, 1998; Wenngren et al., 2002; Treleaven et al., 2005a). Moreover, experimental studies have shown that injection of lidocaine into the soft tissues of the neck at the level of C2/C3 induces ataxia and staggering gait in humans (de Jong et al., 1977). Other studies have found that neck muscle fatigue affects postural control, possibly by altering afferent input to the central nervous system (Schieppati et al., 2003), and that neck muscle vibration, which stimulates muscle spindle afferents, generates illusions of displacement and movement of a visual target as well as sensations of head displacement (Biguer et al., 1988; Taylor and McCloskey, 1991; Han and Lennerstrand, 1995). Finally, restraining cervical mobility affects oculomotor control, presumably as a consequence of decreased cervical somatosensory input (Karlberg et al., 1991).

The Cause-and-Effect Relationship between Pain and Neuromuscular Changes

Although altered neural control of the cervical muscles may initiate neck pain, compelling evidence from experimental studies shows an effect of pain on muscle activation. For example, activation of chemoreceptive and nociceptive afferent fibers from neck muscles and joints affects the proprioceptive activity of muscle spindle afferent fibers (Pedersen et al., 1997; Thunberg et al., 2001; Hellstrom et al., 2002). In addition, excitation of cervical nociceptors induces an immediate, yet complex, reorganization of motor strategies (Falla et al., 2007a,b).

During voluntary contraction, cervical muscles consistently demonstrate pain-induced inhibition when acting as agonists (Madeleine et al., 2006; Falla et al., 2007a,b). For example, during cervical flexion, pain induced by injection of hypertonic saline into the sternocleidomastoid muscle results in a force-dependent reduction of sternocleidomastoid EMG amplitude (Falla et al., 2007b). Likewise, during cervical extension, local excitation of splenius capitis nociceptive afferents reduces splenius capitis muscle activity (Falla et al., 2007b). Even though an inhibition of the painful muscle is observed, mechanical output can remain unchanged in painful conditions. This finding suggests that nociception induces a redistribution of load in the various muscles performing a task to allow motor output to be maintained. Consistent with this hypothesis, pain induced in the sternocleidomastoid muscle results in decreased sternocleidomastoid EMG activity with a concomitant bilateral reduction of splenius capitis and trapezius muscle activity (Falla et al., 2007b). Similarly, reduced sternocleidomastoid muscle activity occurs during cervical rotation following hypertonic saline-evoked pain in the splenius capitis muscle (Svensson et al., 2004). However, the observed alterations in muscle activity are not fully predicted by current models of pain and motor control (Johansson and Sojka, 1991; Lund et al., 1991) but rather appear to be task-dependent modifications in motor control strategies (Fig. 2). For example, experimentally induced splenius capitis pain has no effect on the sternocleidomastoid (antagonist) muscle during isometric cervical extension but rather induces an increase in synergistic muscle activity (Falla et al., 2007b).

Taken together, these observations suggest a dynamic reorganization of muscle coordination in order to minimize the use of the painful muscle and avoid disruption of the task (Falla and Farina, 2008). In the short term, this reorganization may be interpreted as an efficient and effective strategy that is consistent with the notion of redundancy

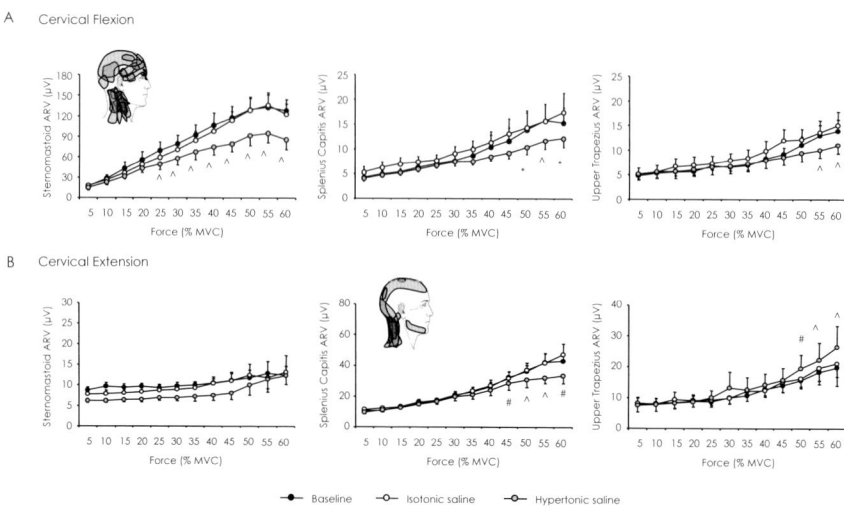

Fig. 2. (A) Mean and standard error of EMG average rectified value (ARV) of the sternal head of the sternocleidomastoid (sternomastoid), splenius capitis, and upper trapezius muscles across a linearly increasing cervical flexion force contraction from 0 to 60% of the maximum voluntary contraction (MVC) at baseline (pre-injection), and following the injection of isotonic (control) and hypertonic (pain condition) saline into the ster-nomastoid. (B) Mean and standard error of EMG ARV of the sternomastoid, splenius capitis, and upper trapezius muscles across a linearly increasing cervical extension force contraction from 0 to 60% MVC at baseline (pre-injection), and following the injection of isotonic (control) and hypertonic (pain condition) saline into the splenius capitis. Note the consistent reduction in EMG amplitude for the painful muscle when acting as an agonist and variable changes for synergist/antagonist muscles depending on the task. Significant difference of hypertonic saline condition compared to baseline: * $P < 0.05$; # $P < 0.01$; ^ $P < 0.001$. Reprinted with permission from Falla et al. (2007b).

of the cervical muscle system, which holds that specific forces may be produced by several combinations of muscle actions. However, in the long term, pain-induced altered neural control may cause some muscles to experience overload and, and as a consequence, injury, while caus-ing other muscles to have reduced activity with consequent atrophy of specific fiber types. Thus, changes in muscle control may be initiated in the presence of pain and/or tissue injury; however, they appear to be sus-tained beyond the acute pain phase and may contribute to the chronicity of neck pain. Moreover, long-term alterations in motor control may par-tially explain the morphological and histological changes documented in the cervical muscles in persons with neck pain (Falla and Farina, 2007).

Likewise, biochemical and morphological changes in the cervical muscles may perpetuate both altered motor control and pain. For example, impaired intramuscular microcirculation may alter metabolite concentration in the intercellular muscle interstitium, thus activating group III and IV muscle afferents, which in turn can exert reflex actions on spinal neurons.

Rehabilitation

If pain alters the motor control of the cervical spine, then does muscle function recover spontaneously in patients with chronic neck pain if their pain is reduced? With regard to proprioception, improvements in head relocation and pain have been demonstrated with manipulative therapy (Heikkila et al., 2000; Palmgren et al., 2006), with training of the craniocervical flexor muscles (Jull et al., 2007b), and with specific proprioception rehabilitation programs (Revel et al., 1994; Jull et al., 2007b). However, clinical trials of interventions that have shown efficacy for reducing neck pain have not shown spontaneous recovery of other aspects of cervical neuromuscular control. For example, altered activation of the deep and superficial cervical flexor muscles persists despite the alleviation of symptoms (Jull et al., 2002; Sterling et al., 2003) (Fig. 3A). These findings suggest that specific retraining may be required to restore changes in cervical neuromuscular function—an approach that finds support in a series of clinical trials (Jull et al., 2005; Falla et al., 2006, 2007c). These studies show that a low-intensity exercise regime designed to train the deep craniocervical flexors—longus colli and longus capitis—is effective at increasing the activation of the deep cervical flexor muscles, enhancing the speed of their activation when challenged by a postural perturbation (Jull et al., 2005) and improving the ability to maintain an upright posture of the cervical spine during prolonged sitting (Falla et al., 2007c). Similar benefits did not accrue from 6 weeks of higher-intensity strength and endurance training for the cervical muscles (Jull et al., 2005; Falla et al., 2007c). However, higher-intensity exercise to challenge the neck flexor muscles is required to reduce the fatigability of the sternocleidomastoid and anterior scalene muscles and to improve the strength of the cervical

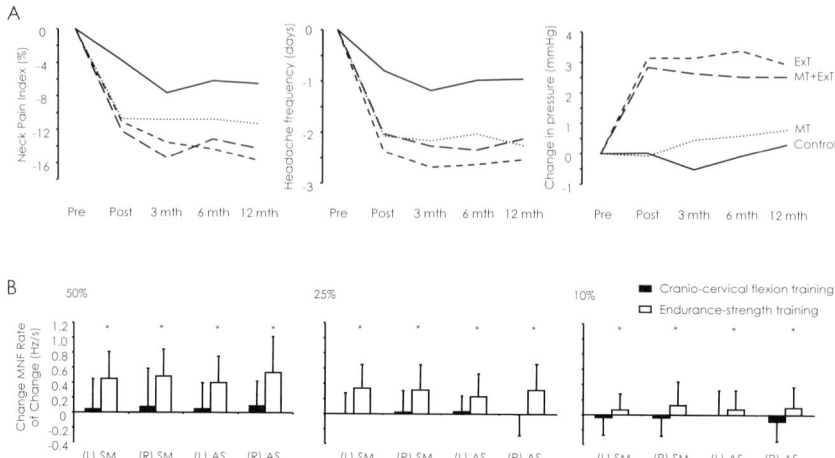

Fig. 3. (A) Data from participants with cervicogenic headache randomized into four groups: the manipulative therapy group (MT), exercise therapy group (ExT), combined therapy group (MT+ExT), and control group. Mean values for the Northwick Park Neck Pain Questionnaire, headache frequency, and change in pressure on the clinical test of craniocervical flexion recorded at baseline, in the week immediately after treatment (week 7) and 3, 6, and 12 months (mth) after the intervention. Although each intervention group demonstrated reduced neck pain intensity and headache frequency, only the groups that received specific muscle rehabilitation (ExT or MT+ExT) improved their performance on the craniocervical flexion test (clinical test of deep cervical flexor muscle activation). Reprinted with permission from Jull et al. (2002). (B) Data (mean and standard deviation) are shown for the change (pre- to postintervention) in the rate of change of the mean spectral frequency (MNF) for the left (L) and right (R) sternocleidomastoid (SM) and anterior scalene (AS) muscles at 50%, 25%, and 10% of the maximum voluntary contraction. Patients with chronic neck pain were randomized into two groups that received either endurance and strength training of the cervical flexors or low-load craniocervical flexion retraining. After 6 weeks of exercise intervention, both groups demonstrated a significant reduction in neck pain intensity; however, cervical muscle fatigue was reduced only in patients who participated in the strength and endurance training program. An asterisk (*) indicates $P < 0.05$ between groups. Reprinted with permission from Falla et al. (2006).

muscles in persons with neck pain (Falla et al., 2006), an outcome that did not occur following lower-load muscle retraining (Fig. 3B).

In summary, recent evidence emphasizes the need for early and effective rehabilitation of cervical neuromuscular function, which should be selected based on careful examination and thus be specific to the impairments of the individual patient. Although the suggestion has not yet been confirmed, adequate rehabilitation of cervical motor control may be effective at reducing the recurrence of neck pain symptoms (Gore et al., 1987).

Acknowledgment

Deborah Falla is supported by the National Health and Medical Research Council of Australia (ID 351678).

References

Barton PM, Hayes KC. Neck flexor muscle strength, efficiency, and relaxation times in normal subjects and subjects with unilateral neck pain and headache. Arch Phys Med Rehabil 1996;77:680–687.

Behrsin JF, Maguire K. Levator scapulae action during shoulder movement. A possible mechanism of shoulder pain of cervical origin. Aust J Physiother 1986;32:101–106.

Biguer B, Donaldson IM, Hein A, Jeannerod M. Neck muscle vibration modifies the representation of visual motion and direction in man. Brain 1988;111:1405–1424.

Borghouts AJ, Koes BW, Bouter LM. The clinical course and prognostic factors of non-specific neck pain: a systematic review. Pain 1998;77:1–13.

Boyd Clark LC, Briggs CA, Galea MP. Muscle spindle distribution, morphology, and density in longus colli and multifidus muscles of the cervical spine. Spine 2002;27:694–701.

Chiu TT, Law E, Chiu TH. Performance of the craniocervical flexion test in subjects with and without chronic neck pain. J Orthop Sports Phys Ther 2005;35:567–571.

Dall'Alba P, Sterling M, Treleaven J, Edwards S, Jull G. Cervical range of motion discriminates between asymptomatic persons and those with whiplash. Spine 2001;26:2090–2094.

de Jong PT, de Jong JM, Cohen B, Jongkees LB. Ataxia and nystagmus induced by injection of local anesthetics in the neck. Ann Neurol 1977;1:240–246.

Dutia MB. The muscles and joints of the neck: their specialisation and role in head movement. Prog Neurobiol 1991;37:165–178.

Elliott J, Jull G, Noteboom JT, Darnell R, Galloway G, Gibbon WW. Fatty infiltration in the cervical extensor muscles in persistent whiplash-associated disorders: a magnetic resonance imaging analysis. Spine 2006;31:847–855.

Falla D. Unravelling the complexity of muscle impairment in chronic neck pain. Man Ther 2004;9:125–133.

Falla D, Bilenkij G, Jull G. Patients with chronic neck pain demonstrate altered patterns of muscle activation during performance of a functional upper limb task. Spine 2004a;29:1436–1440.

Falla D, Farina D. Muscle fiber conduction velocity of the upper trapezius muscle during dynamic contraction of the upper limb in patients with chronic neck pain. Pain 2005;116:138–145.

Falla D, Farina D. Neural and muscular factors associated with motor impairment in neck pain. Curr Rheumatol Rep 2007;9:497-502.

Falla D, Farina D. Neuromuscular adaptation in experimental and clinical neck pain. J Electromyogr Kinesiol 2008;18:255–261.

Falla D, Farina D, Graven-Nielsen T. Experimental muscle pain results in reorganization of coordination among trapezius muscle subdivisions during repetitive shoulder flexion. Exp Brain Res 2007a;178:385–393.

Falla D, Farina D, Kanstrup Dahl M, Graven-Nielsen T. Muscle pain induces task-dependent changes in cervical agonist/antagonist activity. J Appl Physiol 2007b;102:601–609.

Falla D, Jull G, Edwards S, Koh K, Rainoldi A. Neuromuscular efficiency of the sternocleidomastoid and anterior scalene muscles in patients with neck pain. Disabil Rehabil 2004b;26:712–717.

Falla D, Jull G, Hodges P, Vicenzino B. An endurance-strength training regime is effective in reducing myoelectric manifestations of cervical flexor muscle fatigue in females with chronic neck pain. Clin Neurophysiol 2006;117:828–837.

Falla D, Jull G, Hodges PW. Feedforward activity of the cervical flexor muscles during voluntary arm movements is delayed in chronic neck pain. Exp Brain Res 2004c;157:43–48.

Falla D, Jull G, Hodges PW. Patients with neck pain demonstrate reduced electromyographic activity of the deep cervical flexor muscles during performance of the craniocervical flexion test. Spine 2004d;29:2108–2114.

Falla D, Jull G, Russell T, Vicenzino B, Hodges P. Effect of neck exercise on sitting posture in patients with chronic neck pain. Phys Ther 2007c;87:408–417.

Falla D, Rainoldi A, Merletti R, Jull G. Myoelectric manifestations of sternocleidomastoid and anterior scalene muscle fatigue in chronic neck pain patients. Clin Neurophysiol 2003;114:488–495.

Feipel V, Salvia P, Klein H, Rooze M. Head repositioning accuracy in patients with whiplash-associated disorders. Spine 2006;31:E51–58.

Fejer R, Kyvik KO, Hartvigsen J. The prevalence of neck pain in the world population: a systematic critical review of the literature. Eur Spine J 2006;15:834–848.

Field S, Treleaven J, Jull G. Standing balance: a comparison between idiopathic and whiplash-induced neck pain. Man Ther 2007; in press.

Fredin Y, Elert J, Britschgi N, Nyberg V, Vaher A, Gerdle B. A decreased ability to relax between repetitive muscle contractions in patients with chronic symptoms after whiplash trauma of the neck. J Musculoskel Pain 1997;5:55–70.

Gerdle B, Lemming D, Kristiansen J, Larsson B, Peolsson M, Rosendal L. Biochemical alterations in the trapezius muscle of patients with chronic whiplash associated disorders (WAD): a microdialysis study. Eur J Pain 2008;12:82–93.

Gore DR, Sepic SB, Gardner GM, Murray MP. Neck pain: A long term follow-up of 205 patients. Spine 1987;12:1–5.

Hagg GM, Anstrom A. Load pattern and pressure pain threshold in the upper trapezius muscle and psychosocial factors in medical secretaries with and without shoulder/neck disorders. Int Arch Occup Environ Health 1997;69:423–432.

Hallgren RC, Greenman PE, Rechtien JJ. Atrophy of suboccipital muscles in patients with chronic pain: a pilot study. J Am Osteopath Assoc 1994;94:1032–1038.

Han Y, Lennerstrand G. Eye movements in normal subjects induced by vibratory activation of neck muscle proprioceptors. Acta Ophthalmol Scand 1995;73:414–416.

Heikkila H, Astrom P. Cervicocephalic kinesthetic sensibility in patients with whiplash injury. Scand J Rehabil Med 1996;28:133–138.

Heikkila H, Johansson H, Wenngren BI. Effects of acupuncture, cervical manipulation and NSAID therapy on dizziness and impaired head repositioning of suspected cervical origin: a pilot study. Man Ther 2000;5:151–157.

Heikkila HV, Wenngren B. Cervicocephalic kinesthetic sensibility, active range of cervical motion, and oculomotor function in patients with whiplash injury. Arch Phys Med Rehabil 1998;79:1089–1094.

Hellstrom F, Thunberg J, Bergenheim M, Sjolander P, Djupsjobacka M, Johansson H. Increased intra-articular concentration of bradykinin in the temporomandibular joint changes the sensitivity of muscle spindles in dorsal neck muscles in the cat. Neurosci Res 2002;42:91–99.

Johansson H, Sojka P. Pathophysiological mechanisms involved in genesis and spread of muscular tension in occupational muscle pain and in chronic musculoskeletal pain syndromes: a hypothesis. Med Hypotheses 1991;35:196-203.

Jull G, Amiri M, Bullock-Saxton J, Darnell R, Lander C. Cervical musculoskeletal impairment in frequent intermittent headache. Part 1: Subjects with single headaches. Cephalalgia 2007a; 27:793–802.

Jull G, Barrett C, Magee R, Ho P. Further clinical clarification of the muscle dysfunction in cervical headache. Cephalalgia 1999;19:179–185.

Jull G, Falla D, Hodges P, Vicenzino B. Cervical flexor muscle retraining: physiological mechanisms of efficacy. 2nd International Conference on Movement Dysfunction. Edinburgh, 2005.

Jull G, Falla D, Treleaven J, Hodges P, Vicenzino B. Retraining cervical joint position sense: the effect of two exercise regimes. J Orthop Res 2007b;25:404–412.

Jull GA. Deep cervical flexor muscle dysfunction in whiplash. J Musculoskel Pain 2000;8:143–154.

Jull G, Trott P, Potter H, Zito G, Niere K, Shirley D, Emberson J, Marschner I, Richardson C. A randomized controlled trial of exercise and manipulative therapy for cervicogenic headache. Spine 2002;27:1835–1843.

Karlberg M, Magnusson M, Johansson R. Effects of restrained cervical mobility on voluntary eye movements and postural control. Acta Otolaryngol 1991;111:664–670.

Karlberg M, Persson L, Magnusson M. Impaired postural control in patients with cervico-brachial pain. Acta Otolaryngol Suppl 1995;520:440–442.

Knox J, Beilstein DJ, Charles SD, Aarseth GA, Rayar S, Treleaven J, Hodges PW. Changes in head and neck position have a greater effect on elbow joint position sense in people with whiplash-associated disorders. Clin J Pain 2006;22:512–518.

Kristjansson E, Dall'Alba P, Jull G. A study of five cervicocephalic relocation tests in three different subject groups. Clin Rehabil 2003;17:768–774.

Larsson B, Bjork J, Kadi F, Lindman R, Gerdle B. Blood supply and oxidative metabolism in muscle biopsies of female cleaners with and without myalgia. Clin J Pain 2004;20:440–446.

Larsson R, Cai H, Zhang Q, Oberg PA, Larsson SE. Visualization of chronic neck-shoulder pain: impaired microcirculation in the upper trapezius muscle in chronic cervico-brachial pain. Occup Med (London) 1998a;48:189–194.

Larsson SE, Bengtsson A, Bodegard L, Henriksson KG, Larsson J. Muscle changes in work-related chronic myalgia. Acta Orthop Scand 1998b;59:552–556.

Lund JP, Donga R, Widmer CG, Stohler CS. The pain-adaptation model: a discussion of the relationship between chronic musculoskeletal pain and motor activity. Can J Physiol Pharmacol 1991;69:683–694.

Madeleine P, Leclerc F, Arendt-Nielsen L, Ravier P, Farina D. Experimental muscle pain changes the spatial distribution of upper trapezius muscle activity during sustained contraction. Clin Neurophysiol 2006;117: 2436–2445.

Madeleine P, Prietzel H, Svarrer H, Arendt-Nielsen L. Quantitative posturography in altered sensory conditions: a way to assess balance instability in patients with chronic whiplash injury. Arch Phys Med Rehabil 2004;85:432–438.

McPartland JM, Brodeur RR, Hallgren RC. Chronic neck pain, standing balance, and suboccipital muscle atrophy--a pilot study. J Manipulative Physiol Ther 1997;20:24–29.

Michaelson P, Michaelson M, Jaric S, Latash ML, Sjolander P, Djupsjobacka M. Vertical posture and head stability in patients with chronic neck pain. J Rehabil Med 2003;35:229–235.

Moore KL, Dalley AF. Clinically orientated anatomy. Philadelphia: Lippincott; 1999.

Nederhand MJ, Hermens H, Ijzerman MJ, Turk D, Zilvold G. Cervical muscle dysfunction in the chronic whiplash associated disorder grade 2: the relevance of the trauma. Spine 2002;27:1056–1061.

Nederhand MJ, Ijzerman MJ, Hermens HJ, Baten CTM, Zilvold G. Cervical muscle dysfunction in the chronic whiplash associated disorder grade II (WAD-II). Spine 2000;25:1938–1943.

O'Leary S, Jull G, Kim M, Vicenzino B. Cranio-cervical flexor muscle impairment at maximal, moderate, and low loads is a feature of neck pain. Man Ther 2007;12:34–39.

Palmgren PJ, Sandstrom PJ, Lundqvist FJ, Heikkila H. Improvement after chiropractic care in cervicocephalic kinesthetic sensibility and subjective pain intensity in patients with nontraumatic chronic neck pain. J Manipulative Physiol Ther 2006;29:100–106.

Pedersen J, Sjolander P, Wenngren BI, Johansson H. Increased intramuscular concentration of bradykinin increases the static fusimotor drive to muscle spindles in neck muscles of the cat. Pain 1997;70:83–91.

Placzek JD, Pagett BT, Roubal PJ, Jones BA, McMichael HG, Rozanski EA, Gianotto KL. The influence of the cervical spine on chronic headache in women: a pilot study. J Manual Manipulative Ther 1999;7:33–39.

Revel M, Andre Deshays C, Minguet M. Cervicocephalic kinesthetic sensibility in patients with cervical pain. Arch Phys Med Rehabil 1991;72:288–291.

Revel M, Minguet M, Gergoy P, Vaillant J, Manuel JL. Changes in cervicocephalic kinesthesia after a proprioceptive rehabilitation program in patients with neck pain: a randomized controlled study. Arch Phys Med Rehabil 1994;75:895–899.

Roatta S, Windhorst U, Ljubisavljevic M, Johansson H, Passatore M. Sympathetic modulation of muscle spindle afferent sensitivity to stretch in rabbit jaw closing muscles. J Physiol 2002;540:237-248.

Roberts TDM. Neurophysiology of postural mechanisms. London: Butterworths; 1978.

Rosendal L, Larsson B, Kristiansen J, Peolsson M, Sogaard K, Kjaer M, Sorensen J, Gerdle B. Increase in muscle nociceptive substances and anaerobic metabolism in patients with trapezius myalgia: microdialysis in rest and during exercise. Pain 2004;112:324–334.

Sandlund J, Djupsjobacka M, Ryhed B, Hamberg J, Bjorklund M. Predictive and discriminative value of shoulder proprioception tests for patients with whiplash-associated disorders. J Rehab Med 2006;38:44–49.

Schieppati M, Nardone A, Schmid M. Neck muscle fatigue affects postural control in man. Neuroscience 2003;121:277–285.

Schor RH, Kearney RE, Dieringer N. Reflex stabilization of the head. In: Peterson BW, Richmond FJR, editors. Control of head movement. Oxford: Oxford University Press;1988. p. 141–166.

Sjostrom H, Allum JH, Carpenter DM, Adkin AL, Honegger F, Ettlin T. Trunk sway measures of postural stability during clinical balance tests in patients with chronic whiplash injury symptoms. Spine 2003;28:1725–1734.

Sterling M, Jull G, Vicenzino B, Kenardy J, Darnell R. Development of motor dysfunction following whiplash injury. Pain 2003;103:65–73.

Svensson P, Wang K, Sessle BJ, Arendt-Nielsen L. Associations between pain and neuromuscular activity in the human jaw and neck muscles. Pain 2004;109:225–232.

Szeto GP, Straker LM, O'Sullivan PB. A comparison of symptomatic and asymptomatic office workers performing monotonous keyboard work 1: Neck and shoulder muscle recruitment patterns. Man Ther 2005;10:270–280.

Taylor JL, McCloskey DI. Proprioception in the neck. Exp Brain Res 1988;70:351–360.

Taylor JL, McCloskey DI. Illusions of head and visual target displacement induced by vibration of neck muscles. Brain 1991;114:755–759.

Thunberg J, Hellstrom F, Sjolander P, Bergenheim M, Wenngren B, Johansson H. Influences on the fusimotor-muscle spindle system from chemosensitive nerve endings in cervical facet joints in the cat: Possible implications for whiplash induced disorders. Pain 2001;91:15–22.

Tjell C, Rosenhall U. Smooth pursuit neck torsion test: a specific test for cervical dizziness. Am J Otol 1998;19:76–81.

Treleaven J, Jull G, LowChoy N. The relationship of cervical joint position error to balance and eye movement disturbances in persistent whiplash. Man Ther 2006;11:99–106.

Treleaven J, Jull G, LowChoy N. Smooth pursuit neck torsion test in whiplash-associated disorders: relationship to self-reports of neck pain and disability, dizziness and anxiety. J Rehabil Med 2005a;37:219–223.

Treleaven J, Jull G, LowChoy N. Standing balance in persistent whiplash: a comparison between subjects with and without dizziness. J Rehabil Med 2005b;37:224–229.

Treleaven J, Jull G, Sterling M. Dizziness and unsteadiness following whiplash injury: characteristic features and relationship with cervical joint position error. J Rehabil Med 2003;35:36–43.

Veiersted KB, Westgaard RH, Andersen P. Pattern of muscle activity during stereotyped work and its relation to muscle pain. Int Arch Occup Environ Health 1990;62:31–41.

Vernon HT, Aker P, Aramenko M, Battershill D, Alepin A, Penner T. Evaluation of neck muscle strength with a modified sphygmomanometer dynamometer: reliability and validity. J Manipulative Physiol Ther 1992;15:343–349.

Watson DH, Trott PH. Cervical headache: an investigation of natural head posture and upper cervical flexor muscle performance. Cephalalgia 1993;13:272–284.

Wenngren BI, Pedersen J, Sjolander P, Bergenheim M, Johansson H. Bradykinin and muscle stretch alter contralateral cat neck muscle spindle output. Neurosci Res 1998;32:119–129.

Wenngren BI, Pettersson K, Lowenhielm G, Hildingsson C. Eye motility and auditory brainstem response dysfunction after whiplash injury. Acta Otolaryngol 2002;122:276–283.

Wilson VJ. Organisation of reflexes evoked by stimulation of neck receptors. Exp Brain Res 1984;9:63–71.

Zwart JA. Neck mobility in different headache disorders. Headache 2007;37:6–11.

Correspondence to: Deborah Falla, PhD, Center for Sensory-Motor Interaction, Department of Health Science and Technology, Aalborg University, Fredrik Bajers Vej 7, D-3, DK-9220 Aalborg, Denmark. Tel: +45 99 40 74 59; fax: +45 98 15 40 08; email: deborahf@hst.aau.dk.

27

Pain and Jaw Motor Function

Peter Svensson

*Department of Clinical Oral Physiology, School of Dentistry, University of Aarhus, Aarhus, Denmark;
Department of Oral and Maxillofacial Surgery, Aarhus University Hospital, Aarhus, Denmark; Orofacial Pain
Laboratory, Center for Sensory-Motor Interaction, Aalborg University, Aalborg, Denmark*

From a clinical perspective it is of great importance to understand how pain and jaw motor functions are interrelated. One possibility is that a dysfunction of the jaw motor system leads to overloading of the musculoskeletal tissue, setting up a microenvironment capable of activating nociceptors and thereby leading to pain. The other possibility is that if pain occurs (for example, due to tissue or nervous system injuries), then the jaw motor system changes in response to nociceptive activity. In the first scenario, treatment would logically be directed toward the dysfunction, which in turn should resolve the pain problem. In the second scenario, the emphasis would be on management of pain, which should then normalize the jaw motor function. This controversy has continued for many years in relation to orofacial musculoskeletal pain conditions known as temporomandibular disorders (TMDs). This chapter highlights recent findings related to the many interactions between pain and jaw motor function. For further discussion, the reader is referred to additional reviews on this topic (e.g., Stohler, 1999; Sessle, 2000; Svensson and Graven-Nielsen, 2001; Lobbezoo et al., 2006; Schindler and Svensson, 2007; Svensson, 2007).

Fundamentals of Musculoskeletal Pain
edited by Thomas Graven-Nielsen, Lars Arendt-Nielsen, and Siegfried Mense
IASP Press, Seattle, © 2008

Special Characteristics of the Trigeminal System

Normal jaw motor functions involve fast, precise, highly coordinated, and pain-free movement of the mandible during mastication, swallowing, speech, yawning, and so on. Features particularly pertinent to the jaw motor system include frequent activity and use both during the day and at night, the fact that jaw movements rely on only one joint (the temporomandibular joint [TMJ]), the unique muscle fiber composition, the functional partitioning of the jaw muscles, and bilateral activity (Miles, 2004). Deviation from normal jaw movements can be recognized in the clinic as altered range of motion, irregular movements, tremor, postural changes of the mandible, and eventually TMJ noises such as clicking or grating sounds. Thus, despite a number of similarities in the organization and behavior of the spinal and trigeminal motor systems, the special biomechanical, neurophysiological, and psychological characteristics of the trigeminal area discourage direct extrapolations of research findings pertaining to the spinal system to the trigeminal system. In the following paragraphs, I will review the interaction between pain and jaw motor function when the mandible is in its relaxed position (postural position), during tooth-clenching or grinding, during repetitive dynamic movements such as mastication, and finally in terms of reflex activity.

Postural Position of the Mandible

With the mandible in its resting or postural position (Woda et al., 2001), which normally means the teeth are about 2–3 mm apart, some studies, in particular the older literature, have suggested increased electromyographic (EMG) activity—frequently referred to as muscle hyperactivity—in the jaw-closing muscles of TMD pain patients when compared to control subjects (see Svensson and Graven-Nielsen, 2001). The hypothesis was that muscle hyperactivity would lead to decreased blood flow, changes in metabolism, and release of substances capable of sensitizing nociceptive endings in the tissue, creating a local vicious cycle (Simons,

2004). However, muscle hyperactivity has proven difficult to demonstrate, and many of the original studies had flaws and possible confounding factors such as "cross-talk" from facial muscles, as well as control groups that were inadequate in terms of size, gender, and age; bruxism was also prevalent among subjects. Some of the best-controlled studies have shown very small (1–2 μV) EMG increases, representing a small percentage of the maximum voluntary EMG activity. Therefore, the diagnostic and pathophysiological significance of such findings for musculoskeletal pain remains unclear.

A recent clinical study showed increased EMG activity in the jaw-closing muscles in patients with myofascial TMD pain as well as in patients with orofacial trigeminal neuropathic pain; the increased activity was independent of pain intensity or location (Bodéré et al., 2005). This finding indicates that a local vicious cycle in the muscle is unlikely to be the main underlying pathophysiological mechanism of pain and that central factors, perhaps in response to an afferent nociceptive barrage, may be involved. Nevertheless, caution remains necessary with such low levels of absolute EMG activity, which can hardly be differentiated from background EMG "noise" in the jaw muscles (e.g., Graven-Nielsen et al., 1997; Svensson et al., 1998b).

Interestingly, the human mandible trembles at about 3–8 Hz when it is in its resting position with the jaw muscles relaxed, although the amplitude of this movement is too low to be detected visually (Junge et al., 1998; Jaberzedah et al., 2003; Miles, 2004). There is good evidence that the mandible in the resting position is under a "pulsatile control"—a term used to describe alternating bursts of activity in central neural pulse generators in the brainstem leading to activation of jaw-opening and jaw-closing alpha-motoneurons (Miles, 2004). Experimental pain in the masseter muscle, invoked by hypertonic saline (HS), can reduce the power of the resting jaw tremor (Jaberzadeh et al., 2003). This finding indicates that jaw muscle pain is capable of tonically modulating the amplitude of the outputs from central "pulsatile control" generators in the brainstem, which drive the alternating activation of antagonistic muscles that produce jaw tremor at rest and during jaw movements. It can be speculated that different mechanisms might account for this pain-induced modulation of the amplitude of resting tremor of the mandible and for the pulsatile discontinuities of the mandible during movement (Jaberzadeh et al., 2003).

Experimental pain could tonically decrease either the excitability of trigeminal motoneurons or the output from the central generator in the brainstem that drives the alternating activity in the jaw-closing and jaw-opening muscles. Several studies have reported different outcomes when they have looked for changes in tonic activity of masticatory muscles during experimental pain. Stohler et al. (1996) described a weak (<1 μV), but significant, increase in resting EMG activity in the masseter muscle during tonic saline-evoked pain, and a similar increase when subjects were recalling a memory of pain. My colleagues and I (Svensson et al. 1998b) also reported a transient increase lasting about 30–60 seconds in resting EMG activity in the masseter, but the increase did not correlate with pain intensity or duration of pain. More recently, we showed that experimental pain in the neck muscles is associated with a local increase in EMG activity and with significantly increased activity in the jaw-closing muscles (Svensson et al., 2004). However, the conventional methods for monitoring tonic EMG would not be able to distinguish between a change in the very low level of continuous EMG and a change in the very low-amplitude rhythmic pulses (Jaberzadeh et al., 2003). That is, the operational definition of tonic resting EMG in the earlier studies did not incorporate the idea arising from Junge et al. (1998) that "tonic" EMG in the resting jaw muscles is not necessarily a constant signal (Jaberzadeh et al., 2003).

The relatively small EMG changes in the human jaw-closing muscles with the mandible at rest contrast with the robust increases of 200–300% above baseline observed in animal studies using intramuscular EMG electrodes to record nocifensive reflex jaw responses following noxious stimulation of temporomandibular joint or muscle tissue (e.g., Hu et al., 1993; Cairns et al., 1998). The facilitation of EMG activity in both jaw-closing and jaw-opening muscles of rats and cats following injection of various algesic substances into the deep craniofacial tissues indicates that nociceptive afferents supplying these tissues activate excitatory pathways projecting to the alpha-motoneuron pools of these muscles (see Sessle, 2000). The co-contraction of the jaw-opening and jaw-closing muscles may serve as a "splinting" effect and reduce jaw movements (Sessle, 2000).

Thus, it seems clear that pain itself has the ability to influence the motor programs associated with the control of the mandible in its resting position, but so far no studies have been able to provide sufficient evidence that such shifts in position may be a critical etiological factor for TMD pain.

Tooth Clenching and Grinding

Tooth clenching and grinding, normally termed bruxism, is considered to be an involuntary activity of the jaw muscles either during sleep or when awake (Lavigne et al., 2003). The associated jaw muscle activity can be classified as either rhythmic (phasic), sustained (tonic), or a mixture of both types (Lavigne et al., 2003). It is estimated that about 8% of the adult population are sleep bruxers, but as many as 60% will demonstrate some form of rhythmic masticatory muscle activity. Thus, sleep bruxism is viewed as an exaggerated normal behavior, which in some cases can be associated with significant attrition and eventually destruction of the teeth. Researchers eagerly discuss whether sleep bruxism is related to TMD pain (van der Meulen et al., 2006). About 20–30% of sleep bruxers report jaw muscle pain, which could be due to a kind of localized post-exercise muscle soreness; alternatively, it might indicate a generalized muscle pain condition like fibromyalgia. However, several studies have now found that patients with the most jaw muscle EMG activity during sleep are those with the fewest muscle symptoms (Lavigne et al., 1997; Arima et al., 2001). One consideration is that protective or adaptive mechanisms in painful conditions prevent the overuse of muscles during sleep.

Human experimental studies have nevertheless clearly shown that sustained voluntary EMG activity (grinding or clenching) of a certain intensity and duration can lead to symptoms both in jaw muscles and in the TMJ (e.g., Arima et al., 1999; Torisu et al., 2007). However, the pain is of rather low intensity and is short-lived, in accordance with the notion that the jaw muscles are extremely fatigue resistant. The current view is therefore that self-reported bruxism and other parafunctional jaw activities are relatively modest risk factors for the development or maintenance of TMD pain (Johansson et al., 2006). However, there may be a need to better understand potential differences between the effects of bruxism in the waking state versus the sleep state and to differentiate between self-reported measures and EMG-based recordings of bruxism.

When subjects are asked to clench as hard or as long as they can, either in the intercuspal position or on a bite force meter, it is a consistent finding that TMD pain patients can produce less force and EMG activity in their jaw-closing muscles and have less endurance than control subjects (see Svensson and Graven-Nielsen, 2001). With experimental jaw muscle pain, similar findings can be demonstrated in healthy subjects (Wang et al., 2000a) (Fig. 1). When the EMG activity is examined at the single motor unit level, it can be shown that during sustained low-level tooth-clenching at a constant force level, the firing frequency of single motor unit action potentials is decreased (Sohn et al., 2000). A follow-up study showed that the associated twitch force increased during experimental pain (Sohn et al., 2004). The authors suggested that this increase might represent a peripheral compensatory mechanism to maintain constant force despite decreased firing rates, although other explanations can be suggested (see Chapter 29 by Farina).

Recent findings support the view that types of pain other than musculoskeletal pain can influence the EMG activity of jaw-closing muscles during tooth clenching. For example, Ernberg et al. (2007) showed that postoperative pain following third molar removal is associated with significant decreases in EMG activity in both the jaw-closing and jaw-opening muscles during maximal voluntary contractions.

In summary, the findings related to tooth clenching and grinding suggest that pain and soreness may develop as a consequence, but that pain itself is a strong modifier that generally inhibits jaw motor function.

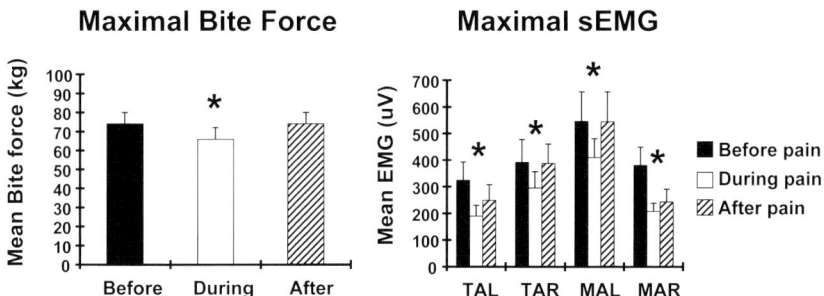

Fig. 1. Maximal voluntary bite force recordings and surface electromyographic (sEMG) activity in 12 healthy subjects before, during, and after painful stimulation of the left masseter muscle (MAL). MAR = right masseter muscle; TAL and TAR = left and right anterior temporalis muscle. Pain was induced by infusion of 5% hypertonic saline for up to 15 minutes using a computer-controlled microinfusion pump. Asterisks (*) indicate significantly lower values compared to before pain ($P < 0.05$). Mean values (+ SEM) from three different clenching conditions (right molar, left molar, or incisor). Modified from Wang et al. (2000).

Dynamic Contractions

The interaction between pain and jaw motor function has classically been explained by the vicious cycle concept mentioned above, where muscle hyperactivity leads to pain, and pain reinforces the hyperactivity (Travell et al., 1942). However, researchers who reviewed this theory in a series of papers came to the conclusion that the vicious cycle was not supported by valid scientific research (Lund et al., 1991). The reviewers instead proposed the pain-adaptation model, which strongly contrasts with the vicious cycle model (Lund et al., 1991). The pain-adaptation model predicts that trigeminal nociceptive inputs to premotoneurons in the brainstem facilitate inhibitory pathways to alpha-motoneurons during agonist function and enhance excitatory pathways during antagonist function. The essential prerequisite for the model is a collection of premotoneurons constituting the "central pattern generator" in the brainstem along with groups of inhibitory and excitatory interneurons (Lund and Kolta, 2006). The pain-adaptation model explains many of the motor effects of TMD pain but does not provide any explanation for the cause of pain. Nevertheless, the pain-adaptation model has facilitated the understanding that no causal link between pain and changes in jaw motor function (mandibular dysfunction) can be derived from cross-sectional clinical studies because pain in itself has a significant influence on jaw motor function. Johansson and Sojka (1991) presented an alternative model, which integrates the gamma-motoneuron system, to explain muscle tension and spread of muscle pain, and more recently the sympathetic nervous system has been implicated in the pathophysiological mechanisms of muscle pain (Passatore and Roatta, 2007). Further research will be necessary to test the hypotheses and pivotal features of these different models.

Human experimental pain studies have helped to clarify the interaction between trigeminal nociceptive inputs and jaw motor function. Injections of HS into the human masseter muscle reduced the agonist EMG burst during jaw-opening and jaw-closing movements with the mouth empty and during gum chewing (Lund et al., 1991; Svensson et al., 1996). Experimental masseter pain also reduces the maximum displacement of the mandible in the lateral and vertical axes and reduces the maximum velocity during opening and closing of the jaw. Türp et al. (2002) showed that there were differential effects of HS-induced jaw muscle pain on EMG activity in jaw-closing muscles depending on the position of the recording electrodes. Thus, studies using experimental jaw muscle pain have consistently shown a decrease in agonist EMG activity in the range of 10–15%, a small increase in antagonist EMG activity, and modest reductions in maximum displacement. These findings from the trigeminal system are in accordance with other experimental pain studies in the spinal system and with recordings of muscle activity during walking and repetitive shoulder movements in humans (Graven-Nielsen et al., 2000). So far, the experimental studies have mainly examined the influence of masseter muscle pain on jaw motor function, but studies are in progress to describe the effects of pain in, for example, the lateral pterygoid muscle, using more accurate and sensitive tools to assess jaw movements (Sae-Lee et al., 2006).

The experimental findings in humans are supported by observations in animals. In rabbits with cortically driven mastication, noxious pressure applied to the zygoma or intramuscular HS injection caused a significant reduction in the agonist EMG burst, significant increases in the duration of the masticatory cycle, and significantly smaller amplitudes of jaw movements (Westberg et al., 1997). This finding clearly indicates that the "central pattern generator" controlling the rhythmic jaw movements in mastication is also influenced by nociceptive inputs, but in a manner that is qualitatively different from its effect on the tremor generator.

In summary, many aspects of sensory-motor integration in patients with TMD pain seem to apply to the pain-adaptation model. Several human experimental pain studies and animal trials substantiate this hypothesis, but there is a need for further studies on how pain interferes with types of dynamic function other than mastication and for better understanding of the complex coordination between multiple muscle groups in the trigeminal area.

Reflex Studies

This section considers the inhibitory reflex response, consisting of a "silent" or exteroceptive suppression period in the jaw-closing muscles, and the excitatory reflex response, such as the jaw jerk or jaw stretch reflex.

Numerous human studies have examined the influence of various types of experimental pain on inhibitory reflexes in the jaw-closing muscles (Wang et al., 1999; van der Glas et al., 2000; Torisu et al., 2007). The duration of the late inhibitory period and the magnitude of the suppression of EMG activity are decreased by trigeminal painful inputs (e.g., Wang et al., 1999). This finding can be interpreted as a disinhibition or a net facilitation of the reflex response (Svensson and Graven-Nielsen, 2001). This effect of painful jaw muscle stimulation is shown not only in surface EMG activity but also in the reflex responses of single motor unit action potentials (Svensson et al., 1999). Thus, there is solid evidence to suggest that experimental jaw muscle pain disinhibits the output of trigeminal motoneuron activity, particularly on the painful side, but also to a lesser extent on the contralateral nonpainful side (e.g., Wang et al., 2000a). It is therefore clear that activity in trigeminal nociceptors affects the reflex pathways underlying the inhibitory reflex circuits, which may affect various jaw movement patterns. Similar effects can also be observed when the arms or legs are painfully stimulated, which suggests that pain-evoked stress responses may trigger endogenous pain modulatory systems that may play an additional role in modulating these reflex pathways (Cadden, 2007).

A series of systematic studies from the Orofacial Pain Laboratory at Aalborg University have provided good evidence that the human jaw stretch reflex is facilitated during experimental jaw muscle pain (e.g., Peddireddy et al., 2005; Wang et al., 2000b). A similar finding has also been reported for stretch reflexes in the limb muscles during HS-evoked pain in the soleus and tibialis anterior muscles (Matre et al., 1998). Interestingly, there are significant sex-related differences in these responses: men have significantly greater facilitation of the stretch reflex responses than women during pain (Cairns et al., 2003). It has subsequently been suggested that experimental muscle pain causes increased activity in the gamma-motoneuron system. This suggestion fits with the observations of increased muscle spindle activity evoked by intramuscular injection of algesic substances (arachidonic acid, bradykinin, or serotonin) in some animal experiments (Hellström et al., 2000). However, other researchers have also observed either excitatory or inhibitory effects. For example, we found that experimental muscle pain inhibits the stretch reflex excitation of low-threshold motor units (Svensson et al., 2000), and Bodéré et al. (2005) showed a decreased amplitude of the jaw jerk reflex in myofascial TMD pain patients and also in patients with orofacial neuropathic pain. Direct recordings of the heteronymous H-reflex (Svensson et al., 1998a) and of the recovery cycle (Truini et al., 2006) suggest that the excitability of the motoneuron pool is not changed during acute ongoing muscle pain. This variety of effects may reflect the flexibility and complexity of the jaw motor system in the interaction between nociceptive activity and motor reflexes. An increased stretch reflex could indicate greater stiffness of the jaw system in painful conditions, which might be associated with impaired motor performance in patients with jaw muscle pain.

Discussion

This review of human experimental and clinical pain research related to jaw motor function does not support the general view that pain is simply due to a dysfunction or overuse of the jaw muscles. The literature shows that different types and conditions of jaw motor function are critically influenced and modulated by nociceptive activity. Thus, many important issues remain to be explored in future studies. For example, the pain-adaptation model cannot explain the origin of pain. Moreover, the long-term consequences of an adaptation of jaw motor function to a chronic painful input are unknown, and there might be conditions in which the jaw muscles are unable to adapt, such as when the same load or work is required. Experimental pain studies only have examined pain at a single muscle site, whereas most TMD pain patients have pain in multiple sites in the craniofacial region. Thus, the influence of spatial summation on sensory-motor integration needs to be established. The different duration of pain between acute experimental studies and persistent clinical conditions should be kept in mind when data are interpreted.

Human and animal studies are in general agreement with each other and have not been able to reject the pain-adaptation model. However, these studies differ in many aspects. For example, human pain studies are performed in conscious human beings, and the influence of higher-order brain centers and psychological effects cannot be excluded. The finding that chewing sometimes increases the perceived intensity of pain also suggests that higher-order brain centers could contribute to pain-induced changes in chewing. Furthermore, human studies are performed with a food bolus in the mouth, whereas the animal studies look at empty open-close jaw movements evoked by electrical stimulation of the corticobulbar tract. The central pattern generator and associated motor programs related to such different types of jaw movements could also be differentially influenced by pain.

In summary, nociceptive inputs and pain have various impacts on jaw motor function in terms of changes in postural position, force, reflexes, and activation patterns of jaw muscles during static and dynamic contractions. On the other hand, jaw muscle contractions can also lead to fatigue and pain and feed new afferent information into the complex neurocircuitry that controls jaw motor function. The translation of the findings from animal and human experimental pain research into recommendations for best management approaches of TMD pain is far from evident. A cautious suggestion would be to focus on pain management rather than on correction of a mandibular dysfunction involving extensive oral rehabilitation.

References

Arima T, Svensson P, Arendt-Nielsen L. Experimental grinding in healthy subjects: a model for postexercise jaw muscle soreness. J Orofac Pain 1999;13:104–114.

Arima T, Arendt-Nielsen L, Svensson P. Effect of jaw muscle pain and soreness evoked by capsaicin before sleep on orofacial motor activity during sleep. J Orofac Pain 2001;15:245–256.

Bodéré C, Tèa SH, Giroux-Metges MA, Woda A. Activity of masticatory muscles in subjects with different orofacial pain conditions. Pain 2005;116:33–41.

Cadden SW. Modulation of human jaw reflexes: heterotopic stimuli and stress. Arch Oral Biol 2007;52:370–373.

Cairns BE, Sessle BJ, Hu JW. Evidence that excitatory amino acid receptors within the temporomandibular joint region are involved in the reflex activation of the jaw muscles. J Neurosci 1998;18:8056–8064.

Cairns BE, Wang K, Hu JW, Sessle BJ, Arendt-Nielsen L, Svensson P. The effects of glutamate-evoked masseter muscle pain on the human jaw-stretch reflex differs in men and women. J Orofac Pain 2003;17:317–325.

Ernberg M, Schopka JH, Fougeront N, Svensson P. Changes in jaw muscle EMG activity and pain after third molar surgery. J Oral Rehabil 2007;34:15–26.

Graven-Nielsen T, McArdle A, Phoenix J, Arendt-Nielsen L, Jensen TS, Jackson MJ, Edwards RH. In vivo model of muscle pain: quantification of intramuscular chemical, electrical, and pressure changes associated with saline-induced muscle pain in humans. Pain 1997;69:137–143.

Graven-Nielsen T, Svensson P, Arendt-Nielsen L. Effect of muscle pain on motor control: a human experimental approach. Adv Physiother 2000;2:26–38.

Hellström F, Thunberg J, Bergenheim M, Sjölander P, Pedersen J, Johansson H. Elevated intramuscular concentration of bradykinin in jaw muscle increases the fusimotor drive to neck muscles in the cat. J Dent Res 2000;79:1815–1822.

Hu JW, Yu X-M, Vernon H, Sessle BJ. Excitatory effects on neck and jaw muscle activity of inflammatory irritant applied to cervical paraspinal tissues. Pain 1993;55:243–250.

Jaberzadeh S, Svensson P, Nordstrom MA, Miles TS. Differential modulation of tremor and pulsatile control of human jaw and finger by experimental muscle pain. Exp Brain Res 2003;150:520–524.

Johansson H, Sojka P. Pathophysiological mechanisms involved in genesis and spread of muscular tension in occupational muscle pain. Med Hypoth 1991;135:196–203.

Johansson A, Unell L, Carlsson GE, Soderfeldt B, Halling A. Risk factors associated with symptoms of temporomandibular disorders in a population of 50- and 60-year-old subjects. J Oral Rehabil 2006;33:473–481.

Junge D, Rosenberg JR, Halliday DM. Physiological tremor in human jaw-muscle system. Arch Oral Biol 1998;43:45–54.

Lavigne GJ, Kato T, Kolta A, Sessle BJ. Neurobiological mechanisms involved in sleep bruxism. Crit Rev Oral Biol Med 2003;14:30–46.

Lavigne GJ, Rompre PH, Montplaisir JY, Lobbezoo F. Motor activity in sleep bruxism with concomitant jaw muscle pain. A retrospective pilot study. Eur J Oral Sci 1997;105:92–95.

Lobbezoo F, van Selms MK, Naeije M. Masticatory muscle pain and disordered jaw motor behaviour: literature review over the past decade. Arch Oral Biol 2006;51:713–720.

Lund JP, Donga R, Widmer CG, Stohler CS. The pain-adaptation model: a discussion of the relationship between chronic musculoskeletal pain and motor activity. Can J Physiol Pharmacol 1991;69:683–694.

Lund JP, Kolta A. Generation of the central masticatory pattern and its modification by sensory feedback. Dysphagia 2006;21:167–174.

Matre DA, Sinkjaer T, Svensson P, Arendt-Nielsen L. Experimental muscle pain increases the human stretch reflex. Pain 1998;75:331–339.

Miles TS. Masticatory muscles. In: Miles TS, Nauntofte B, Svensson P, editors. Clinical oral physiology. Copenhagen: Quintessence; 2004. p 199–218.

Passatore M, Roatta S. Modulation operated by the sympathetic nervous system on jaw reflexes and masticatory movement. Arch Oral Biol 2007;52:343–346.

Peddireddy A, Wang K, Svensson P, Arendt-Nielsen L. Effect of experimental posterior temporalis muscle pain on human brainstem reflexes. Clin Neurophysiol 2005;116:1611–1620.

Sae-Lee D, Wanigaratne K, Whittle T, Peck CC, Murray GM. A method for studying jaw muscle activity during standardized jaw movements under experimental jaw muscle pain. J Neurosci Methods 2006;157:285–293.

Schindler H, Svensson P. Myofascial temporomandibular disorder pain. In: Turp JC, Sommer C, Hugger A, editors. The puzzle of orofacial pain. Pain and Headache. Basel: Karger; 2007. p 91–123.

Sessle BJ. Acute and chronic craniofacial pain: brainstem mechanisms of nociceptive transmission and neuroplasticity, and their clinical correlates. Crit Rev Oral Biol Med 2000;11:57–91.

Simons DG. Review of enigmatic MTrPs as a common cause of enigmatic musculoskeletal pain and dysfunction. J Electromyogr Kinesiol 2004;14:95–107.

Sohn MK, Graven-Nielsen T, Arendt-Nielsen L, Svensson P. Inhibition of motor unit firing during experimental muscle pain in humans. Muscle Nerve 2000;23:1219–1226.

Sohn MK, Graven-Nielsen T, Arendt-Nielsen L, Svensson P. Effects of experimental muscle pain on mechanical properties of single motor units in human masseter. Clin Neurophysiol 2004;115:76–84.

Stohler CS. Craniofacial pain and motor function: pathogenesis, clinical correlates, and implications. Crit Rev Oral Biol Med 1999;10:504–518.

Stohler CS, Zhang X, Lund JP. The effect of experimental jaw muscle pain on postural muscle activity. Pain 1996;66:215–221.

Svensson P. What can human experimental pain models teach us about clinical TMD? Arch Oral Biol 2007;52:391–394.

Svensson P, Arendt-Nielsen L, Houe L. Sensory-motor interactions of human experimental unilateral jaw muscle pain: a quantitative analysis. Pain 1996;64:241–249.

Svensson P, De Laat A, Graven-Nielsen T, Arendt-Nielsen L. Experimental jaw-muscle pain does not change heteronymous H-reflexes in the human temporalis muscle. Exp Brain Res 1998a;121:311–318.

Svensson P, Graven-Nielsen T. Craniofacial muscle pain: review of mechanisms and clinical manifestations. J Orofac Pain 2001;15:117–145.

Svensson P, Graven-Nielsen T, Matre D, Arendt-Nielsen L. Experimental muscle pain does not cause long-lasting increases in resting electromyographic activity. Muscle Nerve 1998b;21:1382–1389.

Svensson P, McMillan AS, Graven-Nielsen T, Wang K, Arendt-Nielsen L. Modulation of an inhibitory reflex in single motor units in human masseter by tonic painful stimulation. Pain 1999;83:441–446.

Svensson P, Miles TS, Graven-Nielsen T, Arendt-Nielsen L. Modulation of stretch-evoked reflexes in single motor units in human masseter muscle by experimental pain. Exp Brain Res 2000;132:65–71.

Svensson P, Wang K, Sessle BJ, Arendt-Nielsen L. Associations between pain and neuromuscular activity in the human jaw and neck muscles. Pain 2004;109:225–232.

Torisu T, Wang K, Svensson P, De Laat A, Fujii H, Arendt-Nielsen L. Effect of low-level clenching and subsequent muscle pain on exteroceptive suppression and resting muscle activity in human jaw muscles. Clin Neurophysiol 2007;118:999–1009.

Travell J, Rinzler S, Herman M. Pain and disability of the shoulder and arm. Treatment by intramuscular infiltration with procaine hydrochloride. JAMA 1942;120:417–422.

Truini A, Romaniello A, Svensson P, Galeotti F, Graven-Nielsen T, Wang K, Cruccu G, Arendt-Nielsen L. Experimental skin pain and muscle pain induce distinct changes in human trigeminal motoneuronal excitability. Exp Brain Res 2006;174:622–629.

Türp JC, Schindler HJ, Pritsch M, Rong Q. Antero-posterior activity changes in the superficial masseter muscle after exposure to experimental pain. Eur J Oral Sci 2002;110:83–91.

van der Glas HW, Cadden SW, van der Bilt A. Mechanisms underlying the effects of remote noxious stimulation and mental activities on exteroceptive jaw reflexes in man. Pain 2000;84:193–202.

van der Meulen MJ, Lobbezoo F, Aartman IH, Naeije M. Self-reported oral parafunctions and pain intensity in temporomandibular disorder patients. J Orofac Pain 2006;20:31–35.

Wang K, Arima T, Arendt-Nielsen L, Svensson P. EMG-force relationships are influenced by experimental jaw-muscle pain. J Oral Rehabil 2000a;27:394–402.

Wang K, Svensson P, Arendt-Nielsen L. Effect of tonic muscle pain on short-latency jaw-stretch reflexes in humans. Pain 2000b;88:189–197.

Wang K, Svensson P, Arendt-Nielsen L. Modulation of exteroceptive suppression periods in human jaw-closing muscles by local and remote experimental muscle pain. Pain 1999;82:253–262.

Westberg KG, Clavelou P, Schwartz G, Lund JP. Effects of chemical stimulation of masseter muscle nociceptors on trigeminal motoneuron and interneuron activities during fictive mastication in the rabbit. Pain 1997;73:295–308.

Woda A, Pionchon P, Palla S. Regulation of mandibular postures: mechanisms and clinical implications. Crit Rev Oral Biol Med 2001;12:166–178.

Correspondence to: Peter Svensson, DDS, PhD, Dr Odont., Department of Clinical Oral Physiology, School of Dentistry, University of Aarhus, Vennelyst Boulevard 9, DK-8000 Aarhus C, Denmark. Fax: + 45 8619 5665, email: psvensson@ odont.au.dk.

Changes in Sensorimotor Control in Low Back Pain

Paul W. Hodges

NHMRC Centre of Clinical Research Excellence in Spinal Pain, Injury and Health,
School of Health and Rehabilitation Sciences,
The University of Queensland, Brisbane, Australia

There is wide variability in reported changes in sensorimotor control of the trunk muscles in low back and pelvic pain. Different studies have reported increased muscle activity (Arendt-Nielsen et al., 1996), decreased activity (Soderberg and Dostal, 1978), and no change (Cohen et al., 1986; Alexiev, 1994). Inconsistent and incomplete understanding of the motor adaptations in spinal pain has led to the assumption that there are no consistent responses to pain. However, despite the variable results, a theoretical framework is emerging to rationalize the complex changes in sensorimotor control. This chapter addresses the changes that occur in low back pain, considers the possible underlying mechanisms, and discusses the consequences of adaptation in the sensorimotor system with pain.

Changes in Muscle Control in Low Back Pain

Low back pain (LBP) is associated with a vast array of changes in trunk muscle activity. Many of these changes are likely to affect the movement and stability of the spine and pelvis, but the nature of these changes is complicated; some changes suggest reduced muscle activity, but others indicate increased activity. For instance, increased co-contraction of flexor and extensor muscles has been reported when a load is released from the trunk (Radebold et al., 2000), activity of erector spinae muscles is increased during the swing phase in gait (Arendt-Nielsen et al., 1996), and bracing of the abdominal muscles is increased during an active straight leg raise (O'Sullivan et al., 2002). Furthermore, activity of the obliquus externus abdominis is increased in association with shoulder movements during experimentally induced pain (Hodges et al., 2003b) and when there is a threat of pain (Moseley et al., 2004). These findings suggest augmented control of the spine and pelvis. This proposal is supported by findings of reduced motion of the spine in individuals with back pain. For instance, individuals with LBP are less likely to prepare the spine with movement prior to arm movement (Mok et al., 2004). In these individuals, intervertebral motion is decreased during trunk flexion (Kaigle et al., 1998), and counter-rotation of the shoulders and pelvis is reduced during locomotion (Lamoth et al., 2002). However, numerous studies have found no change in activity of the large superficial muscles in LBP (Cohen et al., 1986; Alexiev, 1994).

Other data tend to indicate that the control of the spine is compromised in pain. For instance, activity of the transversus abdominis (Hodges et al., 1996) and multifidus muscles (MacDonald et al., 2004) is delayed during arm movements, and tonic activity of the transversus abdominis is reduced both during walking (Saunders et al., 2004) and during repetitive arm movements in experimentally induced pain (Hodges et al., 2003b). Furthermore, there is evidence for decreased cross-sectional area (Hides et al., 1994), increased fatigability (Roy et al., 1989), and increased intramuscular fat in the paraspinal muscles (Alaranta et al., 1993). These latter measures, although not directly indicating changes in control, suggest functional changes in the muscles. Given that in vivo and in vitro evidence suggests a contribution of these muscles to spinal control (Kaigle et al., 1997; Hodges et al., 2003a; Barker et al., 2005), such changes are likely to lead to impairment. Other data from specific LBP populations provide direct evidence of impaired intervertebral control.

For instance, intervertebral translation is abnormal in patients with spondylolisthesis (Schneider et al., 2005), and buckling has been observed with fluoroscopy in a single subject during a weight-lifting task (Cholewicki and McGill, 1996).

Taken together, these data provide evidence for both augmented and impaired control of the spine. How can these findings be rationalized? Most studies have recorded from only a small subset of muscles. As such, they have failed to recognize the redundancy in the trunk muscle system, which means that many muscles can achieve a similar goal. Radebold et al. (2000) hint that investigation of multiple muscles may help understand the changes in control. Their data show that although most subjects with LBP had increased activation of at least one superficial abdominal or paraspinal muscle in a postural task, the pattern varied among individuals. If recordings had been made from only a subset of muscles, this variation would have been missed.

There may be a common goal that underpins the adaptation to pain. Despite the variability, one underlying principle could be adaptation to pain or injury by increasing muscle activity to increase the safety margin and protect the part from pain and injury (or re-injury). However, due to the system's redundancy, different strategies can be used to achieve this goal. With a strategy of increased activity of large muscles, the nervous system would decrease the potential for error, limit the impact of unanticipated disturbances to the spine, and reduce the potential for further injury. In effect, rather than selecting a strategy from a spectrum of dynamic possibilities that are perfectly matched to the demands of the task, the nervous system may select a simple solution that provides reasonable (but perhaps not optimal) quality of control that satisfies the demands of a range of conditions. However, because many muscles can achieve the same goal, different individuals may select different combinations of muscle activity to achieve this goal, and the strategy may also differ between tasks.

To test the idea that a range of different strategies of muscle activation achieve a similar outcome for the spine, van Dieen et al. (2003a) conducted a model using simulation of a range of strategies adopted by persons with LBP. Stability of the spine was increased by each permutation of muscle activation, regardless of whether the strategy involved increased co-contraction of flexors and extensors, increased activity of the flexors alone, or increased activity of the extensors. Recent data from a study of experimental pain suggest that when pain is induced in healthy individuals, most of them adopt a pattern of increased activity, but again the pattern varies among individuals (Hodges et al., 2006a); in each case a there was a different pattern of increased and decreased muscle activity.

Individuals with LBP often show impaired activity of the deep muscles. For example, an individual may present with changes in the deep muscles that would be consistent with compromised control, yet with increased activity of the superficial muscles, consistent with protection of the spine. Thus, despite the increased activity, control of intervertebral motion may be compromised due to impaired activity of the deep muscles. In summary, available data suggest that the goal of increased stability of the spine may be achieved to varying degrees by different individuals. It is likely, if not probable, that subgroups of individuals with LBP could be identified from this variability.

Mechanisms for Changes in Muscle Control in Low Back Pain

Why is control of the spine modified in individuals with LBP? There are several key issues to consider. An initial consideration is which came first—the pain or the motor control changes? There is evidence for both. Changes in the control of the trunk muscles can lead to the development of pain. Cholewicki et al. (2005) reported that delayed offset of activity of the superficial abdominal muscles is associated with the development of acute LBP in athletes. In this case, the challenge is to identify factors that would lead to the initial change in control. Potential candidates include habitual postures or movement patterns, impaired proprioception, and other comorbid disorders (e.g., incontinence) that may compromise trunk muscle control (Smith et al., 2006). Conversely, a large literature argues that pain and injury lead to changes in control and structure of the trunk muscles. For instance, experimental LBP changes trunk muscle activity during walking (Arendt-Nielsen et al., 1996) and during arm movement tasks (Hodges et al., 1996), and experimental injury in pigs leads to rapid atrophy of the multifidus muscles (Hodges et al., 2006b). These changes are similar to those identified in patients with clinical pain. If pain and injury lead to changes in the structure and behavior of the trunk muscles, what is the mechanism? Pain can affect control at multiple levels of the nervous system, involving all levels including motor planning, spinal mechanisms, and proprioception (Fig. 1).

Changes in the Corticospinal System in Pain

Among the changes implicated in pain are changes in excitability of the corticospinal system at the level of the motor cortex (Valeriani et al., 1999) or the motoneuron (Le Pera et al., 2001), peripheral effects such as changed muscle spindle sensitivity (Pedersen et al., 1997), and effects "upstream" of the motor cortex (Butler et al., 2003) (e.g., in the premotor

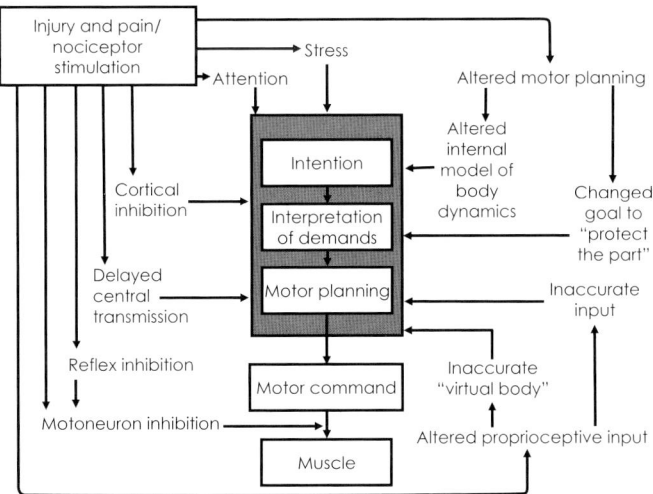

Fig. 1. Possible mechanisms by which pain affects the planning of movement and the activation of trunk muscles. Pain and nociceptor stimulation can affect motor output at any level of the nervous system. Major potential mechanisms include the possible effect of pain on motoneurons and descending motor pathways, proprioception (leading to inaccurate interpretation of body position and movement and therefore poor ability to plan movement and respond), cognition (due to stress and fear), and a change in motor strategy.

cortex). Findings on the effect of pain on the motor cortex are conflict-
ing. Transcranial magnetic stimulation (TMS) over the motor cortex has
been used to assess motor cortex excitability, but reduced (Valeriani et
al., 1999), increased (Rossi and Decchi, 1997) and unchanged (Romaniello et al., 2000) responses have been reported. However, the response to
TMS alone is difficult to interpret because it can be affected by other factors such as motoneuron excitability (Taylor et al., 2000). The response
of the superficial paraspinal muscles to TMS has been investigated in
persons with LBP (Strutton et al., 2005). Although these data suggest increased threshold to evoked potentials in LBP, for the reasons described
above it is not possible to determine whether these changes are occurring at the level of the cortex or motoneuron. Recent findings in pigs
suggest that cortical excitability, but not motoneuron excitability of the
multifidus muscle (assessed by evaluation of the response to descending volleys evoked by stimulation at the level of the medullary pyramids;
Ugawa et al., 1991), may be increased immediately after injury to the intervertebral disk (Hodges et al., 2007).

  The effects of pain on motoneuron excitability have also been debat-
ed. Motoneuron excitability is commonly estimated from the H-reflex—the
electrical equivalent of a stretch reflex that involves electrical stimulation of
the muscle afferents to elicit a largely monosynaptic reflex response in
the muscle. If motoneuron excitability is modulated, the response to this
stimulus changes. Results are variable with pain. Although decreased H-
reflex amplitude has been identified at rest (Rossi and Decchi, 1997), this
finding is not apparent in other studies using different paradigms (Matre
et al., 1998). However, among other problems, these responses are affected by presynaptic inhibitory effects on type Ia afferent endings (Rudomin, 2002), which may change the muscle response without any change
occurring in the motoneuron. Thus, it is unclear whether changes in motoneuron excitability occur with pain. In contrast, data from animal studies indicate that injury to joint structures such as the ligaments and joint
capsule can change motoneuron excitability (Ekholm et al., 1960). Human studies show a reduction in maximal force (Stokes and Young, 1984)
and decreased H-reflex amplitude (Spencer et al., 1984). However, these
latter findings do not permit interpretation of motoneuron changes.

Other authors have evaluated the stretch reflex, which is affected by muscle spindle sensitivity, presynaptic inhibition, and motoneuron excitability. A popular argument is that pain influences the sensitivity of muscle spindles (Johansson and Sojka, 1991), increasing the stretch reflex response (Matre et al., 1998). Stimuli that excite pain afferents have been shown to increase excitability of gamma-motoneurons, which innervate muscle fibers of the muscle spindle and modulate its sensitivity (Jovanovic et al., 1990). It has been argued that stretch reflex gain would increase due to increased sensitivity of the muscle spindle during pain (Johansson and Sojka, 1991). In line with this reasoning, the stretch reflex has been shown by some investigators (Matre et al., 1998), but not others (Zedka et al., 1999), to be facilitated during experimental pain. However, changes at multiple sites may explain the change in reflex gain (e.g., motoneuron excitability, spindle sensitivity, and presynaptic effects), and these changes may have opposite effects on the evoked response (e.g., if the motoneuron is inhibited, but spindle sensitivity is increased, the net effect may be no change). Thus, although the stretch reflex amplitude of the erector spinae muscles has been argued to be unchanged by experimental muscle pain (Zedka et al., 1999), this finding is difficult to interpret. Pain may also affect the contraction properties of the muscle, but with unclear effects on motor control. This possibility is reviewed in detail elsewhere (Farina et al., 2008).

In summary, although pain may cause changes in excitability along the motor pathway, data are inconsistent, and the exact nature of changes is difficult to identify from the available literature. However, it is reasonable to expect that changes in the motor pathway will influence motor control and contribute to the variable changes observed in people with LBP.

Changes in Motor Planning

Although the evidence for changes in motor pathway excitability is not clear, there is good evidence that motor planning is changed in the presence of pain. As mentioned earlier, pain is often associated with activity of muscles that would tend to increase protection for the spine; that is, the nervous system appears to switch its strategy to protect the affected part of the body from pain and injury (or re-injury).

Several authors have argued that this strategy is adopted to compensate for reduced osseoligamentous stability of the spine (Panjabi, 1992; van Dieen et al., 2003a). However, similar changes can be replicated when pain is induced experimentally by injection of hypertonic saline (Hodges et al., 2003b), when osseoligamentous stability is not changed. Furthermore, changes can be induced when pain is anticipated, but not present (Moseley et al., 2004). Thus, adaptation may occur in a number of situations when the real or perceived stability of the spine is decreased, when there is a real or perceived risk of further injury, or when there is a real or perceived threat of pain.

The proposal that trunk muscle activity adapts to "protect the part" from threat has many similarities with the "pain-adaptation" model of Lund et al. (1991). That is, the adaptation aims to prevent painful movements. However, although the original model proposed that the changes in muscle activity could be explained by inhibition and facilitation at the spinal cord or brainstem, several pieces of evidence suggest that the adaptation is likely to involve higher levels of processing. First, the adaptation occurs in the absence of nociceptor input if there is the threat of pain (Moseley et al., 2004). Although descending pain systems may influence spinal networks, these data suggest that spinal and brainstem circuits cannot explain the effects. Second, as mentioned above, the trunk system has a high degree of redundancy. Although during simple limb movements it may be possible to hypothesize simple integratory networks that inhibit the agonist and facilitate the antagonist muscles, this scenario is difficult to rationalize for the trunk. In the trunk it is difficult to partition muscles as agonists or antagonists in many tasks. Furthermore, the patterns of change in activity are complex, requiring interpretation of the net outcome of contraction of multiple fascicles. Such changes would seem to require more complex integration. Third, several studies have shown that the organization of motor patterns changes (Hodges, 2001). In summary, although spinal and brainstem mechanisms may contribute to the changes in control of the trunk muscles in pain, it is likely that many of the changes represent a decision by the nervous system to move differently (i.e.,. change to a different strategy) in order to meet a different goal: "protection of the part."

Sensory Changes

Motor control may change as a result of deficits in sensation. If accurate sensory information is not available, control of movement is unlikely to be accurate. There is considerable evidence of abnormal sensory function in LBP. For instance, the ability to reposition the spine to a target angle is reduced (Gill and Callaghan, 1998), and the amount of displacement required to detect movement is increased (Leinonen et al., 2003). The nervous system may also ignore sensory information from the lumbar spine. When vibration is applied to the back muscles in healthy individuals, there is a perception of muscle lengthening and a resultant postural correction. However, when the back muscles are vibrated in people with LBP, the postural reaction is reduced (Brumagne et al., 2004). This finding suggests that the weighting of proprioceptive information from the spine is reduced in LBP. Reduced acuity or weighting of proprioceptive information from the spine is likely to lead to abnormal movement coordination and may contribute to a shift in response strategy to protect the trunk.

Summary

Multiple factors have the potential to lead to changes in the control of the trunk muscles before and after pain and injury. Thus, the variable response to LBP is likely to be due to the net outcome of the multiple changes that affect sensorimotor control in pain. However, the net effect appears to be "protection of the part."

Consequences of Changes in Sensorimotor Control in the Spine and Pelvis

After an acute injury or onset of pain, the strategy to "protect the part" may be ideal to prevent worsening of symptoms and provide an opportunity for tissue healing. However, when the pain is prolonged, this strategy may no longer be appropriate. Changes in strategy that lead to both increased and decreased muscle activity may have consequences for the spine. The potential for consequences is significant because motor control changes commonly do not resolve when the pain is resolved (Hides et al., 1996; Hodges et al., 1996).

From one point of view, a strategy to protect the spine and pelvis may be positive because it splints the spine and may prevent pain and re-injury (Panjabi, 1992; van Dieen et al., 2003b). Although this treatment may be beneficial in the short term, if the adaptation is maintained for a long period it is likely to have negative consequences for the spine and pelvis due to increased loading (McGill, 2002; Marras et al., 2004), restriction of movement (Mok et al., 2004), and inadequate fine-tuning of trunk movement.

Loading on the spine is increased as a result of muscle co-contraction, as has been shown in persons with LBP during lifting tasks (Marras et al., 2004). Although there is debate whether increased loading is detrimental to the spine, it is argued that high cumulative load may lead to mechanical and physiological changes (Kumar, 1990). These issues may accelerate degeneration (Ching et al., 2003) and increase the long-term risk for LBP recurrence. Furthermore, increased trunk muscle activity is likely to reduce the availability of movement to absorb and dissipate force. Recent data confirm that persons with LBP are less likely to use movement as a component of their strategy to control the spine. This strategy is associated with a greater perturbation to the trunk (Mok et al., 2004) and more time to recover their balance after the movement of the limb (Mok et al., 2007). Both of these issues are likely to have consequences in the long term.

Finally, impaired activity of the deep muscles, in conjunction with increased activity of the superficial muscles, is likely to have consequences for the control of movement and for stability at the intervertebral level. Deep muscle function is important for spinal control (Kaigle et al., 1997; Hodges et al., 2003a; Barker et al., 2005), and the contribution of these muscles to control of the lumbar spine and pelvis is unlikely to be completely compensated for—or replicated—by activity of the larger, more superficial, muscles. The models of Bergmark (1989) and Crisco and Panjabi (1991) predict that without activity of the deeper muscles, the integrity of the spine cannot be maintained. Thus, impaired function of these muscles is likely to leave the entire spinal system vulnerable. While this impairment may not be a problem in the short term, as the increased activity of the superficial muscles is likely to stiffen and protect the spine, in the long term it is likely to be problematic.

Thus, although changes in sensorimotor control to "protect the part" may have short-term benefit, the risk of back pain recurrence will increase if the almost obligatory use of this strategy does not cease along with the resolution of pain. It is well accepted that previous LBP is a strong predictor of future back injury (Greene et al., 2001). Data from numerous studies of individuals with a history of LBP, but no pain at the time of testing, indicate that changes in motor control persist after the resolution of symptoms (Hodges and Richardson, 1996). The possibility that abnormal muscle activation leads to LBP is supported by recent data showing that delayed offset of activity of the abdominal muscles predicts LBP (Cholewicki et al., 2005). Furthermore, persistent reduction of the cross-sectional area of the multifidus is associated with increased risk of LBP recurrence compared to individuals who received training to restore muscle size (Hides et al., 2001).

A key issue to consider is why some individuals go on to have LBP recurrence while others do not. Although further work is required to determine possible factors, recent data suggest that the failure of resolution of the motor adaptation may be linked to unhelpful attitudes and beliefs about pain (Moseley and Hodges, 2006). Persistence or recurrence of LBP (Burton et al., 1995) and pain-related attitudes are associated with changes in motor strategy (Watson, 1997), providing a physiological link between psychological factors and LBP recurrence.

Conclusion

It is clear that optimal control of the spine and pelvis requires a carefully controlled dynamic system. In such a system, the nervous system matches the strategy of activation of the trunk muscles to the multiple tasks that must be coordinated to achieve optimal control of the spine. Despite the variability described in the literature, data from persons with LBP generally indicate deficits in the ability of the nervous system to select the appropriate strategy, and often a preference to activate simple strategies that involve a net increase in trunk muscle activity to "protect the part" and increase the safety margin. This strategy is associated with changes in deep muscle control and proprioception. In view of the complexity of these changes, comprehensive rehabilitation is likely to require a motor learning approach to restore complex control strategies. Any rehabilitation protocol must be based on comprehensive assessment of the individual patient.

Acknowledgments

Paul Hodges is supported by a fellowship from the National Health and Medical Research Council of Australia.

References

Alaranta H, Tallroth K, Soukka A, Heliaara M. Fat content of lumbar extensor muscles in low back disability: a radiographic and clinical comparison. J Spin Disord 1993;6:137–140.

Alexiev AR. Some differences of the electromyographic erector spinae activity between normal subjects and low back pain patients during the generation of isometric trunk torque. Electromyogr Clin Neurophysiol 1994;34:495–499.

Arendt-Nielsen L, Graven-Nielsen T, Svarrer H, Svensson P. The influence of low back pain on muscle activity and coordination during gait: a clinical and experimental study. Pain 1996;64:231–240.

Barker P, Guggenheimer K, Grkovic I, Briggs C, Jones D, Thomas C, Hodges P. Effects of tensioning the lumbar fasciae on segmental stiffness during flexion and extension. Spine 2005;31:397–405.

Bergmark A. Stability of the lumbar spine. A study in mechanical engineering. Acta Orthop Scand 1989;60:1–54.

Brumagne S, Cordo P, Verschueren S. Proprioceptive weighting changes in persons with low back pain and elderly persons during upright standing. Neurosci Lett 2004;366:63–66.

Burton A, Tillotson K, Main C, Hollis S. Psychosocial predictors of outcome in acute and subchronic low back trouble. Spine 1995;20:722–728.

Butler JE, Taylor JL, Gandevia SC. Responses of human motoneurons to corticospinal stimulation during maximal voluntary contractions and ischemia. J Neurosci 2003;23:10224–10230.

Ching CT, Chow DH, Yao FY, Holmes AD. The effect of cyclic compression on the mechanical properties of the inter-vertebral disc: an in vivo study in a rat tail model. Clin Biomech (Bristol, Avon) 2003;18:182–189.

Cholewicki J, McGill SM. Mechanical stability of the *in vivo* lumbar spine: Implications for injury and chronic low back pain. Clin Biomech 1996;11:1–15.

Cholewicki J, Silfies SP, Shah RA, Greene HS, Reeves NP, Alvi K, Goldberg B. Delayed trunk muscle reflex responses increase the risk of low back injuries. Spine 2005;30:2614–2620.

Cohen MJ, Swanson GA, Naliboff BD, Schlander SL, McArthur DL. Comparison of electromyographic response patterns during posture and stress tasks in chronic low back pain patterns and control. J Psychosom Res 1986;30:135–141.

Crisco JJ, Panjabi MM. The intersegmental and multisegmental muscles of the lumbar spine: a biomechanical model comparing lateral stabilising potential. Spine 1991;7:793–799.

Ekholm J, Eklund G, Skoglund S. On the reflex effects from the knee joint of the cat. Acta Physiol Scand 1960;50:167–174.

Farina D, Arendt-Nielsen L, Roatta S, Graven-Nielsen T. The pain-induced decrease in low-threshold motor unit discharge rate is not associated with the amount of increase in spike-triggered average torque. Clin Neurophysiol 2008;119:43–51.

Gill KP, Callaghan MJ. The measurement of lumbar proprioception in individuals with and without low back pain. Spine 1998;23:371–377.

Greene HS, Cholewicki J, Galloway MT, Nguyen CV, Radebold A. A history of low back injury is a risk factor for recurrent back injuries in varsity athletes. Am J Sports Med 2001;29:795–800.

Hides JA, Jull GA, Richardson CA. Long term effects of specific stabilizing exercises for first episode low back pain. Spine 2001;26:243–248.

Hides JA, Richardson CA, Jull GA. Multifidus muscle recovery is not automatic after resolution of acute, first-episode low back pain. Spine 1996;21:2763–2769.

Hides JA, Stokes MJ, Saide M, Jull GA, Cooper DH. Evidence of lumbar multifidus muscle wasting ipsilateral to symptoms in patients with acute/subacute low back pain. Spine 1994;19:165–177.

Hodges PW. Changes in motor planning of feedforward postural responses of the trunk muscles in low back pain. Exp Brain Res 2001;141:261–266.

Hodges P, Cholewicki J, Coppieters M, MacDonald D. Trunk muscle activity is increased during experimental back pain, but the pattern varies between individuals. International Society for Electrophysiology and Kinesiology, Turin, 2006a.

Hodges PW, Galea M, Kaigle Holm A, Holm S. Corticomotor excitability of the deep paraspinal muscles is increased at a single lumbar level following intervertebral disk lesion. Proceedings of the International Brain Research Organisation Conference, Melbourne, 2007.

Hodges P, Kaigle Holm A, Holm S, Ekstrom L, Cresswell A, Hansson T, Thorstensson A. Intervertebral stiffness of the spine is increased by evoked contraction of transversus abdominis and the diaphragm: in vivo porcine studies. Spine 2003a;28:2594–2601.

Hodges PW, Kaigle Holm A, Hansson T, Holm S. Rapid atrophy of the lumbar multifidus follows experimental disc or nerve root injury. Spine 2006b;31:2926–2933.

Hodges PW, Moseley GL, Gabrielsson AH, Gandevia SC. Acute experimental pain changes postural recruitment of the trunk muscles in pain-free humans. Exp Brain Res 2003b;151:262–271.

Hodges PW, Richardson CA. Inefficient muscular stabilisation of the lumbar spine associated with low back pain: a motor control evaluation of transversus abdominis. Spine 1996;21:2640–2650.

Johansson H, Sojka P. Pathophysiological mechanisms involved in genesis and spread of muscular tension in occupational muscle pain and in chronic musculoskeletal pain syndromes: a hypothesis. Med Hypotheses 1991;35:196–203.

Jovanovic K, Anastasijevic R, Vuco J. Reflex effects on gamma fusimotor neurones of chemically in-
    duced discharges in small-diameter muscle afferents in decerebrate cats. Brain Res 1990;521:89–
    94.
Kaigle AM, Holm SH, Hansson TH. 1997 Volvo Award winner in biomechanical studies. Kinematic
    behavior of the porcine lumbar spine: a chronic lesion model. Spine 1997;22:2796–2806.
Kaigle AM, Wessberg P, Hansson TH. Muscular and kinematic behavior of the lumbar spine during
    flexion- extension. J Spinal Disord 1998;11:163–174.
Kumar S. Cumulative load as a risk factor for back pain. Spine 1990;15:1311–1316.
Lamoth CJ, Meijer OG, Wuisman PI, van Dieen JH, Levin MF, Beek PJ. Pelvis-thorax coordination
    in the transverse plane during walking in persons with nonspecific low back pain. Spine 2002;27:
    E92–99.
Le Pera D, Graven-Nielsen T, Valeriani M, Oliviero A, Di Lazzaro V, Tonali PA, Arendt-Nielsen L.
    Inhibition of motor system excitability at cortical and spinal level by tonic muscle pain. Clin
    Neurophysiol 2001;112:1633–1641.
Leinonen V, Kankaanpaa M, Luukkonen M, Kansanen M, Hanninen O, Airaksinen O, Taimela S.
    Lumbar paraspinal muscle function, perception of lumbar position, and postural control in disc
    herniation-related back pain. Spine 2003;28:842–848.
Lund JP, Donga R, Widmer CG, Stohler CS. The pain-adaptation model: a discussion of the rela-
    tionship between chronic musculoskeletal pain and motor activity. Can J Physiol Pharmacol
    1991;69:683–694.
MacDonald D, Moseley GL, Hodges PW. The function of the lumbar multifidus in unilateral low
    back pain. In Vleeming A, Mooney V, Hodges P, Lee D, McGill S, Ostgaard HC, O'Sullivan P,
    van Tulder M, Triano J. World Congress of Low Back and Pelvic Pain: Effective diagnosis and
    treatment of lumbopelvic pain. Melbourne: ECO; 2004. p. 329.
Marras WS, Ferguson SA, Burr D, Davis KG, Gupta P. Spine loading in patients with low back pain
    during asymmetric lifting exertions. Spine J 2004;4:64–75.
Matre DA, Sinkjaer T, Svensson P, Arendt-Nielsen L. Experimental muscle pain increases the human
    stretch reflex. Pain 1998;75:331–339.
McGill S. Low back disorders: evidence based prevention and rehabilitation. Champaign, IL: Human
    Kinetics; 2002.
Mok NW, Brauer SG, Hodges PW. Hip strategy for balance control in quiet standing is reduced in
    people with low back pain. Spine 2004;29:E107–112.
Mok N, Brauer S, Hodges P. Failure to use movement in postural strategies leads to increased spinal
    displacement in low back pain. Spine 2007;32:E537–543.
Moseley GL, Hodges PW. Reduced variability of postural strategy prevents normalisation of motor
    changes induced by back pain—a risk factor for chronic trouble? Behav Neurosci 2006;120:474–
    476.
Moseley GL, Nicholas MK, Hodges PW. Does anticipation of back pain predispose to back trouble?
    Brain 2004;127:2339–2347.
O'Sullivan PB, Beales DJ, Beetham JA, Cripps J, Graf F, Lin IB, Tucker B, Avery A. Altered motor
    control strategies in subjects with sacroiliac joint pain during the active straight-leg-raise test.
    Spine 2002;27:E1–8.
Panjabi MM. The stabilizing system of the spine. Part I. Function, dysfunction, adaptation, and en-
    hancement. J Spinal Dis 1992;5:383–389.
Pedersen J, Sjolander P, Wenngren BI, Johansson H. Increased intramuscular concentration of bra-
    dykinin increases the static fusimotor drive to muscle spindles in neck muscles of the cat. Pain
    1997;70:83–91.
Radebold A, Cholewicki J, Panjabi MM, Patel TC. Muscle response pattern to sudden trunk loading
    in healthy individuals and in patients with chronic low back pain. Spine 2000;25:947–954.
Romaniello A, Cruccu G, McMillan AS, Arendt-Nielsen L, Svensson P. Effect of experimen-
    tal pain from trigeminal muscle and skin on motor cortex excitability in humans. Brain Res
    2000;882:120–127.
Rossi A, Decchi B. Changes in Ib heteronymous inhibition to soleus motoneurones during cutane-
    ous and muscle nociceptive stimulation in humans. Brain Res 1997;774:55–61.
Roy SH, DeLuca CJ, Casavant DA. Lumbar muscle fatigue and chronic low back pain. Spine
    1989;14:992–1001.

Rudomin P. Selectivity of the central control of sensory information in the mammalian spinal cord. Adv Exp Med Biol 2002;508:157–170.

Saunders S, Coppieters M, Hodges P. Reduced tonic activity of the deep trunk muscle during locomotion in people with low back pain. In: Vleeming A, Mooney V, Hodges P, Lee D, McGill S, Ostgaard HC, O'Sullivan P, van Tulder M, Triano J. World Congress of Low Back and Pelvic Pain: Effective diagnosis and treatment of lumbopelvic pain. Melbourne: ECO; 2004. p. 261.

Schneider G, Pearcy MJ, Bogduk N. Abnormal motion in spondylolytic spondylolisthesis. Spine 2005;30:1159–1164.

Smith MD, Russell A, Hodges PW. Disorders of breathing and continence have a stronger association with back pain than obesity and physical activity. Aust J Physiother 2006;52:11–16.

Soderberg GL, Dostal WF. Electromyographic study of three parts of the gluteus medius muscle during functional activities. Phys Ther 1978;58:691–696.

Spencer JD, Hayes KC, Alexander IJ. Knee joint effusion and quadriceps reflex inhibition in man. Arch Phys Med Rehabil 1984;65:171–177.

Stokes M, Young A. The contribution of reflex inhibition to arthrogenous muscle weakness. Clin Sci (Lond) 1984;67:7–14.

Strutton PH, Theodorou S, Catley M, McGregor AH, Davey NJ. Corticospinal excitability in patients with chronic low back pain. J Spinal Disord Tech 2005;18:420–424.

Taylor JL, Butler JE, Gandevia SC. Changes in muscle afferents, motoneurons and motor drive during muscle fatigue. Eur J Appl Physiol 2000;83:106–115.

Ugawa Y, Rothwell JC, Day BL, Thompson PD, Marsden CD. Percutaneous electrical stimulation of corticospinal pathways at the level of the pyramidal decussation in humans. Ann Neurol 1991;29:418–27.

Valeriani M, Restuccia D, Di Lazzaro V, Oliviero A, Profice P, Le Pera D, Saturno E, Tonali P. Inhibition of the human primary motor area by painful heat stimulation of the skin. Clin Neurophysiol 1999;110:1475–1480.

van Dieen JH, Cholewicki J, Radebold A. Trunk muscle recruitment patterns in patients with low back pain enhance the stability of the lumbar spine. Spine 2003a;28:834–841.

van Dieen JH, Selen LP, Cholewicki J. Trunk muscle activation in low-back pain patients, an analysis of the literature. J Electromyogr Kinesiol 2003b;13:333–51.

Watson PJ, Booker CK. Evidence for the role of psychological factors in abnormal paraspinal activity in patients with chronic low back pain. J Musculoskel Pain 1997;5:41–56.

Zedka M, Prochazka A, Knight B, Gillard D, Gauthier M. Voluntary and reflex control of human back muscles during induced pain. J Physiol (Lond) 1999;520:591–604.

Correspondence to: Paul W. Hodges, MD, PhD, BPhty(Hons), NHMRC Centre of Clinical Research Excellence in Spinal Pain, Injury and Health, School of Health and Rehabilitation Sciences, The University of Queensland, Brisbane, Queensland 4072, Australia. Tel: +61 7 3365 2008; fax: +61 7 3365 2775; email: p.hodges@uq.edu.au.

Effect of Experimental Muscle Pain on Motor Unit Properties

Dario Farina

Center for Sensory-Motor Interaction, Department of Health Science and Technology, Aalborg University, Aalborg, Denmark

A motor unit consists of a motor neuron in the ventral horn of the spinal cord, its axon, and the muscle fibers it innervates (Sherrington, 1925). The population of motor units in a muscle is heterogeneous. Different motor units are characterized by differences in size, excitability, and distribution of input of the motor neurons, and by the number of muscle fibers innervated and the force they generate during contraction and resistance to fatigue (Burke et al., 1970).

The motor unit transforms synaptic input received by the motor neuron into mechanical output produced by the muscle fibers (Heckman and Enoka, 2004). Muscle force is generated by recruitment of motor units and modulation of their discharge rates (De Luca et al., 1982). The neural output from the spinal cord that constitutes the drive to the muscles results from the interaction between descending and afferent input at the spinal and supraspinal level.

A major proportion of small-diameter group III and IV muscle afferents are sensitive to noxious mechanical and chemical stimuli (Mense and Stahnke, 1983, 1985). Noxious stimuli can be delivered by intramuscular injection of chemical substances (Graven-Nielsen, 2006) to create experimental pain models that share many of the characteristics of clinical muscle pain conditions (Arendt-Nielsen et al., 1996). Experimental muscle pain causes changes in motor control that are detectable in individual muscles (e.g., Farina et al., 2005b; Madeleine et al., 2006) and in the coordination among muscles (e.g., Graven-Nielsen et al., 1997; Ciubotariu et al., 2004; Falla et al., 2007a,b). The adaptation of muscle activity during muscle pain reflects an altered strategy in the control of individual motor units. This new strategy allows submaximal motor tasks to be performed in a similar way in painful and nonpainful conditions, but it alters the coordination and load sharing among muscles.

This chapter briefly reviews the experimental evidence of the effect of muscle pain on the control of motor units and the force they generate.

Measuring Motor Unit Activity

There is a direct association between the generation of an action potential in the motor neuron and in the innervated muscle fibers. The detection of electric signals from muscles thus provides a window into the neural output from the spinal cord. Electromyographic (EMG) signals can be detected in muscles with either surface or intramuscular electrodes. Although the surface EMG signal is the sum of the action potentials of the active motor units and is thus directly associated with the neural output from the spinal cord, there are limitations in its interpretation in terms of individual motor unit activity (Farina et al., 2004a). Thus, intramuscular EMG is classically used to detect single motor units (Adrian and Bronk, 1929). The selectivity of intramuscular recordings permits the identification of motor unit action potentials and thus the instants of activation of the associated motor neurons.

In addition to the discharge patterns of motor neurons, electrophysiological techniques allow the measurement of the properties of the muscle fibers in individual motor units. The averaging of the joint torque (Stein et al., 1972) and of the surface EMG (Farina et al., 2002) triggered by the occurrence of action potentials provides an estimate of the force or torque expressed by individual motor units, also called twitch force, and of the electrophysiological fiber membrane properties.

Pain and Motor Unit Control

Motor unit discharge rate has been observed to decrease during painful contractions of constant force compared with control conditions (Farina et al., 2004b, 2005a; Sohn et al., 2000), in accordance with the pain-induced decrease in the amplitude of the surface EMG signal (e.g., Graven-Nielsen et al., 1997). It has also been shown that the change in discharge rate is correlated with pain intensity (Farina et al., 2004b) (Fig. 1) and

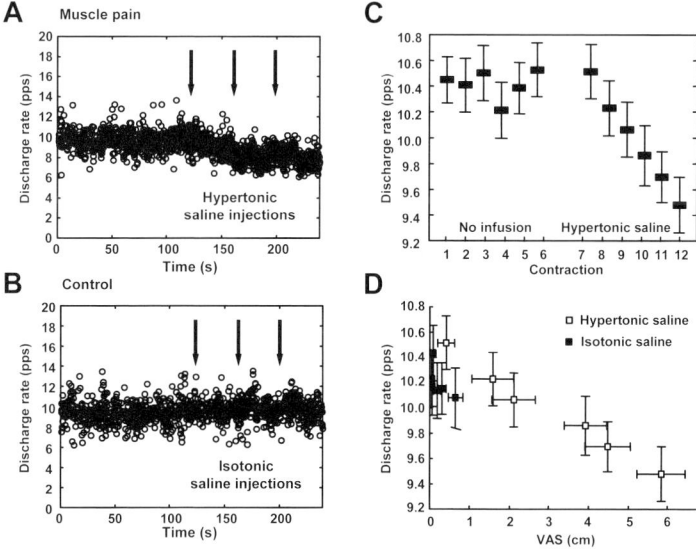

Fig. 1. (A) Instantaneous discharge rate of a motor unit before and during injection of hypertonic saline in the tibialis anterior muscle. The arrows indicate the time instants corresponding to the end of the injection of three boluses (0.2 mL, 0.5 mL, and 0.9 mL) of hypertonic saline. The discharge rate progressively decreases during experimental muscle pain induced by hypertonic saline injection. (B) As in panel A, but with injection of isotonic (nonpainful) saline. (C) Data from 55 motor units recorded from 12 subjects. Hypertonic saline was injected into the tibialis anterior muscle with the same modalities as in panel A. (D) Relation between average discharge rate and visual analogue scale (VAS) scores (±SE) for contractions with infusion of hypertonic saline (N = 55 motor units) and isotonic saline (N = 49 motor units). Adapted from Figs. 6, 7, and 8 in Farina et al. (2004) (used with permission).

that discharge rates return to control values as soon as the pain vanishes (Farina et al., 2008a). There is also evidence that the inhibition in motor neuron output is not identical in all regions of the same muscle (Madeleine et al., 2006). Although muscle pain is also associated with altered contractile muscle fiber properties (see the section "Pain and contractile fiber properties" below), there is no correlation between changes in discharge rate and changes in the force generation capacity of muscle fibers (Farina et al., 2008a). Thus, the decrease in discharge rate is not a direct consequence of altered fiber contractility.

The central mechanisms involved in decreased output from motor neurons with pain are not fully understood, partly because of limitations in the techniques for motor unit assessment (see the section "Limitations of current techniques" below). Inhibition through peripheral reflex circuitries is in agreement with studies that have shown an inhibitory effect of pain on spinal reflexes. For example, the motor potentials evoked by transcranial magnetic stimulation are reduced during muscle pain (Le Pera et al., 2001), with a concomitant decrease in amplitude of the H-reflex in resting conditions that indicates inhibition of spinal motor neurons (Rossi et al., 1997; Le Pera et al., 2001). On the other hand, not all H-reflex studies have shown results in agreement with these observations in conditions of varying pain duration and background muscle activity (Matre et al., 1998; Svensson et al., 1998). In addition, during experimental muscle pain, the stretch reflex is robustly facilitated (Matre et al., 1998; Svensson et al., 1998; Wang et al., 2000), and the long-latency inhibitory reflex (the silent period) is disinhibited, resulting in net facilitation (Wang et al., 1999). These findings seem to contradict a reduced rate of activation of motor neurons during muscle pain. However, most experimental studies assessing the effect of muscle pain on excitatory and inhibitory reflexes have not assessed the potential effect of postsynaptic modulation by nociceptive activity because the motor unit discharge rate or global muscle activity was kept constant before assessment of the reflex, which can be a potential confounding factor.

A recent study has demonstrated facilitation of recurrent inhibition of the soleus muscle during experimental muscle pain, with a close relationship between the temporal aspects of the induced pain and the efficacy of recurrent inhibition (Rossi et al., 2003). Although the functional effects of recurrent inhibition on motor unit discharge rate are complex (Katz and Pierrot-Deseilligny, 1999), the findings of a reduced discharge rate of motor units during static painful contractions may reflect facilitated recurrent inhibition by muscle pain.

A main role of spinal mechanisms in reducing the discharge rate of motor neurons in painful contractions is in accordance with the possible role of small-diameter muscle afferents in the fatigue-induced decrease of motor unit discharge rate during sustained, nonpainful contractions (Bigland-Ritchie et al., 1986). Injection of hypertonic saline at the beginning of a sustained contraction was shown to decrease the initial discharge rate of motor units; however, the total decrease due to fatigue was the same in painful and nonpainful conditions (Farina et al., 2005a) (Fig. 2). This finding indicates that fatigue-induced and pain-induced decreases in discharge rate may share similar underlying mechanisms.

The effect of pain at the spinal level may also be indirect. The sympathetic nervous system is known to be activated as part of the defense reaction to noxious stimuli (Janig, 1985). Increased secretion of epinephrine has been measured in response to acute pain stimuli, such as the cold pressor test (Robertson et al., 1979) and electrical stimulation of the skin (Greisen et al., 1999). The sympathetic system has direct control over muscle spindles via sympathetic innervation (Bombardi et al., 2006). This action, which is particularly pronounced in jaw and neck muscles, is generally characterized by reduced sensitivity to changes in muscle length. The basal discharge of spindles is reduced following sympathetic activation, although it may be enhanced in certain conditions (Roatta et al., 2002). The reduction in spindle sensitivity explains the sympathetically induced decrease in the magnitude of both jaw jerk and tonic vibration reflex in jaw muscles (Grassi et al., 1993a,b). Disfacilitation of spindle afferent activity is associated with decreased output from the motor neurons (Macefield et al., 1991), which can explain the observations in experimental pain studies. Alteration of muscle spindle basal discharge and sensitivity also impairs proprioception and thus influences the coactivation of synergistic and antagonist muscles (Passatore and Roatta, 2006).

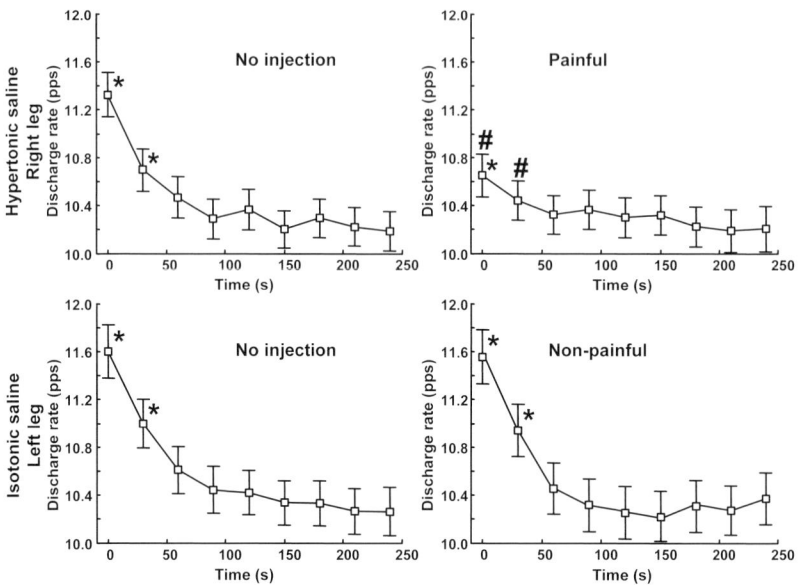

Fig. 2. Mean (± SE) discharge rate of motor units in the tibialis anterior muscle at nine time intervals, separated by 30 seconds, during a 4-minute isometric contraction at 25% of the maximal dorsiflexion torque. Data are reported for the conditions before and following injection of hypertonic and isotonic (0.5 mL) saline. * Significantly different compared to all other time instants within the same contraction ($P < 0.05$). # Significantly different compared to the same time instants of the previous contraction of the same leg without injection ($P < 0.01$). Redrawn from Farina et al. (2005) (used with permission).

In addition to spinal mechanisms, the descending drive to the muscle group involved in the task may also change with pain. It is possible that the central nervous system adopts a different control strategy in painful conditions, aimed at decreasing the activity of the synergistic and/or antagonist muscles. Accordingly, experimental pain in neck muscles determines a complex reorganization of coordination among agonist and antagonist muscles, which depends on the task performed (Falla et al., 2007a). At the single motor unit level, experimental muscle pain modifies the discharge rates of motor units in both painful and nonpainful muscles (Hodges et al., 2004), an action that may be mediated by altered descending drive to the muscle group involved in the task.

Pain and Contractile Fiber Properties

Few studies have assessed the contractile properties of single motor units during experimental muscle pain in humans (Sohn et al., 2004; Farina et al., 2008a). Sohn et al. (2004) observed an increase in twitch amplitude with experimental pain induced by injection of capsaicin into the masseter muscle. The observation was explained by potentiation and was considered a compensatory mechanism for the pain-induced decrease in discharge rate during contractions of constant force. However, potentiation reflects temporary membrane hyperpolarization, which increases muscle fiber conduction velocity and M-wave amplitude (Hicks et al., 1989a,b); these variables were unaffected by pain induced with injection of hypertonic saline (Farina et al., 2004b, 2005a,b). Farina et al. (2008a) observed a similar increase to that reported by Sohn et al. (2004) in the spike-triggered average twitch torque of motor units in the tibialis anterior muscle following injection of hypertonic saline. However, twitch increase was not correlated with the decrease in motor unit discharge rate, showing that the two phenomena were not associated through a compensatory mechanism. Discharge rates returned to control values as soon as the pain vanished, in accordance with the observed correlation between subjective pain ratings and motor unit discharge rate (Farina et al., 2004b), whereas twitch torque remained increased after cessation of pain (Farina et al., 2008a) (Fig. 3). In addition, there were no changes in the membrane electrophysiological properties of the muscle fibers, including the propagation velocity of action potentials. Excluding changes in the electrical membrane properties, it has recently been hypothesized that pain may affect intracellular contractile mechanisms (Farina et al., 2008a; Roatta et al., 2007).

Although activation of nociceptive afferents without damage to contractile structures cannot have a direct effect on fiber contractility, pain may modulate the activity of the sympathetic system. In addition to a direct effect on muscle spindles, as discussed above, the sympathetic nervous system modulates several functions in muscle fibers, mainly

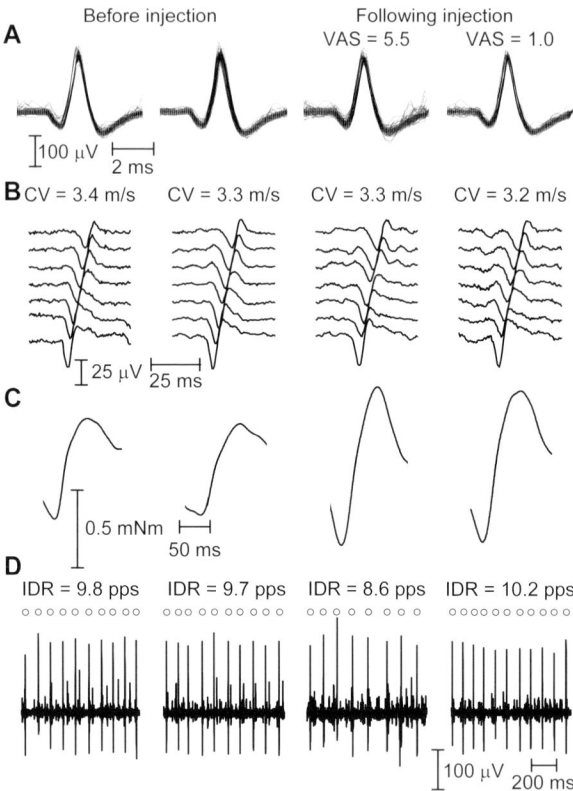

Fig. 3. Analysis of single motor unit properties before and after injection of hypertonic saline in the tibialis anterior muscle. (A) Intramuscular action potentials of the analyzed motor unit for four contractions, two before and two after the injection. (B) Averaged multichannel surface EMG. (C) Spike-triggered averaged twitch torque. The multichannel EMG signals record the propagating action potential and allow estimation of muscle fiber conduction velocity. (D) One-second portion of intramuscular recordings during isometric contraction at 10% of the maximal dorsiflexion torque. CV = conduction velocity. The increased twitch torque following injection of hypertonic saline is maintained when visual analogue scale (VAS) scores of pain intensity decrease and discharge rate returns to preinjection values. Redrawn from Farina et al. (2008a) (used with permission).

through the action of epinephrine on β_2 adrenergic receptors (Bowman, 1980; Roatta and Passatore, in press).

The mechanisms of release and reuptake of Ca^{2+} ions from/into the sarcoplasmatic reticulum and the activity of the Na/K pump across the sarcolemma bear importance in the development of muscle force and are affected by sympathetic activation (reviewed by Bowman, 1980).

The potentiation of the Na/K pump by β_2 agonists induced a substantial increase in the force of fatigued muscles and of isolated muscle fibers. In nonfatigued muscles, epinephrine and β_2 agonists slightly increased the amplitude of the twitch force, particularly in type II muscle fibers, and decreased its duration in type I fibers. These effects are mediated by a potentiation of the mechanisms of Ca^{2+} release and reuptake from or into the sarcoplasmatic reticulum (Ha et al., 1999). Although the positive ionotropic effect could be elicited only at high drug concentrations and could thus be of little physiological significance (Bowman, 1980), the twitch shortening in type I fibers could be observed at much lower drug concentrations as well as in response to reflexively induced secretion of epinephrine in anesthetized animals.

A shortening of twitch duration results in reduced average force and increased amplitude of oscillation of the force developed in a subtetanic contraction. With regard to force production in individual motor units, the amplitude of oscillation in the force produced corresponds to the amplitude of the twitch force. In these conditions, the amplitude of the estimated twitch may exhibit a marked increase (Marsden and Meadows, 1970), as observed in experimental pain studies (Sohn et al., 2004; Farina et al., 2008a).

Although at present it is not possible to fully prove an involvement of sympathetic modulation in the observed alterations of motor unit twitch torque with pain, some considerations make this mechanism plausible. First, the fibers in which an increased twitch torque has been observed belong to type I, given their low recruitment threshold. Second, it has been proven that the sympathetic system is activated by painful stimuli (Robertson et al., 1979; Greisen et al., 1999). Third, in studies in cats, intravenous injection of epinephrine had an effect on electrically evoked contractions of cat soleus muscle that was maintained for more than 10 minutes, when cardiovascular parameters returned to baseline (Bowman, 1980). This finding may explain the long-lasting effect of pain on the motor unit twitch (Farina et al., 2008a) (Fig. 3). Finally, Roatta et al. (2007) have recently shown that sympathetic activation by the cold pressor test affects the properties of low-threshold motor unit twitch torque in a similar way to that observed in studies on experimental muscle pain.

In line with this interpretation, the increased peak value of the averaged twitch torque observed during muscle pain may be a methodological consequence of the reduced half-relaxation time, the main adrenergic effect on low-threshold motor units. Interestingly, the observed change in twitch torque, rather than being an adaptive mechanism to the decrease in discharge rate (or vice versa), would further reduce the force produced by low-threshold motor units due to reduced fusion. This effect may be important in the adjustment of neural strategies in response to changed contractile properties.

Maintaining Motor Output

According to the discussion above, a painful muscle contributes reduced force to a static task by two main effects: (1) reduced neural drive to the muscle (decreased motor unit discharge rates) and (2) reduced force generation capacity of the motor units for a given discharge rate due to force twitch shortening. It cannot be excluded that these two effects might be counteracted by other neural adjustments within the painful muscle, such as increased motor unit synchronization or decreased recruitment threshold of higher threshold motor units. However, there are currently no data to support these hypotheses. Moreover, surface EMG amplitude has been consistently shown to decrease following induction of pain (e.g., Graven-Nielsen et al., 2007; Falla et al., 2007a). Within the limitations in interpretation of surface EMG amplitude (Farina et al., 2004), this finding supports the hypothesis of an overall decrease in neural drive to the painful muscle. Accordingly, muscle pain impairs the performance of maximal tasks (Graven-Nielsen et al., 2007).

Although maximal performance is reduced by muscle pain, submaximal motor tasks can be performed fairly normally in painful conditions (e.g., Falla et al., 2007b). Alterations in the properties of the painful muscle, which are likely to reduce the force contribution to the task, can be counteracted with another activation strategy of the muscle group involved in the task. The new control strategy in painful conditions should compensate for the reduced contribution of the painful muscle, but it depends on the specific processing of pain stimuli at the supraspinal level. The resulting coordination among muscles is constrained by the desired motor output, so the adjustment is task-dependent (Falla et al., 2007a). According to current evidence, it can also be speculated that, because the sympathetic activation may have a weakening effect on muscle contractile properties (Roatta et al., 2007), the overall neural drive to the muscles involved in a task should increase in painful conditions.

Limitations of Current Techniques

Techniques for the investigation of motor units in vivo have many limitations. In vivo identification of extracellular action potentials in multiunit EMG recordings allows the assessment of the discharge pattern of motor neurons from only a small area in the muscle near the recording site of a highly selective electrode. The selectivity of the recording is necessary to identify individual motor units from the multiunit recordings, but it limits the number of motor units that can be concurrently investigated. For this reason, most in vivo studies report results on few motor units that constitute only a small proportion of the population of active motor units (Enoka and Fuglevand, 2001). Most of the knowledge on motor unit physiology is based on the interpretation of ensembles of serially recorded single unit activity from different sessions and subjects. A generalized picture of the mechanisms of muscle control can be derived, though important limitations remain in the development of conceptual schemes of motor unit behavior. Results on the effect of pain on motor unit properties are limited to a few low-threshold units analyzed per subject, and it is not known whether these results can be generalized to high-threshold units. In addition, it is usually impossible to reliably record single motor unit activity during movement, and therefore only the isometric contraction paradigm has been used for single motor unit studies in painful conditions.

Another limitation of methods for assessing motor unit properties is the difficulty in estimating the twitch torque of muscle fibers within individual motor units. The spike-triggered averaging of the joint torque, the only current method for estimating motor unit twitches during voluntary contractions, may be affected by factors difficult to control in experimental conditions (Calancie and Bawa, 1986). Moreover, it is not possible to estimate twitch torque at high discharge rates. As a consequence, it is also not possible to directly associate contractile and control motor unit properties because they are usually assessed in different types of contraction, such as intramuscular EMG feedback for twitch estimation and joint force feedback for control properties.

These limitations reduce the impact of models of the effect of pain on motor unit activity to functionally relevant mechanisms. The development of new methods for motor unit investigation (e.g., Farina et al., 2008b) will be fundamental in furthering our understanding of how pain modulates motor unit properties.

Summary

Experimental muscle pain decreases the discharge rate of motor units in the painful muscle during performance of a static task. It also changes the contractile properties of the muscle fibers in individual motor units. A plausible interpretation of this finding is an effect of the sympathetic nervous system on fiber contractility. Overall, during pain the muscle contributes less to the force produced in a static task than in nonpainful conditions. The altered contribution of the painful muscle to the exerted force is associated with a reorganization of coordination among synergic and antagonist muscles that allows a submaximal motor task to be performed in a similar way in painful and nonpainful conditions. This altered strategy may be optimal in the short term because it allows (almost) unaltered motor output with reduced activation of the painful muscle. However, in the long term it may cause changes in muscle properties due to reduced or increased activity. These long-term changes may in turn affect motor strategy (Falla and Farina, 2007).

Acknowledgments

Part of the work described in this chapter was supported by the Danish Technical Research Council (project "Centre for Neuroengineering (CEN)," contract 26-04-0100) and by the European project "Cybernetic Manufacturing Systems" (CyberManS; contract 016712).

References

Adrian ED, Bronk DW. The discharge of impulses in motor nerve fibres: Part II. The frequency of discharge in reflex and voluntary contractions. J Physiol 1929;67:119–151.

Arendt-Nielsen L, Graven-Nielsen T, Svarrer H, Svensson P. The influence of low back pain on muscle activity and coordination during gait: a clinical and experimental study. Pain 1996;64:231–240.

Bigland-Ritchie BR, Dawson NJ, Johansson RS, Lippold OC. Reflex origin for the slowing of motoneurone firing rates in fatigue of human voluntary contractions. J Physiol 1986;379:451–459.

Bombardi C, Grandis A, Chiocchetti R, Bortolami R, Johansson H, Lucchi ML. Immunohistochemical localization of alpha1a-adrenoceptors in muscle spindles of rabbit masseter muscle. Tissue Cell 2006;38:121–125.

Bowman WC. Effects of adrenergic activators and inhibitors on skeletal muscles. In: Szekeres L, editor. Adrenergic activators and inhibitors. Handbook of Experimental Pharmacology, Vol. 54. New York: Springer-Verlag; 1980. p 47–128.

Burke RE, Jankowska E, Ten Bruggencate G. A comparison of peripheral and rubrospinal synaptic input to slow and fast twitch motor units of triceps surae. J Physiol 1970;207:709–732.

Calancie B, Bawa P. Limitations of the spike-triggered averaging technique. Muscle Nerve 1986;9:78–83.

Ciubotariu A, Arendt-Nielsen L, Graven-Nielsen T. The influence of muscle pain and fatigue on the activity of synergistic muscles of the leg. Eur J Appl Physiol 2004;91:604–614.

De Luca CJ, LeFever RS, McCue MP, Xenakis AP. Behavior of human motor units in different muscles during linearly varying contractions. J Physiol 1982;329:113–128.

Enoka RM, Fuglevand AJ. Motor unit physiology: some unresolved issues. Muscle Nerve 2001;24:4–17.

Falla D, Farina D. Neural and muscular factors associated with motor impairment in neck pain. Curr Rheumatol Rep 2007;9:497–502.

Falla D, Farina D, Dahl MK, Graven-Nielsen T. Muscle pain induces task-dependent changes in cervical agonist/antagonist activity. J Appl Physiol 2007a;102:601–609.

Falla D, Farina D, Graven-Nielsen T. Experimental muscle pain results in reorganization of coordination among trapezius muscle subdivisions during repetitive shoulder flexion. Exp Brain Res 2007b;178:385–393.

Farina D, Arendt-Nielsen L, Graven-Nielsen T. Experimental muscle pain reduces initial motor unit discharge rates during sustained submaximal contractions. J Appl Physiol 2005;98:999–1005.

Farina D, Arendt-Nielsen L, Graven-Nielsen T. Experimental muscle pain decreases voluntary EMG activity but does not affect the muscle potential evoked by transcutaneous electrical stimulation. Clin Neurophysiol 2005;116:1558–1565.

Farina D, Arendt-Nielsen L, Merletti R, Graven-Nielsen T. Assessment of single motor unit conduction velocity during sustained contractions of the tibialis anterior muscle with advanced spike triggered averaging. J Neurosci Methods 2002;115:1–12.

Farina D, Arendt-Nielsen L, Merletti R, Graven-Nielsen T. Effect of experimental muscle pain on motor unit firing rate and conduction velocity. J Neurophysiol 2004;91:1250–1259.

Farina D, Arendt-Nielsen L, Roatta S, Graven-Nielsen T. The pain-induced decrease in low-threshold motor unit discharge rate is not associated with the amount of twitch increase. Clin Neurophysiol 2008a;119:43–51.

Farina D, Merletti R, Enoka RM. The extraction of neural strategies from the surface EMG. J Appl Physiol 2004;96:1486–1495.

Farina D, Yoshida K, Stieglitz T, Koch KP. Multichannel thin-film electrode for intramuscular electromyographic recordings. J Appl Physiol 2008b;104:821–827.

Grassi C, Deriu F, Artusio E, Passatore M. Modulation of the jaw jerk reflex by the sympathetic nervous system. Arch Ital Biol 1993a;131:213–226.

Grassi C, Deriu F, Passatore M. Effect of sympathetic nervous system activation on the tonic vibration reflex in rabbit jaw closing muscles. J Physiol 1993b;469:601–613.

Graven-Nielsen T. Fundamentals of muscle pain, referred pain, and deep tissue hyperalgesia. Scand J Rheumatol Suppl 2006;122:1–43.

Graven-Nielsen T, Svensson P, Arendt-Nielsen L. Effects of experimental muscle pain on muscle activity and co-ordination during static and dynamic motor function. Electroenc Clin Neurophysiol 1997;105:156–164.

Greisen J, Hokland M, Grofte T, Hansen PO, Jensen TS, Vilstrup H, Tonnesen E. Acute pain induces an instant increase in natural killer cell cytotoxicity in humans and this response is abolished by local anaesthesia. Br J Anaesth 1999;83:235–240.

Ha TN, Posterino GS, Fryer MW. Effects of terbutaline on force and intracellular calcium in slow-twitch skeletal muscle fibres of the rat. Br J Pharmacol 1999;126:1717–1724.

Heckman CJ, Enoka RM. Physiology of the motor neuron and the motor unit. In: Eisen A, editor. Clinical neurophysiology of motor neuron diseases. Handbook of Clinical Neurophysiology, Vol. 4. New York: Elsevier; 2004. p. 119–147.

Hicks A, Fenton J, Garner S, McComas AJ. M wave potentiation during and after muscle activity. J Appl Physiol 1989b;66:2606–2610.

Hicks A, McComas AJ. Increased sodium pump activity following repetitive stimulation of rat soleus muscles. J Physiol 1989a;414:337–349.

Hodges P, Ervilha U, Graven-Nielsen T. How is force maintained when motor unit firing rate is decreased during experimental muscle pain? Investigation of synergist muscles. In: Proceedings XV ISEK Congress, Boston, 2004. p. 161.

Janig W. Systemic and specific autonomic reactions in pain: afferent and endocrine components. Eur J Anaesthesiol 1985;2:319–46.

Katz R, Pierrot-Deseilligny E. Recurrent inhibition in humans. Progress Neurobiol 1999;57:325–355.

Le Pera D, Graven-Nielsen T, Valeriani M, Oliviero A, Di Lazzaro V, Tonali PA, Arendt-Nielsen L. Inhibition of motor system excitability at cortical and spinal level by tonic muscle pain. Clin Neurophysiol 2001;112:1633–1641.

Macefield G, Hagbarth KE, Gorman R, Gandevia SC, Burke D. Decline in spindle support to alpha-motoneurones during sustained voluntary contractions. J Physiol 1991;440:497–512.

Madeleine P, Leclerc F, Arendt-Nielsen L, Ravier P, Farina D. Experimental muscle pain changes the spatial distribution of upper trapezius muscle activity during sustained contraction. Clin Neurophysiol 2006;117:2436–2445.

Marsden CD, Meadows JC. The effect of adrenaline on the contraction of human muscle. J Physiol 1970;207:429–488.

Matre DA, Sinkjaer T, Svensson P, Arendt-Nielsen L. Experimental muscle pain increases the human stretch reflex. Pain 1998;75:331–339.

Mense S, Meyer H. Different types of slowly conductive afferent units in cat skeletal muscle and tendon. J Physiol 1985;363:403–417.

Mense S, Stahnke M. Responses in muscle afferent fibres of slow conduction velocity to contractions and aschaemia. J Physiol 1983;342:383–397.

Passatore M, Roatta S. Influence of sympathetic nervous system on sensorimotor function: whiplash associated disorders (WAD) as a model. Eur J Appl Physiol 2006;98:423–449.

Roatta S, Arendt-Nielsen L, Cescon C, Farina D. Sympathetic modulation by cold pressor test alters the spike-triggered average torque and discharge rate of low-threshold motor units. Society for Neuroscience, San Diego, 2007.

Roatta S, Passatore M. Autonomic effects on skeletal muscle. In: Binder MD, Hirokawa N, Windhorst U, editors. Encyclopedia of neuroscience. Berlin: Springer, in press.

Roatta S, Windhorst U, Ljubisavljevic M, Johansson H, Passatore M. Sympathetic modulation of muscle spindle afferent sensitivity to stretch in rabbit jaw closing muscles. J Physiol 2002;540:237–248.

Robertson D, Johnson GA, Robertson RM, Nies AS, Shand DG, Oates JA. Comparative assessment of stimuli that release neuronal and adrenomedullary catecholamines in man. Circulation 1979;59:637–643.

Rossi A, Decchi B. Changes in Ib heteronymous inhibition to soleus motoneurones during cutaneous and muscle nociceptive stimulation in humans. Brain Res 1997;774:55–61.

Rossi A, Mazzocchio R, Decchi B. Effect of chemically activated fine muscle afferents on spinal recurrent inhibition in humans. Clin Neurophysiol 2003;114:279–287.

Sherrington C. Remarks on some aspects of reflex inhibition. Proc R Soc Lond B Biol Sci 1925;B97:19–45.

Svensson P, De Laat A, Graven-Nielsen T, Arendt-Nielsen L. Experimental jaw-muscle pain does not change heteronymous H-reflexes in the human temporalis muscle. Exp Brain Res 1998;121:311–318.

Stein RB, French AS, Mannard A, Yemm R. New methods for analyzing motor function in man and animals. Brain Res 1972;40:187–192.

Wang K, Svensson P, Arendt-Nielsen L. Modulation of exteroceptive suppression periods in human jaw-closing muscles by local and remote experimental muscle pain. Pain 1999;82:253–262.

Wang K, Svensson P, Arendt-Nielsen L. Effect of tonic muscle pain on short-latency jaw-stretch reflexes in humans. Pain 2000;88:189–197.

Correspondence to: Dario Farina, PhD, Center for Sensory-Motor Interaction (SMI), Department of Health Science and Technology, Aalborg University, Fredrik Bajers Vej 7 D-3, DK-9220 Aalborg, Denmark. Tel: +4599408821; fax: +4598154008; email: df@hst.aau.dk.

Index